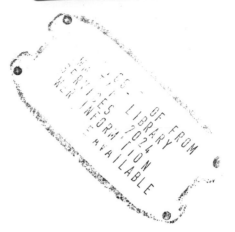

THE YEAR IN HYPERTENSION 2003

www.hypertensionacademy.co.uk
www.sankyo-pharma.co.uk

Sankyo Pharma UK Limited, Repton Place, White Lion Road,
Amersham, Bucks. HP7 9LP.   Tel: 01494 766 866

OLM13.1

THE YEAR IN
HYPERTENSION

2003

GREGORY YH LIP, WAI KAENG LEE

University Department of Medicine, City Hospital, Birmingham, UK

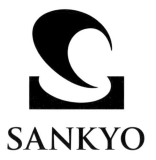

SANKYO

Provided as an
educational service to medicine by
Sankyo Pharma UK Ltd.

CLINICAL PUBLISHING SERVICES
OXFORD

Clinical Publishing Services Ltd

Oxford Centre for Innovation
Mill Street, Oxford OX2 OJX, UK

Tel: +44 1865 811116
Fax: +44 1865 251550
Web: www.clinicalpublishing.co.uk

Distributed by:

CRC Press LLC
2000 NW Corporate Blvd
Boca Raton, FL 33431, USA
E-mail: orders@crcpress.com

CRC Press UK
23–25 Blades Court
Deodar Road
London SW15 2NU, UK
E-mail: crcpress@itps.co.uk

A catalogue record for this book is available from the British Library

ISBN 1 904392 13 X

**The publisher makes no representation, express or implied, that the dosages in this
book are correct. Readers must therefore always check the product information and
clinical procedures with the most up-to-date published product information and data
sheets provided by the manufacturers and the most recent codes of conduct and
safety regulations. The authors and the publisher do not accept any liability for any
errors in the text or for the misuse or misapplication of material in this work**

Commissioning editor: Jonathan Gregory
Project manager: Rosemary Osmond
Typeset by Footnote Graphics Limited, Warminster, Wiltshire, UK
Printed in Spain by T G Hostench SA, Barcelona

Contents

Part IV

Pharmacological

Authors

PROFESSOR GREGORY YH LIP, MD, FRCP. FACC. FESC, Consultant
Cardiologist and Professor of Cardiovascular Medicine, Director-Haemostasis
Thrombosis and Vascular Biology Unit, University Department of Medicine,
City Hospital, Birmingham, UK.

DR WAI KAENG LEE, MB, BCh, MRCP, Cardiology Research Fellow,
University Department of Medicine, City Hospital, Birmingham, UK.

Part I

Pathophysiology

1

Aldosterone in hypertension: gaining more recognition … more than just a 'ratio'

Introduction

The prevalence of primary aldosteronism (PA) was previously thought to be low, being less than 1% in the hypertensive clinic population, with aldosterone-producing adrenal adenoma (APA) accounting for approximately two-third of cases. The use of the aldosterone-to-renin ratio (ARR) has led to the diagnosis of a higher prevalence of PA in both hypertensive clinic and primary care populations.

However, the main difficulty is in determining the gold standard diagnostic criteria, although many accepted that when a ratio of 750 or more, more than 90% of patients do not suppress plasma aldosterone with salt loading and fludrocortisone. Similarly, if aldosterone is expressed as ng/dl and given the low limit for plasma renin in 0.3 ng/ml per h, then an ARR value higher than 25 is suggestive of a pathological disorder. The diagnostic test of salt loading with the addition of low-dose fluorocortisone is used in hypertensive subjects who have a raised ARR to look for evidence of autonomous aldosterone production, as occurs in PA. The clinical evidence is accumulating, many now screening all hypertensive patients for aldosteronism with the use of ARR given the high efficacy of spironolactone in treating the disorder. However, spironolactone is not licensed for essential hypertension in the UK; hence ARR profiling is useful in targeting those who would most likely respond to spironolactone.

At least 10 genes have been shown to increase blood pressure (BP), the pathogenesis of steroid hypertension has been shown to be primarily linked to mutations that result in ectopic production of the adrenal corticosterone, or aldosterone. Furthermore, patients with raised ARR have inappropriate aldosterone activity, and animal studies suggest an important interaction between excess salt and excess aldosterone in producing target organ damage in the heart. Recently, a more selective aldosterone receptor antagonist has been developed, eplerenone, and it shows considerable promise in managing and preventing the complications of hypertension. It may have a role both being antifibrotic and antineurohormonal in mild to moderate heart failure, in post-myocardial infarct left ventricular (LV) dysfunction and in progressive renal disease.

Cautions over the current epidemic of primary aldosteronism.

Kaplan NM. *Lancet* 2001; **357**: 953–4.

B ACKGROUND . Over the past 10 years, published literature have reported a much higher frequency of PA than the previously accepted percentage of less than 1% of the population with hypertension. Such percentages, ranging from 2.7% to 32%, are all based on the findings of raised plasma ARR. The previous lower estimates and the more recent higher ones were largely derived from selected population, so the frequency of PA in the overall hypertensive population remains uncertain.

INTERPRETATION . With time, more certainty of the true frequency of PA will be obtained, in part by wider application of the ARR in truly unselected patients with hypertension. For now, the ARR should not be done as a routine procedure on patients with hypertension and the diagnosis of hyperaldosteronism should not be based solely on the finding of a raised ARR. Such a conservative approach will keep to a minimum the costs and dangers of unnecessary work-ups and surgery while providing the full benefits of antihypertensive treatment.

Comment

This viewpoint article by Kaplan drew our attention that PA is probably over-diagnosed. This could be almost certainly due to the overuse of ARR clinically since the report by Gordon *et al.* (|**1**| Hamlet *et al.* [1985]) that ARR could be used as a screening test for PA. Kaplan has urged caution that the criteria for a raised ARR was invalid, as a raised ARR does not necessarily prove the diagnosis. This may be due to several sources of error that may be listed as follows: (i) most ARR data from the USA report plasma aldosterone concentrations (PAC) in ng/dl, whereas most other data are in SI units of pmol/l (almost all investigators report plasma renin activity in ng/ml per h); (ii) other diseases (e.g. chronic renal disease) can cause raised plasma aldosterone and a low renin activity in the absence of PA; (iii) upright posture and sodium intake can also cause ARR to increase; (iv) the effects of antihypertensive drugs are variable (some authorities recommend that patients should be off all drugs for at least 3 weeks before measuring ARR); and (v) almost all reports equated a raised ARR to PA.

Kaplan recommended that ARR should only be used just as a preliminary screen-ing test and only when ARR is raised then additional work-up such as a suppression test (measuring urinary aldosterone after 3 days of salt-loading) is done, preferably before computed tomography (CT) or magnetic resonance (MR) scan.

Validity of the aldosterone–renin ratio used to screen for primary aldosteronism.

Montori VM, Schwartz GL, Chapman AB, Boerwinkle E, Turner ST. *Mayo Clin Proc* 2001; **76**(9): 877–82.

BACKGROUND. PA may be more common in patients with presumed essential hypertension than previously thought. The recent higher prevalence rates of PA (10–15%) have been attributed to an increased use of the ARR to distinguish patients with PA from those with essential hypertension.

INTERPRETATION. In patients with previously diagnosed essential hypertension, calculation of the ARR does not provide a renin-independent measure of circulating aldosterone that is suitable for determining whether PAC is elevated relative to plasma–renin activity (PRA). Because elevation of the ARR is predominantly an indicator of low PRA, its perceived value in screening for PA most likely derives from additional diagnostic tests being done in patients with low-renin hypertension.

Comment

The objective of this study was to determine whether the calculated ratio of PAC to PRA, a proposed screening test for PA, provides a renin-independent measure of circulating aldosterone that is suitable to judge whether PAC is inappropriately elevated relative to PRA. The study was meticulously carried out on 221 black subjects and 276 white subjects (i.e. biracial sample) with previously diagnosed essential hypertension—a population in whom screening for PA has been advocated. Interestingly, their data clearly showed that the ARR is dependent on variations in PRA levels, thus, 'elevation of the ARR was predominantly a sign of low PRA, rather than a measure of elevated PAC relative to PRA'. As discussed in the article by Kaplan (2001) above, there are numerous reasons why we should be more cautious about the use of ARR in clinical practice, and about the current epidemic of PA. The result of this study is timely; perhaps, it has served to reinforce Kaplan's message.

However, such data do not, by themselves, negate the value of ARR as a screening test for PA if, as Montori *et al.* (2001) pointed out, there is a requirement for an absolute elevation in PAC. Only then, more expensive additional work-up to document mineralocorticoid hypersecretion is indicated. This approach should minimize the risk of unnecessary tests, and more importantly, the risk of unnecessary surgery as according to Kaplan, more patients are likely to have adrenal 'incidentalomas' than APAs!

Screening for primary aldosteronism without discontinuing hypertensive medications: plasma aldosterone–renin ratio.

Gallay BJ, Ahmad S, Xu L, Toivola B, Davidson RC. *Am J Kidney Dis* 2001; **37**(4): 699–705.

BACKGROUND. The traditional work-up for PA is cumbersome and requires discontinuing antihypertensive medications, which is inconvenient and potentially dangerous. A simple and accurate screening test that can be used without modifying medications is needed. The plasma ARR is a valid screening assay for PA, but antihypertensives are usually discontinued before obtaining this ratio, limiting its utility.

INTERPRETATION. Data suggest that the ARR is a valid screening assay for PA in patients with poorly controlled BP, and discontinuation of antihypertensive medications is not needed for this test.

Comment

The present prospective study is designed to examine the validity of the ARR as a screening test for PA if the ratio is measured randomly while patients continue anti-hypertensive therapy. The patients tested were being treated with antihypertensive agents from several classes, most notably angiotensin-converting enzyme inhibitors (ACEI), calcium antagonists, beta-blockers and diuretics. During the 18-month study period, 15 of the 90 patients with poorly controlled BP who were screened by

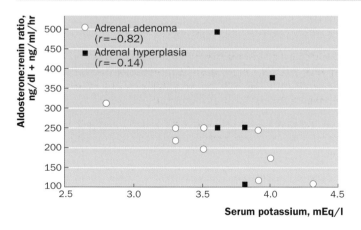

Fig. 1.1 Correlation between ARR and serum potassium level for patients with adrenal adenoma (Δ; $r = -0.82$) and adrenal hyperplasia (•; $r = -0.14$). Source: Gallay *et al.* (2001).

random blood sample while maintaining their prescribed antihypertensive medications had an elevated ARR (>100 ng/dl/ng/ml/h, defined as PA by the authors). All patients with elevated ARRs underwent further diagnostic work-up, including adrenal CT and/or MR imaging and adrenal iodine 131 norcholesterol uptake scan. Ten of the patients were found to have adrenal adenoma on diagnostic work-up, and adenoma was later confirmed by histological examination after surgical removal in these 10 patients. Five patients were found to have adrenal hyperplasia by CT and adrenal scan; all five patients responded to antialdosterone treatment. No patient showed a falsely elevated ARR. All 15 patients had good control of BP after surgery and/or antialdosterone medications.

Quite rightly, the authors did point out that there may a selection bias in their patients as they all have severe, poorly controlled hypertension. As a whole, however, the data suggested that ARR could be used to screen for PA in all normokalaemic, as well as hypokalaemic, patients with severe, poorly controlled hypertension who may be administered several antihypertensive medications. Importantly, antihypertensive medications do not need to be discontinued to determine the ARR. Importantly, five of the 15 patients (33%) had normal serum potassium levels (>3.5 mEq/l); thus, using hypokalaemia as an indication to initiate work-up would have missed the diagnosis in these patients. Impressively, there were no false-positive results. However, it is noteworthy that in the remaining 75 patients with normal ARRs, the possibility of false-negative results cannot be ruled out because no further studies were performed on these patients. Thus, sensitivity cannot be determined from these data.

A review of the medical treatment of primary aldosteronism.

Lim PO, Young WF, MacDonald TM. *J Hypertens* 2001; **19**(3): 353–61.

BACKGROUND. Use of the ARR has suggested that at least 1 in 10 hypertensive subjects have PA. There is thus a timely need to review the literature for effective drug therapies and to speculate on other therapeutic options by taking into account recent advances in understanding the PA disease pathophysiological process.

INTERPRETATION. The diagnosis of PA allows appropriate management with resultant BP control in many hypertensive subjects who otherwise have resistant hypertension despite multiple drug therapy.

Comment

This excellent systematic review on the topic is timely! The role of aldosterone in hypertension has received little attention until recently. As already discussed, the prevalence of hyperaldosteronism is apparently on the increase as the ARR has increasingly been recognized as a screening tool for aldosteronism in suspected hypertensive patients.

A select number of subjects with APA can be expected to respond well to surgical treatment. For the majority of PA cases, especially subjects with idiopathic hyper-aldosteronism, long-term medical treatment is now safe and feasible, although no randomized controlled trials have been carried out to date. The best therapeutic response is obtained by directly antagonizing aldosterone at the receptor level using medium- to low-dose spironolactone and this response can be predicted by a raised ARR. The response to other potassium-sparing diuretics and calcium channel block-ers are modest. Idiopathic hyperaldosteronism responds better than angiotensin II (Ang II)-unresponsive APA to ACEIs and this may also be true with Ang II receptor blockers (ARBs). The discovery of the aldosterone synthase gene (CYP11B1 and CYP11B2, located in tandem on chromosome 8) opens up the possibility for gene therapy.

Insights into glucocorticoid-associated hypertension: review.
Brem AS. *Am J Kidney Dis* 2001; **37**: 1–10.

BACKGROUND. The hypertension that often develops after chronic glucocorticoid exposure has been well described, but poorly understood. The exact incidence of hypertension after prolonged glucocorticoid administration is difficult to determine. Clinical circumstances vary to such a degree that the contribution made by the steroid to the elevated BP is difficult to assess in many cases. The clearest examples of glucocorticoid-associated hypertension exist in patients with known excess adrenal cortisol production.

INTERPRETATION. Glucocorticoids modify multiple intracellular and extracellular biochemical processes but have limited direct effects on BP. In the proximal tubule, glucocorticoids do not induce a change in sodium transport directly but serve to enhance the activity of many existing pathways and transporters. Conversely, the distal tubule and collecting duct are responsive to glucocorticoids. Glucocorticoids are able to bind to mineralocorticoid and glucocorticoid receptors and stimulate sodium reabsorption. Protein binding of the glucocorticoids in serum and the metabolic activity of local 11β-hydroxysteroid dehydrogenase (11β-HSD) limit access of these steroids to both mineralocorticoid receptors and glucocorticoid receptors. In blood vessels, glucocorticoids do not directly affect vascular tone but increase vascular sensitivity to circulating vasoactive agents. Hypertensive and antihypertensive pathways can be affected to variable degrees, leading to varied clinical presentations. Finally, local tissue-specific glucocorticoid metabolism is a critical determining factor in whether a hypertensive effect is observed.

Comment

The purpose of this review is to present new insights and possible mechanisms that may explain how chronic glucocorticoid exposure puts one at risk for hypertension.

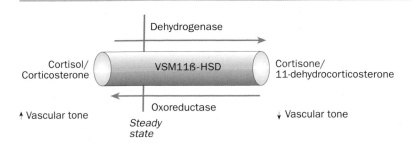

Fig. 1.2 Vascular tissue contains 11β-HSD and shows both dehydrogenase and oxoreductase activity. Inhibition of the dehydrogenase reaction is associated with an enhanced contractile response to pressors, whereas suppression of the oxoreductase reaction is linked to a diminished contractile response to the same pressors. Source: Brem *et al.* (2001).

The association between excess glucocorticoids and hypertension has been much discussed but poorly understood. From both clinical observations and laboratory studies, it is clear that glucocorticoids exert their effects at many different sites responsible for BP regulation. Isoforms of the enzyme 11β-HSD, located in steroid-responsive tissues, metabolize endogenously produced glucocorticoids. These enzymes limit steroid access to mineralocorticoid receptors and/or glucocorticoid receptors. In the kidney, synthetic and endogenous glucocorticoids are capable of enhancing transepithelial sodium transport in the presence of 11β-HSD inhibition. Proximal tubule reabsorption of sodium can be indirectly augmented after chronic exposure to glucocorticoids. In this segment, steroids have a permissive effect, increasing the expression of both Na^+, K^+ adenosine triphosphatase along the basolateral membrane and Na^+–H^+ exchanger along the apical membrane of epithelial cells.

Although glucocorticoids themselves produce no increase in sodium reabsorption in this segment, Ang II-stimulated sodium transport is significantly greater in proximal tubular cells pre-treated with glucocorticoids. The increased transport in distal renal segments is more direct and stems in part from glucocorticoid cross-over binding to mineralocorticoid receptors. In vascular tissue, synthetic and endogenous glucocorticoids, after inhibition of the dehydrogenase reaction, magnify the response to circulating vasoconstrictors. The effects of glucocorticoids in vascular tissue is indirect, upregulating the expression of receptors to many vasoconstrictors and downregulating the effects of potential vasodilators. Thus, glucocorticoids have the potential to alter both circulating volume and vascular resistance.

The neurohormonal natural history of essential hypertension: towards primary or tertiary aldosteronism?

Lim PO, Struthers AD, MacDonald TM. *J Hypertens* 2002; **20**: 11–15.

BACKGROUND. Use of the ARR has controversially suggested that approximately 10% of hypertensives have PA, and most of these individuals are thought to have idiopathic hyperaldosteronism. The usual renin–angiotensin system control is intact in these individuals and is similar to that in low renin and essential hypertensives, differing only in the degree of sensitivity.

INTERPRETATION. There is recent evidence suggesting that hyperaldosteronism relates to aldosterone synthase genetic polymorphism, and also that increased Ang II stimulation of the adrenal glands appears paradoxically to upregulate the receptors increasing Ang II sensitivity. Taken together, the possibility arises that, in susceptible hypertensives, hyperaldosteronism could be acquired. Indeed, it is well known that renin-driven renovascular hypertension is associated with the development of hyperaldosteronism. Hypothetically, within the wider hypertensive population, these findings set the scene that Ang II adrenal sensitivity increases over time until the secretion of aldosterone becomes 'autonomous' and hence 'tertiary' aldosteronism in a significant proportion of hypertensives.

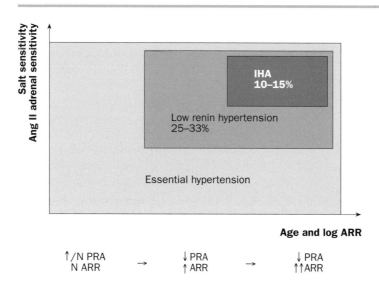

Fig. 1.3 Neurohormonal stages in hypertension. Ang II, angiotensin II; PRA, plasma–renin activity; IHA, idiopathic hyperaldosteronism; N, normal; LogARR, logarithm of aldosterone-to-renin ratio. Source: Lim *et al.* (2002).

Comment

Many now believed that hyperaldosteronism is a continuous pathological disorder that at one end there is low renin essential hypertension and at the other classic autonomous secretion of large quantities of aldosterone with suppressed renin and associated biochemical abnormalities. That is, the so-called 'essential hypertension' (raised BP in the absence of an easily identifiable aetiology), may progress with time to a state of 'low renin hypertension' and 'idiopathic hyperaldosteronism' (a form of PA that is clinically indistinguishable from an APA). It is interesting that the authors explore this hypothesis in several novel ways, that the underlying mechanisms for

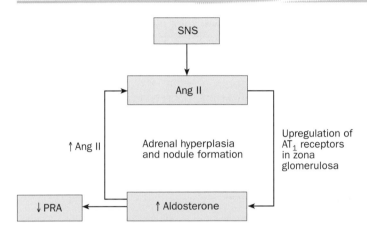

Fig. 1.4 The renin–angiotensin system stimulation of the adrenal gland. SNS, Sympathetic nervous system; Ang II, angiotensin II; AT1, angiotensin II receptor type 1; PRA, plasma–renin activity. Source: Lim *et al.* (2002).

Table 1.1 Circumstantial evidence supporting neurohormonal progression in hypertension

- Animal studies reproducing low renin hypertension
- Documented cases of renovascular diseases in human in which high renin hypertension progresses to low renin hypertension with tertiary hyperaldosteronism
- Prevalence of salt sensitivity increases with age
- Increasing prevalence of low renin hypertension with age
- Increasing incidence of adrenal sensitivity to Ang II with age
- Increasing serum sodium concentration and ARR with age in hypertensive individuals
- There may be a rank order of increasing salt sensitivity, adrenal sensitivity and aldosterone activity from normotension > hypertension > low renin hypertension > idiopathic hyperaldosteronism

Source: Lim *et al.* (2002).

this progression may be due to a persistent stimulation of the adrenal gland by excessive Ang II and thus aldosterone overproduction, and finally evolves into the 'tertiary hyperaldosteronism' state.

The question is how such inappropriate neurohumoral progression can be maintained, which seems in conflict with our usual understanding in the concept of negative feedback regulation of the renin–angiotensin system? Lim *et al.* (2002) proposed a 'vicious cycle' concept where Ang II paradoxically upregulates adrenocortical type 1 Ang II receptors, and thereby increase adrenal sensitivity to Ang II. Furthermore, Lim *et al.* (2002) also explained that certain individuals may be more susceptible to the development of tertiary hyperaldosteronism and has related this to polymorphisms of the aldosterone synthase gene.

Aldosterone antagonists in the treatment of hypertension and target organ damage.

Rajagopalan S, Pitt B. *Curr Hypertens Rep* 2001; **3**(3): 240–8.

BACKGROUND. Mineralocorticoids mediate a number of effects besides regulation of fluid and electrolyte balance. Recent evidence has revealed several non-traditional roles, sites of synthesis and action for these steroids. Aldosterone, the principal mineralocorticoid in humans, appears to be synthesized in physiologically relevant amounts in both the heart and the vasculature, and plays an important part in vessel wall and myocardial remodelling.

INTERPRETATION. The genomic effects of aldosterone are mediated through activation of the classic mineralocorticoid receptor, whereas rapid non-genomic effects seem to involve a distinct receptor and result in activation of multiple downstream signalling pathways. Recently, several lines of evidence seem to suggest an important interaction between the nitric oxide (NO) and the aldosterone pathway in the adrenal gland and vasculature. The evolution of selective aldosterone receptor antagonists will help us understand the role that mineralocorticoids play in the pathogenesis of hypertension, heart failure and atherosclerosis.

Comment

Aldosterone has been implicated in the effects of Ang II in the vasculature. Recent experimental and clinical studies have revealed more evidence that excessive circulating levels of aldosterone can lead to deleterious cardiovascular sequelae independent of the effects on BP and its classical action on epithelial cells. For example, excess plasma aldosterone has been linked to the development of myocardial and vascular fibrosis in uninephrectomized, salt-loaded rats infused with mineralocorticoids and similarly, in humans, an association of aldosterone with LV hypertrophy, impaired diastolic and systolic function, salt and water retention causing aggravation of congestion in patients with established heart failure, reduced vascular compliance and an increased risk of arrhythmias (resulting from intracardiac fibrosis, hypokalaemia, hypomagnesaemia, reduced baroreceptor sensitivity and potentiation of catechola-mine effects). These sequelae of aldosterone excess may contribute to the pathogenesis and worsen the prognosis of congestive heart failure and hypertension. Indeed, the evolution of selective aldosterone receptor antagonists (spironolactone and epleren-one) will help us understand the part that mineralocorticoids play in the patho-genesis of hypertension, heart failure and atherosclerosis. Many clinical trials are now underway in all these settings.

Primary aldosteronism: factors associated with normalization of blood pressure after surgery.

Sawka AM, Young WF, Thompson GB, *et al. Ann Intern Med* 2001; **135**(4): 258–61.

B A C K G R O U N D . **Hypertension often persists after adrenalectomy for PA.**

I N T E R P R E T A T I O N . Resolution of hypertension after adrenalectomy for PA is independently associated with a lack of family history of hypertension and pre-operative use of two or fewer antihypertensive agents.

Comment

The objective of this brief retrospective report was to determine factors associated with resolution of hypertension after adrenalectomy for PA. They included 97 patients who underwent adrenalectomy for PA between 1 January 1993 and 31 December 1999 in a tertiary care referral centre. Pre-operative plasma renin activity, plasma and urinary aldosterone concentrations, and adrenal imaging were measured. Follow-up BP, measured at a clinic visit or at home, was also reviewed. Hypertension was resolved at follow-up (BP $<140/90$ mmHg) without use of antihypertensive agents in 31 of 93 patients (33%). Stepwise multivariable logistic regression analysis adjusted for duration of follow-up, resolution of hypertension was independently associated with family history of hypertension (odds ratio [OR] 10.9, $P <0.001$) and pre-operative use of two or fewer antihypertensive agents (OR 4.7, $P = 0.005$). Additional factors associated with resolution of hypertension based on univariate analysis included younger age, shorter duration of hypertension, higher pre-operative ratio of PAC to plasma renin activity, and higher urine aldosterone level ($P <0.05$). The main limitation of this was unequal follow-up among the patients and thus may have underestimated the proportion of patients in whom hypertension may ultimately have resolved during longer follow-up. Another shortfall was that of a retrospective nature of the study. More importantly, the mechanisms for persistence of hyper-tension post-adrenalectomy could not be addressed. It is possible that many of these patients may concurrently have essential hypertension. Regardless of the result, clinicians should always be wary of BP control in these patients, as longer follow-up may be needed.

Though family history of hypertension and pre-operative use of two or fewer antihypertensive agents may be predictive of persistence of hypertension post-adrenalectomy, the possible underlying mechanism for this phenomenon should be investigated.

Cause of residual hypertension after adrenalectomy in patients with primary aldosteronism.

Horita Y, Inenaga T, Nakahama H, *et al. Am J Kidney Dis* 2001; **37**(5): 884–9.

BACKGROUND. **Although surgical adrenalectomy frequently cures hypertension in patients with PA, as many as 30–40% of these patients have persistent hypertension post-operatively. The reason for this residual hypertension remains unclear. Hypertension causes renal vascular and glomerular injuries (so-called nephrosclerosis), and both hypokalaemia and metabolic alkalosis cause renal tubular atrophy. There has been growing interest in the topic of hypertension and renal injury during the past decade, mostly in response to data provided by the end-stage renal disease registries. PA also injures the renal tissue.**

INTERPRETATION. Severity of glomerulosclerosis and arteriolosclerosis and LV mass is related to BP after adrenalectomy in patients with PA. It was postulated that residual hypertension is renal hypertension.

Comment

The above study was performed to evaluate the clinical value of renal biopsy in patients undergoing surgical adrenalectomy for PA. They included 26 patients with PA caused by a unilateral adrenal cortical adenoma (Conn's syndrome) who under-went unilateral adrenalectomy with concurrent open-wedge renal biopsy. The patients were categorized into two groups: (i) those with normotension with diastolic BP <90 mmHg who were not administered antihypertensive drugs, and (ii) those with residual hypertension with diastolic BP of ≥90 mmHg who were administered medication for 6 months after surgery. The comparison of renal histopathological findings in the two groups are summarized in Fig. 1.5. The results of this study support the position that renal histopathological changes could account for the residual hypertension seen in some patients with PA who have undergone unilateral adrenalectomy for an adrenal cortical adenoma. It was therefore advocated that early detection of PA and its cure might prevent structural renal injury and restore normal BP.

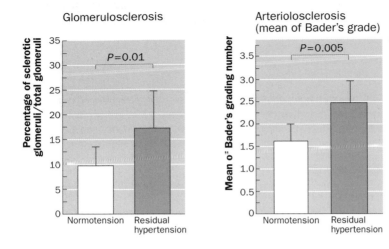

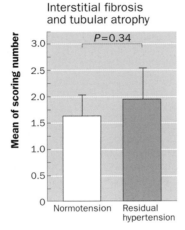

Fig. 1.5 Comparison of renal histopathological findings in patients with PA with normotension and those with hypertension after adrenalectomy. Source: Horita *et al.* (2001).

Efficacy of an angiotensin II receptor antagonist in managing hyperaldosteronism.

Stokes GS, Monaghan JC, Ryan M, Woodward M. *J Hypertens* 2001; **19**(6): 1161–5.

BACKGROUND. Spironolactone is the mainstay of treatment for hypertension secondary to non-adenomatous primary hyperaldosteronism. However, at the dose required for the control of hypertension, spironolactone is commonly limited by its side-effects. There is evidence that Ang II receptors are normally expressed in aldosterone- or cortisol-producing adenomas, and are not involved in the lack of response to Ang II that is characteristic of most patients with hyperaldosteronism caused by adenoma or adrenocortical hyperplasia.

INTERPRETATION. Irbesartan plays a part in combination antihypertensive treatment of patients with hyperaldosteronism.

Comment

This paper described a double-blind randomized placebo-controlled cross-over study of irbesartan in patients receiving long-term medical treatment for hyper-aldosteronism, in order to determine whether an ARB was an effective adjunct in the control of PAC and arterial BP as measured by 24 h ambulatory BP recordings. It has been held that the hypertension associated with primary hyperaldosteronism is salt and water dependent, and thus best managed by diuretics. Spironolactone has been reported to normalize BP in 50% of cases with non-adenomatous primary hyper-aldosteronism. Interestingly, the findings seem to suggest that irbesartan, an ARB could potentially be an adjunct to other therapy for these patients. This may allow dose-sparing of spironolactone in patients with troublesome side-effects from that drug. The mechanism of which ARB achieved such effects is unknown. It is possible that, in patients receiving spironolactone, a reversal of plasma renin activity suppression was induced, resulting in a peripheral vasodepressor response to irbesartan. However, the duration of treatment with irbesartan was too short (only 2 weeks) to allow long-term efficacy of this agent to be assessed in these patients.

Aldosterone to renin ratio as a determinant of exercise blood pressure response in hypertensive patients.

Lim PO, Donnan PT, MacDonald TM. *J Hum Hypertens* 2001; **15**(2): 119–23.

BACKGROUND. ARR is a marker of inappropriate aldosterone activity in hypertension. As aldosterone may adversely affect vascular compliance, we hypothesized that the ARR would relate to exercise BP responses in hypertension.

INTERPRETATION. There was an independent and significant correlation between ARR and exercise systolic BP (SBP).

Comment

This study has further emphasized the importance of inappropriate aldosterone activity as being aetiologically important in the pathogenesis and maintenance of hypertension. The authors hypothesized that ARR would relate to BP responses during exercise more than BPs measured at rest or with ambulatory methods. A total of 119 untreated hypertensive patients were included into the study. Indeed, they demonstrated that the correlation between ARR and exercise SBP was significant, over and above that of office and ambulatory BPs. The ARR was positively related to exercise SBP. It is of note that a previous published study has shown that hypertensive subjects have reduced vascular compliance that causes an impaired reduction in systemic vascular resistance during exercise resulting in a greater rise in exercise SBP in hypertensive compared with normotensive individuals. The finding of this study seems to support the hypothesis that 'inappropriate aldosterone activity' in hypertension contributes to reduced peripheral vascular compliance, which could be unmasked by exercise testing.

Aldosterone receptor antagonism normalizes vascular function in liquorice-induced hypertension.
Quaschning T, Ruschitzka F, Shaw S, Luscher TF. *Hypertension* 2001 Feb; **37**(2 Part 2): 801–5.

BACKGROUND. The enzyme 11β-HSD2 provides mineralocorticoid receptor specificity for aldosterone by metabolizing glucocorticoids to their receptor-inactive 11-dehydro derivatives. This study investigated the effects of the aldosterone receptor antagonists spironolactone and eplerenone on endothelial function in liquorice-induced hypertension.

INTERPRETATION. This is the first study to demonstrate that aldosterone receptor antagonism normalizes BP, prevents upregulation of vascular endothelin-1, restores NO-mediated endothelial dysfunction, and thus, may advance as a novel and specific therapeutic approach in 11b-HSD2-deficient hypertension.

Comment

The data demonstrated for the first time that in 11β-HSD hypertension, chronic aldosterone receptor blockade by either spironolactone or the novel compound eplerenone not only normalizes BP but also prevents upregulation of vascular endothelin-1 and endothelial dysfunction, as reflected by reduced eNOS (endothelial nitric oxide synthase) expression, reduced NO production, and impaired endo-thelium-dependent relaxations. The study also provided the first evidence that impaired NO formation as well as activation of the vascular endothelin-1 system contributes to the development of hypertension induced by administration of the 11β-HSD inhibitor liquorice-derived glycyrrhizic acid. More importantly, recent evidence indicates that elevated aldosterone levels play an important part in the development and progression of myocardial fibrosis and hypertrophy in congestive

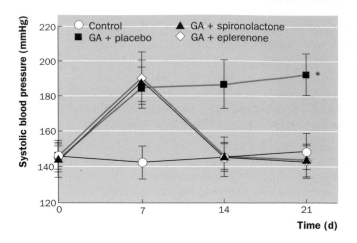

Fig. 1.6 SBP on treatment with different regimens. BP increased after 1 week of glycyrrhetinic acid feeding compared with placebo and returned to baseline after treatment with the aldosterone receptor antagonists spironolactone and eplerenone. Heart rate remained unchanged. *P <0.05 vs control animals. Results are given as mean ± SEM (n = 7 animals per group). Source: Quaschning *et al.* (2001).

heart failure and that sodium retention is not the primary mechanism of cortisol-induced hypertension. These findings may be particularly relevant to this study, because the data suggested that reduced activity of 11β-HSD, due to the generation of endogenous inhibitors or gene defects, could represent an important additional aldosterone-independent mechanism through which inappropriate access of gluco-corticoids to vascular receptors may influence vascular tone. The fact that aldosterone receptor antagonism has recently been proved to decrease mortality in severe heart failure emphasizes the importance of this therapeutic principle and may further contribute to attempts in evaluation of its underlying mechanisms. Because both aldosterone receptor antagonists, spironolactone and eplerenone, normalize BP, prevent upregulation of vascular endothelin-1, and restore NO-mediated endothelial dysfunction, aldosterone receptor antagonism may provide a novel approach in the treatment of cardiovascular disease associated with reduced activity of 11β-HSD.

Liquorice-induced rise in blood pressure: a linear dose–response relationship.

Sigurjonsdottir HA, Franzson L, Manhem K, *et al. J Hum Hypertens* 2001; **15**(8): 549–52.

BACKGROUND. Liquorice has been well known to mankind. Even apparently marginal doses of liquorice as in liquorice-flavoured chewing gum, chewing tobacco and Pontefract cakes have proved to cause hypokalaemia and hypertension.

INTERPRETATION. SBP increased in a linear dose–response but not a time–response relationship. The individual response to liquorice followed the normal distribution. The finding of a maximal effect of liquorice after only 2 weeks has important implications for all doctors dealing with hypertension. There does not seem to be a special group of responders as the degree of individual response to liquorice consumption followed the normal distribution curve.

Comment

Until recently, it has been generally held that one has to consume an almost heroic amount of liquorice to have an effect on the BP. The results of this study interestingly contradicts our traditional belief. The aim of this study was to investigate the dose–response and the time–response relationship between liquorice consumption and rise in BP and explore the interindividual response variability to glycyrrhetinic acid. The studied subjects consisted of three groups of Caucasian volunteers who also served as a control for himself/herself consumed liquorice in various doses, 50–200 g/day, for 2–4 weeks, corresponding to a daily intake of 75–540 mg glycyrrhetinic acid, the active substance in liquorice. BP was measured before, during and after liquorice consumption. The findings indicated that the effects of eating liquorice depends on the dose but prolongation of the consumption from 2 to 4 weeks did not influence the response and the maximal BP rise was reached after the first 2 weeks. Furthermore, there was little interindividual variance in the rise of BP. However, it should be noted that the amount of glycyrrhetinic acid varies between different liquorice products. One should be more wary of liquorice as a cause of secondary hypertension. The easiest way to confirm the diagnosis clinically is to stop the liquorice consumption and follow the patient for several weeks, up to a maximum of 4 months, when the renin suppression should have disappeared.

Healthy, Caucasian volunteers who also served as a control for himself/herself consumed liquorice in various doses, 50–200 g/day, for 2–4 weeks, corresponding to a daily intake of 75–540 mg glycyrrhetinic acid, the active substance in liquorice. The individual response to liquorice followed the normal distribution. As liquorice raised the BP with a linear dose–response relationship, even doses as low as 50 g of liquorice (75 mg glycyrrhetinic acid) consumed daily for 2 weeks can cause a significant rise in BP. The finding of a maximal effect of liquorice after only 2 weeks has important implications for all doctors dealing with hypertension.

Liquorice can lead to a suppressed renin concentration, either secondary to the hypervolaemia or direct inhibition of the renin production. The diagnosis of liquorice-induced hypertension should thus be suspected if the plasma renin concentration or activity is low. The diagnosis is then confirmed by measuring the metabolites of cortisol and cortisone in the urine, as the ratio of the metabolites of cortisol/cortisone in the urine rises with liquorice consumption.

Diagnostic tests for renal artery stenosis in patients suspected of having renovascular hypertension: a meta-analysis.

Vasbinder GB, Nelemans PJ, Kessels A, *et al. Ann Intern Med* 2001; **135**(6): 401–11.

BACKGROUND. As a large proportion of patients with renovascular hypertension are still preferably treated with angioplasty, a valid diagnostic test is needed in the presence of one or more clinical clues. Intra-arterial X-ray angiography is considered the gold standard; however, it is invasive. Many researchers have reported results of other, less invasive diagnostic tests. It is, however, difficult to compare the tests' diagnostic performance.

INTERPRETATION. CT angiography and gadolinium-enhanced three-dimensional MR angiography seem to be preferred in patients referred for evaluation of renovascular hypertension. However, because few studies of these tests have been published, further research is recommended.

Comment

The objective of this meta-analysis was to summarize and compare the validity of CT angiography, MR angiography, ultrasonography, captopril renal scintigraphy, and the captopril test for diagnosis of renal artery stenosis in patients suspected of having renovascular hypertension. Intravenous renal angiography and conventional renography were not considered because earlier studies showed that their accuracy was limited. Data on the accuracy of the different diagnostic methods were analysed and compared by constructing summary receiver-operating characteristic (ROC) curves and by computing areas under the summary ROC curves. The summary ROC curves found that CT angiography and gadolinium-enhanced, three-dimensional MR angiography performed significantly better than the other diagnostic tests. However, the accuracy varied greatly for all diagnostic modalities.

Furthermore, because only a limited number of published studies on CT angiography and gadolinium-enhanced MR angiography could be included in this meta-analysis, further research is recommended. Furthermore, careful selection based on clinical evaluation, which can increase the pre-test probability to 20–40%, is a prerequisite for cost-effective use of these tests in the work-up strategy for patients with possible renovascular hypertension.

Eplerenone: a selective aldosterone receptor antagonist (SARA).

Delyani JA, Rocha R, Cook CS, *et al. Cardiovasc Drug Rev* 2001; **19**(3): 185–200.

BACKGROUND. **Although ACEI and Ang II receptor type 1 receptor antagonists act to suppress the renin–angiotensin–aldosterone system (RAAS), these agents do not adequately control plasma aldosterone levels—a phenomenon termed 'aldosterone synthesis escape'. Spironolactone, a non-selective aldosterone receptor antagonist, is an effective agent to suppress the actions of aldosterone; its use is, however, associated with progestational and antiandrogenic side-effects due to its promiscuous binding to other steroid receptors.**

INTERPRETATION. Eplerenone—the first agent of a new class of drugs known as the selective aldosterone receptor antagonists—is under development. In rodent models, eplerenone provides marked protection against vascular injury in the kidney and heart. In phase II clinical trials, eplerenone demonstrates 24-h control of BP with once or twice daily dosing, and is safe and well tolerated in patients with heart failure when given with standard of care agents. Pharmacokinetic studies reveal that eplerenone has good bioavailability with low protein binding, good plasma exposure, and is highly metabolized to inactive metabolites and excreted principally in the bile. Eplerenone is well tolerated in acute and chronic safety pharmacology studies. Ongoing phase III trials of eplerenone in the treatment of hypertension and heart failure are underway. These studies will extend our understanding of selective aldosterone receptor antagonism in the treatment of chronic cardiovascular disease.

Comment

Despite the impressive clinical benefits derived by inhibiting RAAS with ACE inhibitors and the Ang II receptor type 1 receptor antagonists, it is now well established that 'aldosterone escape' may occur and plays a contributing role in the pathogenesis of a number of deleterious effects beyond its sodium retention properties on the cardiovascular system; these include myocardial necrosis and fibrosis, vascular stiffening and injury, reduced fibrinolysis, endothelial dysfunction, catecholamine release and production of cardiac arrhythmias.

The advent of selective aldosterone receptor antagonists such as eplerenone should prove of great therapeutic value in the prevention of cardiovascular disease and associated end-organ damage. It has been called a 'cleaner, safer' version of spironolactone. The EPlerenone's neuroHormonal Efficacy and SUrvival Study (EPHESUS), a trial of a novel aldosterone antagonist, eplerenone vs placebo, in 6200 patients with myocardial infarction, LV dysfunction and pulmonary congestion will determine whether this approach produces additive clinical benefits in patients already on standard treatment. Primary end-points were all-cause mortality and death or hospitalization from cardiovascular causes. The beneficial effects established by the earliest antineurohormonal agents give confidence that further benefits could be obtained by this intellectual strategy. This and other trial results are eagerly awaited |2,3|.

Eplerenone, a selective aldosterone blocker, in mild-to-moderate hypertension.
Weinberger MH, Roniker B, Krause SL, Weiss RJ. *Am J Hypertens* 2002; **15**(8): 709–16.

BACKGROUND. **Eplerenone, a selective aldosterone blocker that is highly specific for the aldosterone receptor, has the potential to be efficacious in the treatment of hypertension.**

INTERPRETATION. Eplerenone doses of 50–400 mg once daily are well tolerated and effective in reducing BP in patients with mild-to-moderate hypertension during a 24-h period.

Efficacy of eplerenone added to renin-angiotensin blockade in hypertensive patients.
Krum H, Nolly H, Workman D, He W, Roniker B, Krause S, Fakouhi K. *Hypertension* 2002; **40**(2): 117–23.

BACKGROUND. **The efficacy and tolerability of eplerenone, a selective aldosterone blocker, was assessed when added to existing antihypertensive therapy with an ACE inhibitor or an ARB.**

INTERPRETATION. This study demonstrated that in patients whose BP was not controlled with an ACE inhibitor or ARB, the addition of eplerenone over an 8-week period significantly lowered SBP in both groups and diastolic BP in ARB patients. Selective aldosterone blockade with eplerenone, therefore, may be useful add-on therapy in hypertensive patients inadequately controlled on ACE inhibitor or ARB alone.

Comment

This was a multi-centre, placebo run-in, double-blind, randomized, placebo-controlled, parallel-group study. Many patients with hypertension are prescribed an ACE inhibitor or ARB, based on the known benefits of RAAS blockade. If BP is not adequately controlled on either of these agents as monotherapy, additional agent(s) will be required. As eplerenone selectively blocks aldosterone receptors, its use in combination with ACE inhibitor or ARB therapy may confer additional benefits as ACE inhibitors and ARBs target angiotensin production by the RAAS but they do not directly block the effects of aldosterone at the receptor level or its deleterious effects on the cardiovascular system. Aldosterone blockade may result in greater inhibition of sodium reabsorption and expansion of intravascular volume, reduction in cardiac hypertrophy, vascular inflammation, and fibrinoid necrosis of the small arteries and arterioles and decreased aortic collagen accumulation.

Conclusion

A true estimate of the prevalence of PA is uncertain but the disorder is increasingly being recognized. With the increasing use of the plasma aldosterone/PAR ratio as a screening tool for the disorder, several investigators have found prevalence ranging from 3 to 9%, with most patients being normokalaemic.

When evaluating hypertensive patients, physicians should have a high index of suspicion that PA may occur in those with moderate to severe hypertension or with hypertension refractory to standard treatment or in hypertensive patients with disease onset at an early age. The ARR is an easy, inexpensive and rapid means of screening for the disorder but further confirmatory testing is required to clinch the diagnosis. The confirmatory tests may include urinary aldosterone excretion on a high-salt diet, aldosterone suppression after a saline infusion, and the fludrocortisone suppression test is considered the most sensitive. The underlying pathology resulting in PA dictates the treatment strategy. The drug of choice is spironolactone. Surgical intervention should be entertained in those patients with PA in whom imaging studies (high-resolution CT and MR imaging scans) suggest an adenoma.

The significant risk reduction provided by the addition of spironolactone to standard therapy in patients with severe heart failure in the Randomized ALdactone Evaluation Study (RALES) has renewed interest in aldosterone blockade. Indeed, many basic studies have shown that aldosterone contributes to hypertension, myocardial and vascular remodelling, and heart failure. Although ACE inhibitors and ARBs block the RAAS, the reduction in aldosterone is only partial and transient, leaving the potentially deleterious effects of aldosterone unchecked, i.e. 'aldosterone escape'. Unlike spironolactone, eplerenone is a selective aldosterone blocker that has greater selectivity for the mineralocorticoid receptor relative to other steroid receptors. Eplerenone is a once-daily, oral therapy that has been tested in more than 3000 hypertensive patients in 14 clinical trials. Key results with the drug include efficacy in BP lowering across multiple patient populations in both white and black patients with hypertension and is effective and well tolerated when used alone or in combination therapy with agents such as ACEIs or ARBs. Preclinical data have shown that eplerenone is effective in hypertension, proteinuria and nephrosclerosis, LV hypertrophy and fibrosis, and in post-myocardial infarction remodelling.

The recently presented eplerenone, enalapril and eplerenone plus enalapril combination therapy (the '4E' study) for BP reduction and LV mass regression has demonstrated that eplerenone monotherapy was as effective as enalapril monotherapy with regard to regression of LV hypertrophy, and the combination of eplerenone and enalapril produced a significantly greater reduction in LV mass than did eplerenone alone. These data suggest that eplerenone treatment confers cardiovascular benefit and that this benefit is additive with that of an ACE inhibitor.

Confirmation of these provocative observations with respect to LV mass regression would require to advocate the addition of selective aldosterone blocker to the therapeutic regimen used for the management of hypertension complicated by cardiac or renal dysfunction.

References

1. Hamlet SM, Tunny TJ, Woodland E, Gordon RD. Is aldosterone/renin ratio useful to screen a hypertensive population for primary aldosteronism? *Clin Exp Pharmacol Physiol* 1985 May–Jun; **12**(3): 249–52.
2. McMahon EG. Recent studies with eplerenone, a novel selective aldosterone receptor antagonist. *Curr Opin Pharmacol* 2001; 1: 190–6.
3. The Eplerenone, Enalapril and Eplerenone/Enalapril Combination Therapy in Patients with Left Ventricular Hypertrophy (4E) trial, presented at the American College of Cardiology 51st Annual Scientific Session, Atlanta 2002.

2

Endothelial dysfunction and surrogate markers in hypertension

Introduction

A large body of evidence indicates that endothelial dysfunction is a characteristic of patients with essential hypertension. By definition endothelial dysfunction is a functional and reversible alteration of endothelial cells, resulting from an impairment in nitric oxide (NO) availability. Thus endothelial dysfunction must be distinguished from endothelial damage, which is represented by the anatomical disruption of the endothelium.

Endothelial dysfunction is now recognized as a key early event in the pathophysiology of many cardiovascular diseases, such as in coronary artery disease (CAD) and peripheral vascular disease. As the endothelium is the primary target organ for atherosclerosis and is involved in important physiological functions, such as homeostasis of the coagulation/fibrinolysis system and the regulation of vascular tone, good measures of endothelial function are desirable, and function may be assessed by an *in vivo* approach, or by taking a serological approach.

Vascular endothelial cells play a key part in cardiovascular regulation by producing a number of potent vasoactive agents, including the vasodilator molecule NO and the vasoconstrictor peptide endothelin 1. This physiology is exploited in the *in vivo* approach, where changes in blood flow may be monitored by a number of different techniques. These methods have shown impaired endothelium-dependent vasodilatation in asymptomatic subjects with hypercholesterolaemia, insulin-dependent and non-insulin-dependent diabetes mellitus, in both passive and active smokers, in subjects with homocystinuria, and with advancing age in men and post-menopausal women.

Dysfunction of the endothelium has also been implicated in human essential hypertension, although there remains some controversy in this area. Many studies to date have used invasive methods or measurements of forearm blood flow by plethysmography or flow-mediated dilatation (FMD) to assess endothelium-dependent vasodilatation and endothelial function. While endothelial dysfunction has been demonstrated in invasive investigations of patients with risk factors for CAD and angiographically normal coronary arteries, the very (invasive) nature of coronary angiography or other intra-arterial procedures precludes routine use for investigation of endothelial function during the long preclinical stage of atherosclerosis. The possibility also arises that these invasive investigations actually cause the endothelial abnormalities being studied.

Attention has therefore been directed towards non-invasive methods of investigation of endothelial dysfunction. For example, plethysmography can be used to measure alteration in blood flow and peripheral vascular tone in response to stimuli as an indirect assessment of resistance vessel endothelial function. Recently, interest has been focused on non-invasive techniques in assessing conduit artery vascular responses using high resolution external ultrasound, where vascular reactivity in response to endothelium-dependent and endothelium-independent stimuli are compared in large peripheral conduit arteries. For example, augmented shear stress produced by increased blood flow is used as the physiological stimulus to endothelium-dependent dilatation, which is mediated by the release of NO from conduit artery endothelium. Endothelium-dependent dilatation is therefore quantitatively assessed as the change in diameter of the artery (usually the brachial or radial artery in adults and the femoral artery in smaller children) following measurement at rest and following a brief period of reactive hyperaemia induced by suprasystolic inflation for several minutes and release of a cuff distal to site of measurement. By contrast, endothelium-independent dilatation is evoked by sublingual administration of either isosorbide dinitrate or nitroglycerin.

An alternate approach to the *in vivo* physiological methods outlined above is to measure specific products of the endothelial cell. For example, it is known that endothelial dysfunction in hypertension is associated with raised levels of certain specific plasma endothelial markers; some are well-established, such as plasma levels of von Willebrand factor. Use of this marker has demonstrated endothelial injury in essential hypertension (correlating with blood pressure [BP]), hypertension associated with renal disease, and in hypertension associated with pre-eclampsia.

A rapid and reproducible on line automated technique to determine endothelial function.

Sidhu JS, Newey VR, Nassiri DK, Kaski J-C. *Heart* 2002; **88**: 289–92.

BACKGROUND. Endothelial dysfunction plays an important part in atherogenesis and in the pathophysiology of coronary atherosclerosis. Prospective studies have also shown that coronary endothelial dysfunction can predict cardiovascular events. Coronary endothelial function has been shown to correlate with endothelial function in accessible peripheral arteries, such as the brachial artery.

INTERPRETATION. Personal computer-based automated techniques to assess FMD involve image acquisition and recording after which a second (off-line) image interpretation session is required. The need for off-line analysis makes current methods time-consuming and increases the variability of measurement. This paper discusses online, automated analysis technique for FMD assessment, which reduces the variability and greatly increases the speed of measurement. Using this system may mean that fewer patients will be required in clinical trials assessing the effects of interventions on endothelial function. Adopting this method may also facilitate the screening of larger numbers of subjects for endothelial dysfunction.

Comment

Current methods for FMD measurement are limited by the need for off-line analysis, and thus are time-consuming, increases the variability of measurement and requires an image storage system. They have developed an automated, on-line analysis technique whereby images are acquired and arterial diameter is measured simultaneously, making the assessment of FMD more efficient, and may allow widespread use of the technique.

The aim of this small prospective study was to assess the technique's reproducibility and performance in a clinical setting. In this study 12 patients with significant, angiographically documented CAD were compared with 12 healthy volunteers. All subjects had their brachial arteries imaged with a standard vascular ultrasound system with a 5–12 MHz linear transducer. Arterial diameter was measured on-line (in real time) by connecting the ultrasound system to a personal computer equipped with a frame grabber and artery wall detection software (vessel image analysis) specially developed by the authors' group. By using this new technique, FMD was measured following 4.5 min of ischaemia of the proximal forearm in all subjects on two separate days. They showed that the mean ± SD day-to-day variability in FMD measurements was excellent, 0.90 ± 0.48%, in subjects with a wide range of measured FMD and baseline arterial diameters. This compares favourably with the lowest reported variability using current methods. The FMD measurement was available within seconds of completing the scan. The authors conclude that this new method minimizes variability and increases the speed of analysis of FMD, and may therefore facilitate the screening of larger numbers of subjects for endothelial dysfunction. As pointed out, these preliminary data, obtained from 24 subjects, need to be confirmed in a larger number of subjects.

Acute effects of vasoactive drug treatment on brachial artery reactivity.

Gokce N, Holbrook M, Hunter LM, *et al. J Am Coll Cardiol* 2002; **40**(4): 761–5.

BACKGROUND. Ultrasound assessment of brachial artery FMD is emerging as a useful clinical tool. The current practice of withholding cardiac medications before ultrasound studies has unknown utility and would limit the clinical use of the methodology.

INTERPRETATION. Recent administration of commonly used non-nitrate vasoactive drugs has no significant effect on brachial reactivity. These findings suggest that current practice of withholding cardiac medications before testing endothelial function may not be necessary, making this methodology more practical for clinical use.

Comment

Indeed, one pressing methodological issue limiting the clinical and research utility of FMD assessment is the current practice of withholding non-nitrate vasoactive medications for at least 24 h before study. This is because of the concern that concurrent treatment would confound the results. However, there is little evidence to support such common practice. Thus, the aim of this study was to investigate whether concomitant therapy with vasoactive medications alters the results of non-invasive assessment of endothelial function at the brachial artery. Interestingly, no previous studies have examined the specific question addressed in the current study.

The study design was well thought. It comprised of two groups of subjects: (i) 73 normal healthy volunteers (age 27 ± 6 years), and (ii) 72 clinically stable patients (age 57 ± 10 years) with angiographically documented CAD. Normal subjects were studied at baseline and at 3 h after randomized treatment with a single oral dose of placebo, felodipine (5 mg), metoprolol (50 mg) or enalapril (10 mg). Patients with CAD were studied after 24 h of withholding all their vasoactive drugs and again on the next day, 3 h after patients took their clinically prescribed medications.

The results showed that treatment with a single dose of commonly used antihypertensive and antianginal medications lowers BP while metoprolol also lowered heart rate, but these agents have no effect on resting brachial artery size, FMD, nitroglycerin-mediated dilation, and the reproducibility of FMD. These results were obtained when healthy patients received single doses of specific agents for the first time and when patients on chronic therapy for CAD were studied before and after receiving their clinically prescribed medications. These findings suggest that acute alterations in systemic haemodynamics and/or local resting arterial tone induced by these medications do not alter the capacity of the brachial artery to respond to endothelium-derived and exogenous vasodilators, and thus making it more practical for clinical use.

Assessment of endothelial function of the renal vasculature in human subjects.

Delles C, Jacobi J, Schlaich MP, John S, Schmieder RE. *Am J Hypertens* 2002; **15**(1 Pt 1): 3–9.

BACKGROUND. L-Arginine, the substrate of NO synthase, and NG-monomethyl-L-arginine (L-NMMA), a competitive inhibitor of endothelial NO synthase, are used to analyse endothelial function of the renal vasculature. However, little is known about the appropriate dose of L-arginine to be used and the duration of action of L-arginine and L-NMMA.

INTERPRETATION. L-Arginine at a dose of 100 mg/kg is sufficient to analyse endothelial function of the renal vasculature. The prolonged effect of L-NMMA and L-arginine must be taken into account in study protocols using both substances. Thus, stimulation and blockade of NO synthase cannot be examined in the same protocol.

Comment

Infusions of L-arginine and L-NMMA have been widely used to analyse endothelial function of the renal vasculature, but the effective dose, duration of actions and interactions between the two compounds are unclear.

The purpose of this study was to search for an accepted dose of L-arginine to be used in the examination of endothelial function of the renal vasculature in human subjects, and to examine the duration of changes in renal haemodynamics of both L-arginine and L-NMMA. A total of 29 young (mean age 27 years), male, white, healthy volunteers were included in the study. Subjects were divided to participate in two separate protocols. In protocol 1 ($n = 17$), arginine at low-dose (100 mg/kg) and high-dose (250 mg/kg), and high-dose arginine combined either with L-NMMA (total dose, 4.25 mg/kg; $n = 9$) or placebo ($n = 8$) were given. In protocol 2 ($n = 12$), L-NMMA was given before arginine infusion (100 mg/kg). Glomerular filtration rate and renal plasma flow were measured at rest and at the end of each infusion step.

The data suggest that L-arginine at a dose of 100 mg/kg was more appropriate than 250 mg/kg to examine endothelial function of the renal vasculature. Systemic administration of L-NMMA appears to be safe in healthy human subjects. Both L-NMMA and arginine have prolonged effects on renal haemodynamics. However, due to its prolonged effect on renal haemodynamics, systemic L-NMMA may be potentially hazardous in patients with severely impaired renal function.

In studies with the aim of examining both the baseline and stimulated NO synthase activity of the renal vasculature, the authors suggested that L-NMMA and L-arginine should be given on separate days to rule out completely any prolonged effect of either substance. However, other details concerning L-arginine and L-NMMA infusion (in particular, dose–response curves in human subjects) remain to be resolved.

Effect of losartan in aging-related endothelial impairment.

Rajagopalan S, Brook R, Mehta RH, Supiano M, Pitt B. *Am J Cardiol* 2002; **89**(5): 562–6.

BACKGROUND. Ageing is associated with progressive deterioration in endothelial function. It was hypothesized that losartan may represent a useful therapeutic strategy to ameliorate endothelial function in aged subjects.

INTERPRETATION. Administration of losartan for a duration of 6 weeks has favourable effects on inflammatory markers in healthy older subjects, but does not alter peripheral conduit endothelial function.

Comment

Through its effects on the angiotensin type 1 receptor, angiotensin II modulates key molecules involved in early atherogenesis, including adhesion molecules, chemokines and inhibitors of fibrinolysis. Blockade of the renin–angiotensin system with angiotensin-converting enzyme inhibitors or angiotensin II receptor type 1 antagonists may ameliorate these adverse effects and seems particularly attractive in the elderly as a strategy to decrease age-related cardiovascular risk.

In this study, Rajagopalan *et al.* compared the effect of losartan (50 mg/day) with placebo on FMD of brachial artery and plasma levels of vascular cell adhesion molecule-1, intercellular adhesion molecule, monocyte chemoattractant protein-1, and E-selectin in 18 healthy older subjects (mean age 75 ± 3 years) in a 6-week double-blind randomized cross-over study with an intervening 2-week washout period.

The major finding of this study is the demonstration that short-term angiotensin receptor blockade (6 weeks) in a cohort of elderly subjects resulted in a significant reduction in circulating levels of adhesion molecules and the chemokine monocyte chemoattractant protein-1. However, improvement in E-selectin levels did not reach statistical significance. There was no significant different in systolic BP (SBP) lowering and increase of FMD between losartan and placebo. There was a strong negative correlation between baseline endothelial function and change in FMD in response to losartan ($r^2 = -0.75$, $P = 0.0003$), suggesting that the patients likely to improve are those with the poorest response to reactive hyperaemia at baseline.

There may be several reasons why there was no significant improvement in FMD with losartan. A larger sample size, larger dose of losartan and longer duration of treatment may improve the power to detect differences. In addition, the title of 'ageing-related' endothelial impairment is not appropriate as younger healthy subjects was not included for comparison in order to delineate an 'ageing-related' effect on endothelial function.

The only interesting observation in this study was that short-term blockade of angiotensin II with losartan decreases adhesion molecule and chemokine expression suggesting that these molecules are regulated to a significant degree by angiotensin II.

Effects of black race on forearm resistance vessel function.

Kahn DF, Duffy SJ, Tomasian D, *et al. Hypertension* 2002; **40**(2): 195–201.

B A C K G R O U N D . Presentation, response to therapy and clinical outcome in hypertension differ according to race, and these observations could relate to differences in microvascular function.

I N T E R P R E T A T I O N . The present study demonstrates important racial differences in vascular function and a marked impairment in endothelial vasomotor function in black patients with hypertension. Further studies will be required to elucidate the mechanisms and determine whether these insights will lead to more appropriately tailored management of hypertension and its complications.

Comment

Indeed, in their previous study [1] the authors observed no racial differences in endothelial function in the conduit brachial artery of normotensive subjects. They also observed no racial difference in the degree of impairment associated with hypertension. However, they hypothesized that the function of the microvasculature as a resistance vessel (as opposed to function of conduit vessels) is likely to be more relevant to the pathogenesis of the disease, as well as to renal failure associated with hypertension. Therefore, the purpose of the present study was to explore racial differences in the function of resistance vessels of normotensive and hypertensive subjects.

A total of 70 normotensive subjects (34 black and 36 white) and 48 hypertensive subjects (22 black and 26 white) were enrolled in the study. Forearm microvascular function was assessed using intra-arterial agonist infusion (in a randomized fashion) and venous occlusion plethysmography. In normotensive subjects, methacholine-, sodium nitroprusside-, and verapamil-induced vasodilation was equivalent in black and white subjects. In hypertensive subjects, the vasodilator response to methacholine was markedly lower in black subjects compared with white subjects ($P < 0.001$). However, the vasodilator responses to sodium nitroprusside and verapamil were equivalent in black and white hypertensive subjects. Acute ascorbic acid infusion improved the methacholine response equally in black and white hypertensive patients, suggesting that a difference in a rapidly reversible form of oxidative stress does not explain these findings.

This study demonstrated no significant racial differences in resistance vessel function in normotensive subjects. However, in the setting of hypertension, the vasodilator response to methacholine was more severely reduced in black subjects compared with age-matched white subjects, although the responses to sodium nitroprusside and verapamil were similar. These findings suggest that the endothelium may be more susceptible to the adverse effects of hypertension in blacks. Importantly, use of antihypertensive medications, including diuretic did not alter the results.

The racial difference in the response to methacholine, but not to sodium nitroprusside and verapamil, suggests a specific impairment of endothelial function in hypertensive blacks rather than a generalized impairment of vascular function or structure. The ascorbic acid portion of the study provided only limited mechanistic information because ascorbic acid may improve endothelial function by several mechanisms and because other forms of oxidative stress could account for a racial difference in vascular function. Further studies will be required to elucidate the mechanisms for this racial difference in vascular function.

Guidelines for the ultrasound assessment of endothelial-dependent flow-mediated vasodilation of the brachial artery. A report of the International Brachial Artery Reactivity Task Force.

Corretti MC, Anderson TJ, Benjamin EJ, *et al*. International Brachial Artery Reactivity Task Force. *J Am Coll Cardiol* 2002; **39**(2): 257–65.

B A C K G R O U N D . **Endothelial function is thought to be an important factor in the pathogenesis of atherosclerosis, hypertension and heart failure. In the 1990s, high-frequency ultrasonographic imaging of the brachial artery to assess endothelium-dependent FMD was developed. The technique provokes the release of NO, resulting in vasodilation that can be quantitated as an index of vasomotor function.**

I N T E R P R E T A T I O N . The non-invasive nature of the technique allows repeated measurements over time to study the effectiveness of various interventions that may affect vascular health. However, despite its widespread use, there are technical and interpretive limitations of this technique.

Comment

State-of-the-art information is presented and insights are provided into the strengths and limitations of high-resolution ultrasonography of the brachial artery to evaluate vasomotor function, with international guidelines for research application in the study of endothelial physiology.

Table 2.1 Training and quality improvement protocol

Elements	Scanning	Measurement
Manuals	Subjects: written procedure description Sonographers: Succinct protocol flow sheet at station. Longer protocol documentation manual	Explicit written measurement protocol documentation to enhance consistency Manual and automated measurements: Frame and segment selection. Criteria for unmeasurable studies
Worksheets	Record subject factors: If ineligible, why Potential FMD modifiers (e.g., food) Blood pressure and cuff inflation pressure Record-scan factors	Log book to track status of studies Worksheet to record technical quality of study
Training	Scientific Rationale and Physiology of FMD Basic knowledge of ultrasound equipment, two-dimensional and Doppler analysis Demonstrate technical tips and pitfalls	Qualification criteria Training period with close supervision and feedback Formal observer-specific reproducibility assessment

Table 2.1 (*continued*)

Elements	Scanning	Measurement
	Ergonomic issues Qualification criteria Training period with close supervision Periodic review of scan performance Minimum number of studies: At least 100 supervised scans prior to scanning independently At least 100 scans per year to maintain competency	Minimum number of studies: At least 100 supervised scans prior to scanning independently All observers from a given study measure 100 studies together prior to reading independently At least 100 scans per year to maintain competency
Reproducibility	Image variability. In single-site study, each sonographer scans the same participants to assess for systematic differences Statistics Correlations, mean and absolute differences, components of variability (systematic vs random differences) Assess on baseline and peak deflation diameters and FMD Doppler, if assessed	Multisite studies should have core reading laboratory, intra- and interobserver variability, temporal variability
Descriptive Statistics	Assess for systematic differences by sonographer and by site Routine Studies Mean baseline and peak deflation diameters and FMD Doppler data, if reported Per time period and over time to assess for secular drifts in measurements	Assess for systematic differences by observer and by site
Data Cleaning	Missing worksheet or measurement data Criteria to re-evaluate study: range checks, consistency checks	
Laboratory Meetings	Periodic laboratory meetings Review work flow, compliance with scan and measurement protocols Measure random and difficult studies together Review results of data cleaning and reproducibility	

Source: Corretti *et al.* (2002).

Non-invasive assessment of microvascular function in arterial hypertension by transthoracic Doppler harmonic echocardiography.

Bartel T, Yang Y, Muller S, *et al. J Am Coll Cardiol* 2002; **39**(12): 2012–18.

BACKGROUND. Coronary flow velocity reserve (CFVR) measurements by transthoracic Doppler harmonic echocardiography (TTDHE) are useful for assessing epicardial coronary artery stenoses. It remains unclear, however, if microvascular disease can be detected.

INTERPRETATION. The newly described echocardiographic method is suitable for assessing microvascular dysfunction non-invasively and corresponds well to invasive measurements.

Comment

Myocardial ischaemia in patients with hypertensive-related left ventricular hypertrophy (LVH) an important clinical problem. These patients can present with significant myocardial ischaemia without obvious epicardial coronary stenosis. Furthermore, silent myocardial ischaemia has also been reported to be more common in a certain subset of hypertensive patients. Several mechanisms may operate at the same time leading to significant reduction in coronary flow reserve in the absence of significant stenosis of the epicardial coronary arteries.

There are several non-invasive techniques available for the assessment of the degree of myocardial ischaemia in these patients, namely: (i) electrocardiographic exercise stress test with a treadmill or bicycle ergometer; (ii) exercise myocardial perfusion radionuclear imaging looking for perfusion defect; and (iii) stress echocardiography looking for regional wall motion abnormalities or more recently regional perfusion defect using contrast-enhanced tissue Doppler imaging.

Coronary microvascular dysfunction may contribute to impaired coronary flow reserve leading to myocardial ischaemia in these patients. Indeed, intracoronary Doppler assessment of CFVR is gaining importance in the detection of suspected microvascular disorders. TTDHE is an ultrasound approach for the assessment of CFVR. The technique uses contrast Doppler enhancement to measure flows at baseline and during adenosine infusion.

The objectives of this study were to investigate the use of TTDHE to evaluate changes in coronary flow dynamics due to microvascular dysfunction. For this purpose, both intracoronary readings and TTDHE were performed in 25 hypertensive (>160/90 mmHg) and 26 normotensive (<140/85 mmHg, as controls) patients, all without epicardial stenoses on diagnostic coronary angiography and intravascular ultrasound examination. Comparative measurements were performed in the distal left anterior descending coronary artery after intracoronary and intravenous administration of adenosine, and CFVR was calculated. All patients were enrolled prospectively.

As pointed out by the authors, their study is the first to show that TTDHE is capable of measuring CFVR with similar results as intracoronary Doppler in patients with and without arterial hypertension. In both groups, TTDHE-derived CFVR data correlated closely with intracoronary Doppler measurements (group 1: $y = 0.67x + 0.076$, standard error of estimate [SEE] $= 0.25$, $r = 0.87$, $P < 0.001$; group 2: $y = 0.64x + 1.11$, SEE $= 0.26$, $r = 0.87$, $P < 0.001$). Interestingly, CFVR was lower in hypertensives than in normotensive controls (2.44 ± 0.49 vs 3.33 ± 0.40, $P < 0.001$, cut point $= 2.84$), indicate significant microvascular dysfunction in the former group. These findings suggest that TTDHE can be considered a suitable modality to assess both microvascular function and dysfunction. The technique may also become a valuable non-invasive tool for evaluating drug effects on the coronary micro-circulation. As an extension of this work, it would be also interesting to evaluate the relation between the results of stress testing and CFVR in hypertensive patients with normal coronary arteries.

Non-invasive study of endothelial function in white coat hypertension.

Gomez-Cerezo J, Rios Blanco JJ, Suarez Garcia I, *et al. Hypertension* 2002; **40**(3): 304–9.

BACKGROUND. Several studies have demonstrated that endothelial dysfunction is present in patients with essential hypertension. However, the presence of endothelial dysfunction in patients with white coat hypertension (WCH) has not been studied.

INTERPRETATION. FMD was similar in white coat hypertensives and sustained essential hypertensives. The presence of endothelial dysfunction in subjects with WCH suggests that it should not be considered a harmless trait and that WCH has common features with sustained essential hypertension.

Comment

WCH, which may be more appropriately termed as isolated in-office hypertension, is not benign entity. Careful follow-up of these patients has been shown to develop into sustained hypertension at an equal rate as in an age-matched group. Cross-sectional studies examining the effect of WCH on hypertensive organ damage have indicated that patients with WCH develop renal impairment, LV dysfunction, and have a higher LV mass than subjects with normal BP at the clinic and at home. However, various questions regarding its mechanisms and its prognostic relevance are still awaiting answers.

In this study, patients with suspected essential hypertension but no previous anti-hypertensive treatment were recruited. After 24-hour ambulatory BP monitoring, 15 patients were classified with mild to moderate sustained essential hypertension; 14 patients with WCH. Fifteen healthy volunteers were also included. WCH was defined as the observation of high BP levels in the doctor's office but normal average daytime ambulatory SBP <135 mmHg and diastolic BP (DBP) <85 mmHg. FMD at the brachial artery were performed and compared among the three groups.

The study found that basal brachial artery diameter did not differ significantly among the three groups. FMD was higher in the control group while no significant differences were found between the sustained essential hypertension group and the WCH group. Although the percentage of non-dippers was higher in the sustained essential hypertension group than in the WCH group, this difference did not have any effect in the FMD. Thus, the presence of endothelial dysfunction among WCH subjects, to the same degree as in sustained essential hypertension subjects, suggests that this group of patients has early atherosclerosis and therefore may be at an increased cardiovascular risk. Indeed, more studies are needed to find out whether antihypertensive treatment would alter cardiovascular outcomes in WCH patients, and to investigate the potential role of the different antihypertensive drugs in improving endothelial function in this group of patients.

Endothelial function in sustained and white coat hypertension.

Pierdomenico SD, Cipollone F, Lapenna D, Bucci A, Cuccurullo F, Mezzetti A. *Am J Hypertens* 2002; **15**(11): 946–52.

BACKGROUND. Endothelial dysfunction is a frequent finding in essential hypertension. The aim of this study was to assess endothelial function, by evaluating circulating NO metabolites, nitrate plus nitrite (NOx), and endothelium-dependent vasodilation, in WCH in comparison with sustained hypertension and normotension.

INTERPRETATION. The data suggest that middle-aged white coat hypertensive subjects without other cardiovascular risk factors do not show endothelial dysfunction in contrast with sustained hypertensive patients.

Comment

The present study was designed to evaluate circulating levels of NO metabolites, NOx and endothelial dysfunction in subjects with WCH compared with subjects with normotension and those with sustained hypertension.

The study included 22 sustained hypertensive, 22 white coat hypertensive and 22 normotensive subjects matched for age, gender, body mass index and occupation. Women were also matched for menopausal status. Subjects with smoking habit, dyslipidaemia and diabetes mellitus were excluded from the study. Of note, all subjects are white in this study. WCH was defined as clinical hypertension and daytime ambulatory BP <135/85 mmHg. Levels of NOx were measured in all subjects after 2 days of low-nitrate diet. The NOx levels were measured by using the Griess reagent after enzymatic conversion of all nitrate to nitrite. Subjects also underwent brachial artery study by ultrasonography to evaluate endothelial function (FMD) and endothelium-independent vasodilation.

Their data showed that circulating levels of NOx and percentage increase of FMD were higher in white coat hypertensive subjects than in sustained hypertensive patients, whereas no significant difference was found between white coat and normotensive subjects. Endothelium-independent vasodilation was not significantly different among the three groups.

As pointed out by the authors, circulating NOx can be used as an index of endogenous formation of NO, provided that oral intake of nitrate and nitrite is restricted for at least 48 h and other potential confounders are taken into account. Previous studies have reported that NO production may be reduced in essential hypertension. The data of the present study also suggested either a decrease in NO synthesis or an increased NO degradation in sustained hypertensive subjects in comparison with white coat and normotensive subjects. However, the exact reason for these changes in NO metabolism in sustained hypertension is unclear.

Peripheral endothelium-dependent flow-mediated vasodilatation is associated with left ventricular mass in older persons with hypertension.

Sung J, Ouyang P, Bacher AC, Turner KL, *et al. Am Heart J* 2002; **144**: 39–44.

BACKGROUND. Increased LV mass is associated with greater cardiovascular disease risk. Recent studies have also shown an association of increased LV mass with attenuated endothelium-dependent coronary flow reserve. Less is known about the association between LV mass and endothelium-dependent FMD in peripheral arteries, a non-invasive measure of endothelial function.

INTERPRETATION. In addition to the expected influences of body size, impairment of brachial artery FMD was independently related to LV mass in elderly subjects with mild hypertension who did not yet have LVH. Whether mild hypertension is the common mechanism linking LV mass and endothelial function has yet to be determined.

Comment

It is not a surprise that impaired endothelial function is associated with increase LV mass in patients with hypertension given what we have already known about a close relationship exist between high BP and endothelial dysfunction, and high BP with increase LV mass.

One other paper exploring the relation between LV mass and endothelial function is by Perticone *et al.* |2|, which described an association between peripheral endothelial dysfunction (brachial FMD) and increased LV mass in hypertensive patients. Indeed, from the pathophysiological point of view that endothelial function may play a part in mediating vascular tone, which in turn is related to systemic vascular resistance and cardiac workload, it is possible that a common mechanism such as high BP influences endothelial function and LV mass, respectively.

The authors studied 62 subjects (29 male, aged 55–75 years) with untreated mild hypertension who are otherwise healthy. FMD was measured at the brachial artery and LV mass was determined from magnetic resonance imaging and was indexed by body surface area, height and height$^{2.7}$. Lean body mass was measured with dual energy X-ray absorptiometry. In bivariate analysis, LV mass was correlated to lean body mass ($r = 0.63$, $P <0.001$), DBP ($r = 0.35$, $P <0.01$) and FMD ($r = -0.27$, $P <0.05$). In multivariate analysis, 44% of the variance in log-LV mass was explained by lean body mass. An additional 6% of the variance was explained by FMD ($P <0.05$). For each 1% point decrease in FMD, LV mass increased by 1.1%. The association between endothelial function and LV mass was independent of BP.

The authors concluded that endothelial dysfunction is associated with relatively increased LV mass even in a normal LV mass range in subjects with isolated mild hypertension. Endothelial dysfunction may precede measurable LVH and therefore suggested that investigating therapies aimed at normalizing endothelial vasodilator function as a means to limit the development of LVH may be worthwhile. Whether BP or other mechanisms explain the link between endothelial function and LV mass remains to be determined.

Indeed, their results have confirmed the findings of others that lean body mass is a strong correlate of LV mass, accounting for 44% of the variance in log-LV mass. By contrast, only 6% of LV mass variance could be attributed to %FMD, which is relatively small by comparison. Furthermore, although the association was statistically significant between LV mass and %FMD, the correlation was weak. Interestingly, SBP (i.e. LV afterload) was not correlated with LV mass, but DBP was. The authors did not attempt to give explanation. Nevertheless, the use of magnetic resonance imaging for LV mass and dual energy X-ray absorptiometry for lean body mass calculation did provide better 'accuracy' of their data. Certainly, more studies are needed, and as we will see later, the decrease in FMD observed in hypertension may be caused by endothelial dysfunction as well as by structural vascular changes.

Post-ischemic forearm skin reactive hyperemia is related to cardiovascular risk factors in a healthy female population.

Vuilleumier P, Decosterd D, Maillard M, Constantin C, Burnier M, Hayoz D.
J Hypertens 2002; **20**: 1753–7.

B A C K G R O U N D . **The assessment of post-ischaemic skin reactive hyperaemia (SRH) can be used as a sensitive indicator of atherogenesis indicating either diminished vasodilator bioavailability or enhanced vasoconstriction in response to hypoxia. Although the precise pathogenetic mechanisms involved in the alteration of the hyperaemic response following transient ischaemia are not fully understood, preliminary evidences suggest that NO does not play a crucial part in the dilator response of the cutaneous circulation.**

INTERPRETATION. This study shows that in a very low cardiovascular risk female population, a significant correlation can be observed between the weight of cardiovascular risks and the impairment of post-ischaemic forearm SRH. Thus, skin laser Doppler flowmetry (LDF) may represent a valuable, simple and non-invasive tool to assess and monitor microvascular function in future prospective observational and interventional studies.

Comment

This study suggests yet another 'new toy' in the assessment of endothelial dysfunction and thus cardiovascular risk. The objective was to examine whether forearm post-ischaemic SRH measured by LDF can be used to explore microvascular function and whether LDF response is related to cardiovascular risk in a population study. Of note, endothelial dysfunction of the cutaneous microcirculation has recently been demonstrated in the forearm of hypertensive subjects by LDF in response to acetylcholine infusion into the brachial artery.

The technique is easy to use, non-invasive and reproducible. SRH of the forearm was defined as the percentage increase in cutaneous blood flow from resting conditions to peak dilation following a 2 min upper arm occlusion. These were measured prospectively in 862 healthy females (aged 40–75 years) screened for cardiovascular risk factors in the context of a campaign designed to promote the 'control' of cardiovascular risk factors in women.

As in so many previous studies that examined the questions but with different high-tech tools, the Framingham risk score was constructed and relates the score to %SRH change. The cardiovascular risk score is low for this female population (cardiovascular event risk at 10 years 7.89, 95% confidence interval 7.49–8.30), but showed an inverse correlation with SRH of the forearm ($P <0.001$). Hormonal replacement therapy (39.4% of the study population was on hormone replacement therapy) had no significant influence on forearm post-ischaemic SRH in this particular population.

Indeed, this very simple non-invasive method appears to be appropriate to assess microcirculatory functional integrity in a very large population. By contrast, the authors felt that current methods for assessment of endothelial function remains at best a rather challenging task necessitating either invasive procedures for intra-arterial drug infusion or the use of sophisticated ultrasonic devices to measure FMD following distal cuff deflation. However, it should be noted that several important issues require further clarification: the skin circulation is not a major target of atherosclerosis. In this respect, it should be noted that the authors demonstrate a relationship between vascular function and a risk score rather than real cardiovascular events during long-term follow-up.

Accordingly, long-term prospective studies in male subjects at higher risk for cardiovascular events such as diabetics are required. Nevertheless, this study and their new tool look promising—representing a step in the right direction.

Nitric-oxide-mediated relaxations in salt-induced hypertension: effect of chronic 1-selective receptor blockade.

Cosentino F, Bonetti S, Rehorik R, *et al. J Hypertens* 2002; **20**(3): 421–8.

B A C K G R O U N D . Nebivolol is a new 1-selective adrenergic receptor antagonist with a direct vasorelaxant effect that involves activation of the L-arginine–NO pathway. Therefore, treatment with nebivolol may protect against endothelial injury in hypertension.

I N T E R P R E T A T I O N . Despite nebivolol and atenolol having the same BP-decreasing effect, only nebivolol was able to prevent endothelial dysfunction. This study demonstrates for the first time that the acute NO-mediated vasodilatory action of nebivolol is also present during chronic treatment. Hence, nebivolol might become a new therapeutic tool with which to exert vascular protective effects against end-organ damage in conditions associated with NO deficiency.

Comment

In this study Dahl salt-sensitive rats were treated for 8 weeks with standard chow or chow containing 4% NaCl alone or in combination with nebivolol (10 mg/kg per day) or atenolol (100 mg/kg per day). Isometric tension was continuously recorded in isolated aorta and small mesenteric arteries. Constitutive NO synthase activity was determined by [^{3}H]citrulline assay.

They found that chronic salt administration increased SBP by 38 ± 5 mmHg in salt-treated rats as compared with that in control rats. Both nebivolol and atenolol prevented a salt-induced increase in pressure. Constitutive NO synthase activity was significantly decreased by a high-salt diet. The impairment of endothelium-dependent relaxations in response to acetylcholine in salt-treated rats was prevented only by nebivolol, in both large and small arteries. In contrast, the reduced endothelium-independent relaxations and contractions in response to sodium nitroprusside and endothelin-1, respectively, were restored by both drugs. Nebivolol, but not atenolol, restored constitutive NO synthase activity.

Prognostic role of reversible endothelial dysfunction in hypertensive post-menopausal women.

Modena MG, Bonetti L, Coppi F, Bursi F, Rossi R. *J Am Coll Cardiol* 2002; **40**(3): 505–10.

B A C K G R O U N D . Hypertensive post-menopausal women have been shown to have abnormal endothelium-dependent vascular function. However, FMD may change over time, according to antihypertensive treatment; the prognostic value of these changes has not been investigated.

INTERPRETATION. This study demonstrates that a significant improvement in endothelial function may be obtained after 6 months of antihypertensive therapy and clearly identifies patients who possibly have a more favourable prognosis.

Comment

The aim of the present study was to assess (i) whether optimized antihypertensive treatment is effective in modifying endothelial function, and (ii) whether an improvement in FMD in response to treatment, as an expression of reversible endothelial dysfunction, could predict a more favourable prognosis in a population of post-menopausal women.

A total of 400 consecutive post menopausal women with mild-to-moderate hypertension and impaired FMD underwent ultrasonography of the brachial artery at baseline and after 6 months, while optimal control of BP was achieved using anti-hypertensive therapy. They were then followed up for a mean period of 67 months (range 57–78). Endothelial function was measured as FMD of the brachial artery, using high-resolution ultrasound. After 6 months of treatment, FMD had not changed (10% relative to baseline) in 150 (37.5%) of 400 women (group 1), whereas it had significantly improved (>10% relative to baseline) in the remaining 250 women (62.5%) (group 2). During follow-up, there were 32 events (3.50 per 100 person-years) in group 1 and 15 events (0.51 per 100 person-years) in group 2 ($P < 0.0001$).

Conclusion

Where do we go from here? Assessment of endothelial function would allow a greater understanding of the pathophysiology of hypertension and its complications. The increasing recognition of the importance of the endothelium in many vascular disorders and the potential of new therapies specifically directed at the endothelium require the establishment of a 'gold standard' non-invasive assessment of endothelial function. Methods such as high-resolution ultrasound, and plasma endothelial markers are likely to complement each other in providing non-invasive and convenient methods for the serial evaluation of vascular function enabling the study of hypertensive patients and responses to interventions, perhaps providing a better insight into the impact of endothelial function on subsequent clinical vascular events.

References

1. Gokce N, Holbrook M, Duffy SJ, Demissie S, Cupples LA, Biegelsen E, Keaney JF Jr, Loscalzo J, Vita JA. Effects of race and hypertension on flow-mediated and nitroglycerin-mediated dilation of the brachial artery. *Hypertension* 2001; **38**: 1349–54.

2. Perticone F, Maio R, Ceravolo R, Cosco C, Cloro C, Mattioli PL. Relationship between left ventricular mass and endothelium-dependent vasodilation in never-treated hypertensive patients. *Circulation* 1999; **99**: 1991–6.

3

Pulse pressure and arterial stiffness

Introduction

Pulse pressure (PP) has been recognized as an independent predictor of cardio-vascular risk: (i) in people with established cardiovascular disease (CVD); (ii) in subjects with cardiovascular risk factor, such as hypertension, diabetes mellitus; and (iii) in the general population. Its predictive value seems to increase with age, and in particular in those over 60 years of age, the predictive value of PP is superior to that of systolic blood pressure (SBP), diastolic blood pressure (DBP) or mean arterial pressure (MAP). In terms of haemodynamics, PP measures the 'pulsatile component' of BP and can be considered as an indirect marker of arterial stiffness, which is itself an independent predictor of cardiovascular risk, whereas SBP, DBP or MAP measures the 'steady component' BP. Whether PP may be considered as a specific mechanical cardiovascular risk factor or as the surrogate of an underlying vascular disease remains unclear. Over 50 years of age, PP may be regarded as a manifestation of arterial stiffness,

Many terms have emerged during 2002, as research interest in PP and arterial stiffness is growing. Data from comparative studies brachial PP vs central (aortic or carotid) PP, clinic PP vs out-of-office PP measure by 24-hour ambulatory BP monitoring or self (home) BP measurement are emerging. Not unexpectedly, 24-hour mean PP is a better predictor for cardiovascular risk than clinic PP. Central (aortic) PP, from a pathophysiological viewpoint being closer to the heart, coronary arteries and carotid arteries, appears to be superior in predicting cardiovascular risk to that measured at the brachial artery. Indeed, aortic PP, but not brachial PP, has been shown to be independently associated with the presence of coronary artery disease (CAD) in patients undergoing coronary angiography, and also to predict the incidence of restenosis after balloon angioplasty. Therefore, recently published studies of antihypertensive drug efficacy have focused on treatment effects not only on BP but also on PP.

Studies of pulsatile arterial haemodynamics have shown that, PP increases markedly from central (thoracic aorta and carotid artery) to peripheral (brachial) arteries, whereas MAP remains nearly constant along the arterial tree. This increase is due to the propagation of the pressure wave along arterial vessels with a progressive decline in artery diameter and an increase in arterial stiffness resulting in a modification in the timing of wave reflection, making aortic PP physiologically lower than brachial PP and thus leading physiologically to PP amplification. With ageing, or in patients with hypertension and/or end-stage renal disease (ESRD) or diabetes, the conduit arteries become stiffer, the PP increases more rapidly in the thoracic aorta than in peripheral arteries, thus producing an attenuation of the physiological increase in PP from central to peripheral arteries. Such attenuation or disappearance of PP amplification from the carotid or aorta to the brachial artery may be a marker of cardiovascular and overall mortality.

Superiority for either SBP and PP has been difficult to establish, most likely because of their high degree of correlation and the marked interaction with age. From the physiological viewpoint, increased arterial stiffness increases pulse wave velocity (PWV) and causes the reflected wave to arrive early, increasing aortic pressure in late systole. The augmented ascending aortic systolic pressure not only leads to an elevated left ventricular (LV) afterload and thus decreases in stroke volume and cardiac output, an increase in myocardial mass/LV hypertrophy (LVH) and oxygen demand, but also compromise diastolic coronary perfusion/filling pressure. The ill effects of early wave reflection also necessarily include a loss of PP amplification between central and peripheral arteries.

Aortic stiffness is the major determinant of central PP, and aortic PWV is the classic index of aortic stiffness, measured non-invasively with ultrasound methods of high reproducibility. Recent epidemiological studies have shown that, independently of confounding factors, such as age, BP and cardiac mass, aortic PWV is a predictor of cardiovascular mortality in populations of hypertensive subjects, whether they have ESRD or not. In all these studies, the odds ratio was higher for PWV than for the latter two predictors.

Many computerized devices are now available to provide a more direct evaluation of arterial stiffness based on three main methodologies, i.e. analysis of: (i) pulse transit time; (ii) wave contour of the arterial pulse; and/or (iii) direct measurement of arterial geometry and pressure. Different indices can be derived from these methods to provide estimates of arterial stiffness at different levels: regional, systemic (or global) and local vascular stiffness. They are increasingly used in clinical laboratory and/or in clinical departments.

Arterial stiffness is emerging as the most important determinant of increased SBP and PP in our ageing community, regardless of whether this mechanical factor plays a causative role in cardiovascular risk or merely serves as a marker of vascular disease already present. Estimates of arterial stiffness has been shown to have additive predictive value for cardiovascular risk to conventional risk factors commonly used in risk scoring algorithms, such as the Framingham risk scoring equation. Determinations of arterial stiffness and/or PP (central or brachial) are therefore an attractive way to refine further our assessment of global cardiovascular risk. This allows identification of the subjects at highest risk and thus selection for therapeutic intervention with a favourable impact on cost-effectiveness in cardiovascular prevention. The techniques are non-invasive and could be carried out at the patient's bedside.

Table 3.1 Relationship between components of arterial pressure and coronary heart disease risk at different ages; Framingham initial cohort and offspring study |1|

	Age <40	40–49 Years	50–59 Years	60 Years
DBP	1.54†	1.28†	1.14*	1.12
SBP	1.16*	1.15†	1.09†	1.17†
PP	0.84† §	1.16	1.12*	1.24†

* $P < 0.05$.
† $P < 0.01$.
‡ $P < 0.001$.
§ in males 0.71 (negative relation $P < 0.05$).
DBP = diastolic blood pressure; SBP = systolic blood pressure; PP = pulse pressure.
Hazard ratio/10 mmHg.
Source: Franklin et al. (2000).

For the same BP reduction, antihypertensive drugs do not cause the same arterial changes in hypertensive patients. However, the benefit of correcting isolated systolic hypertension (ISH), and by inference PP, to avoid clinical cardiovascular events is established. It is still unknown, however, whether conventional antihypertensives reduce cardiovascular events primarily by altering arterial stiffness and/or PP per se.

Angiotensin II (Ang II) is a powerful factor in the development of elevated BP and tissue damage and its blockade should play a major part in remodelling the vascular wall by reversing damage in patients with essential hypertension (EH). Indeed, a number of clinical studies have demonstrated that Ang II blockade afforded by angiotensin-converting enzyme (ACE) inhibitors and angiotensin receptor blockers (ARBs) reduce aortic stiffness (aortic PWV) beyond their effect on BP lowering per se. It is unknown whether these were achieved by blocking the angiotensin system at a systemic level or locally at the vascular level. It may not be possible to establish whether the benefit derives more from a reduction in SBP or a narrowing of PP because it is difficult to modify one without affecting the other.

Novel compounds such as ALT-711 (see below), which break down established advanced glycation end-products (AGEs) cross-links between proteins, have been demonstrated to reduce arterial stiffness. AGEs can lead to stiffening of the blood vessels, including the large arteries. Unlike ALT-711, OPB-9195 is a specific inhibitor of AGEs formation. Indeed, OPB-9195 has been investigated in hypertension and oxidative damage in stroke-prone spontaneously hypertensive rats (SHRSP). These preliminary studies look promising, and thus, it is possible to influence arterial stiffness without affecting systemic BP. Certainly, to establish the impact of such drugs on arterial stiffness and/or PP, we will need more studies in the coming years.

Which pulse pressure: clinic or home, central or peripheral?

Clinic, home and ambulatory pulse pressure: comparison and reproducibility.
Stergiou GS, Efstathiou SP, Argyraki CK, Gantzarou AP, Roussias LG, Mountokalakis TD. *J Hypertens* 2002; **20**(10): 1987–93.

BACKGROUND. Recent evidence suggests that PP is an independent predictor of cardiovascular risk. With regard to PP, there is some evidence showing that, as for BP, ambulatory PP is also lower than clinic PP. Recently, one study suggested that ambulatory PP may be superior to clinic PP in predicting cardiovascular events. Data are lacking on PP values obtained using home measurements.

INTERPRETATION. Although differences among mean values of clinic PP, home PP and ambulatory PP are small, differences in their reproducibility are important and should be taken into account in the design of trials assessing drug effects on PP.

Comment

Out-of-office BP measurement, using ambulatory or home monitoring, generally provides lower and more reproducible BP values than clinic measurements. In most of the studies, PP has been obtained using measurements of BP in the clinic. However, there is some evidence showing that, as for BP, ambulatory PP is also lower than clinic PP. Indeed, clinical studies have suggested that ambulatory PP may be superior to clinic PP in predicting cardiovascular events. Data are lacking on PP values obtained using home measurements.

In this study, a total of 393 hypertensive subjects' (mean age 52 years, 59% men, 35% treated) PP values were compared using all three methods (clinic, home and ambulatory). The reproducibility of PP was also assessed using the SD of differences (SDD) between measurements in 133 untreated subjects who had repeated clinic PP (five visits), home PP (6 days) and ambulatory PP measurements (two occasions).

The data show that the differences in PP among the three methods were surprisingly small. In particular, clinic PP seemed to provide the higher and ambulatory PP the lower levels, but 95% confidence intervals (CI) excluded any difference greater than 3 mmHg among these values. A reasonable explanation for this discrepancy would be that the parallel changes in SBP and DBP result in more similar levels of PP between measurement methods, compared with those usually observed for both SBP and DBP. The authors pointed out that there is some evidence showing that clinic measurements may overestimate the levels of PP, but the study was small and included older subjects with higher SBP. A study by Verdecchia *et al.* [2] included 2010 untreated hypertensives of similar age to the subjects also indicated higher clinic PP than ambulatory PP but these differences may be attributed to a larger white-coat effect in that study.

On the other hand, the analysis on reproducibility among the three methods, found important differences. For example, the SD was higher for clinic PP compared with home PP or 24-hour ambulatory PP, suggesting that the most variable PP values are provided by clinic measurements and the most stable by ambulatory measurements. Furthermore, clinic PP appears to have the poorest reproducibility even after excluding the 'unstable' measurements of the initial visit. Thus, in this respect, the behaviour of PP in the clinic appears to be similar to that known to exist for clinic BP.

One of the criticisms of the present study would be that mostly middle-aged subjects were included, rather than elderly subjects known to have higher PP values. The poor reproducibility of clinic PP compared with home and ambulatory PP warrants attention when designing trials aiming to assess drug effects on PP.

Diabetes, pulse pressure and cardiovascular mortality: the Hoorn Study.

Schram MT, Kostense PJ, Van Dijk RA, *et al. J Hypertens* 2002; **20**(9): 1743–51.

BACKGROUND. **Type 2 diabetic patients have an increased arterial stiffness and a very high risk of cardiovascular death. However, it is not known whether PP is positively associated with cardiovascular mortality in these patients, nor whether any such relationship is similar in diabetic and non-diabetic individuals. In addition, it is not known whether the increase of PP in diabetes is related to the accelerated vascular ageing that is thought to occur in diabetes, in which case one would expect a stronger association between age and PP than in non-diabetic individuals.**

INTERPRETATION. In type 2 diabetes, PP is positively associated with cardiovascular mortality. The association between age and PP is influenced by the presence of type 2 diabetes and by the height of the MAP. These findings support the concept of accelerated vascular ageing in type 2 diabetes.

Comment

The Hoorn Study is a population-based cohort study on glucose intolerance in a Dutch population conducted from 1989 until 1992. Data on the vital status of the subjects on 1 January 2000 were collected from the mortality register of the municipality of Hoorn.

This study investigated the relationship between PP, an indicator of vascular stiffness, and risk of cardiovascular mortality among type 2 diabetic and non-diabetic individuals. The study also attempts to determine the relationship between PP and its main determinant (i.e. age), and the influence of diabetes and MAP on this relationship.

The prospective cohort comprised of 2484 individuals, including 208 type 2 diabetic patients. Mean age and median follow-up for non-diabetic and diabetic individuals, respectively, were 61 and 66 years, and 8.8 and 8.6 years. There were 116 non-diabetic and 34 diabetic individuals who died of cardiovascular causes. The results showed that PP was associated with cardiovascular mortality among the diabetic with 27% increased risk of cardiovascular death per 10 mmHg increase of PP compared with non-diabetics (adjusted relative risk [RR] [95% CI] per 10 mmHg increase, 1.27 [1.00–1.61] and 0.98 [0.85–1.13], P interaction = 0.07). Among non-diabetics, PP was significantly associated with cardiovascular mortality in crude analysis, but this relationship disappeared after adjustment for age, gender and MAP. The lack of association between PP and cardiovascular mortality in non-diabetics seem rather surprising. The authors pointed out that MAP is an important confounder of this association. Failure to adjust for this confounder can lead to higher estimated levels of RR, and thus to an overestimation of the influence of PP on mortality risk in other studies. However, their study had a relatively short follow-up and very low mortality rate. Studies with a longer follow-up and higher mortality rates generally report stronger associations between PP and mortality (7.2 per 1000 person-years for cardiovascular mortality in this study, compared with 1.7–48.6 per 1000 person-years in other studies).

Interestingly, the PP increase typically observed in diabetics was, in part, related to a stronger association of PP with age compared with non-diabetics. This finding supports the concept of accelerated vascular ageing in type 2 diabetes. Accelerated vascular ageing in diabetes is biologically plausible. During ageing, collagen in large arteries becomes more prominent, while elastin fibres become disrupted, leading to stiffer vessel walls. In diabetes, increases in oxidative stress, carbonyl stress and AGEs may combine to exaggerate these alterations in collagen and elastin structure and function, with resultant loss of vascular elasticity.

As pointed out, PP or arterial stiffness is a target for therapeutic intervention in these patients. However, it is not clear how PP or arterial stiffness can be reduced. Current antihypertensive treatments often focus on reduction of the extracellular volume or smooth muscle cell tone, thereby reducing both SBP and DBP. When both pressures are reduced, PP may not have changed. Some evidence exists that ACE inhibitors or ARBs may have a direct effect on large artery wall properties beyond BP lowering, thereby reducing arterial stiffness (see below). In addition, novel therapeutic drugs, such as ALT-711, which breaks down established AGE cross-links between proteins, have been demonstrated to reduce arterial stiffness, but more evidence is necessary to establish the impact of such drugs.

Isolated diastolic hypertension, pulse pressure, and mean arterial pressure as predictors of mortality during a follow-up of up to 32 years.

Strandberg TE, Salomaa VV, Vanhanen HT, Pitkala K, Miettinen TA.
J Hypertens 2002; **20**(3): 399–404.

BACKGROUND. Both PP and MAP have been implicated as independent predictors of risk, but there are few truly long-term studies. During the 1990s, ISH has emerged as an important modifiable risk factor in the elderly, but despite several studies—most notably the Framingham Study—showing the importance of SBP, many physicians still consider DBP the most important of the two measurements.

INTERPRETATION. The results of this study demonstrate the often neglected role of SBP in predicting long-term CVD risk in middle-aged men. When SBP is less than 140 mmHg, isolated diastolic hypertension is not associated with significantly increased risk of mortality. Administrative guidelines, which affect population health, should also take due note of SBP.

Comment

This is yet another long-term prospective cohort studies on the associations between mortality and various BP components. They studied 3267 initially healthy men, aged 30–45 years, who participated in health check-ups in Helsinki from 1964 onwards, and were followed up for up to 32 years. The results showed that of the different BP variables, MAP, SBP and DBP were quite similar predictors of long-term CVD mortality risk. PP was a significant predictor when adjusted for DBP, but was not significant when adjusted for MAP or SBP in these middle-aged men. Of the different BP subgroups with 160/90 mmHg as the cut-off value for hypertension, only systolic–diastolic hypertension significantly predicted mortality. The present study is reassuring in showing that mortality risk is not significantly increased in isolated diastolic hypertension when SBP is less than 140 mmHg. Conversely, risk is increased when SBP is greater than 140 mmHg and DBP less than 90 mmHg. Use of antihypertensive medications during follow-up did not explain the results.

There are a few limitations of this study. For example, the study population was selective, with all participants being men from the highest social class. Thus generalization of the results to other populations (and especially to women) should be made cautiously. There were no strict procedural guidelines at baseline, and there was only a single BP measurement recorded.

Several of the statistical findings they reported are not completely new. However, it is important to note that Strandberg *et al.* are the first to propose that, when SBP is below 140 mmHg, isolated diastolic hypertension is not associated with a significantly increased mortality risk. In addition, these authors are also the first to state clearly that the data should encourage a reconsideration of the drug-reimbursement policy in Finland, because the diagnosis and treatment of hypertension still rely heavily on DBP. They even went so far as to accuse these DBP-based administrative decisions of being detrimental to public health and potentially jeopardizing research on drug treatment of hypertension.

Prognostic value of treatment-induced changes in twenty-four-hour mean and pulse pressures in adult hypertensive patients.

Schillaci G, Pasqualini L, Vaudo G, *et al. Am J Cardiol* 2002; **90**(8): 896–9.

BACKGROUND. Antihypertensive therapy may lead to a decrease in PP, which does not necessarily parallel that of SBP and DBP. A spontaneous increase in PP over time has been associated with subsequent cardiovascular events. However, the prognostic benefits of treatment-induced PP reduction compared with the reduction in steady BP components (SBP, DBP and MAP) remain to be determined in prospective outcome studies.

INTERPRETATION. Treatment-induced reduction in the 24-hour steady BP components of SBP, DBP and MAP is associated with a significant reduction in the rate of future cardiovascular events in adult hypertensive subjects, whereas changes in 24-hour PP confer no significant prognostic benefit.

Comment

The Progetto Ipertensione Umbria Monitoraggio Ambulatoriale (PIUMA) study was established in 1986 as an observational registry in initially untreated subjects with EH. The purpose of the present analysis was to assess the prognostic significance of changes in PP and MAP induced by antihypertensive treatment in 743 initially untreated hypertensive subjects (age 48 ± 11 years, men 56%) who attended the pre-treatment and follow-up visits and were free of CVD in the PIUMA Study. All subjects had 24-hour ambulatory BP at baseline and after a mean follow-up of 3.5 ± 2 years. Treatment was aimed at reducing office BP to <140/90 mmHg. At the follow-up visit, 30% of the subjects were being treated with life-style measures alone and 70% ($n = 515$) were being treated with antihypertensive drugs. Of these, 257 received monotherapy with diuretics ($n = 20$), beta-blockers ($n = 41$), ACE inhibitors ($n = 99$), ARBs ($n = 17$), calcium channel blockers (CCB)s ($n = 61$) or other drugs ($n = 19$). The remaining subjects were treated with various drug combinations. On average, 24-hour MAP decreased by 6.9 ± 11 mmHg, and 24-hour PP decreased by 2.7 ± 7 mmHg (both P <0.01). After the follow-up examination, patients were further followed for a time window of 1.5 ± 2 years for cardiovascular events. The study population was divided according to their treatment-induced reduction in 24-hour mean and PP, respectively.

The results showed that the cardiovascular event rate was higher in the group in which treatment-induced reduction in 24-hour MAP was below the median value. In contrast, the event rate did not differ in the groups defined by treatment-induced reduction in 24-hour PP.

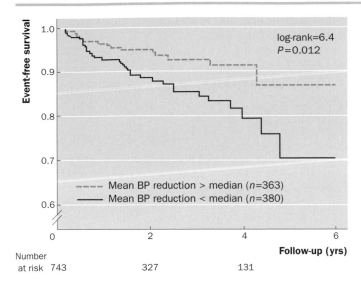

Fig. 3.1 Event-free survival in hypertensive patients with treatment-induced reduction in 24-hour MAP above (broken line) or below (continuous line) the median value. Source: Schillaci *et al.* (2002).

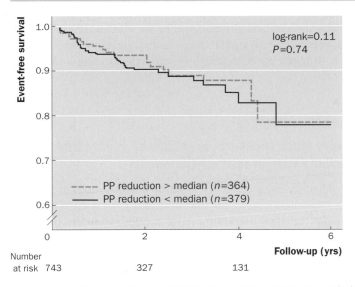

Fig. 3.2 Event-free survival in hypertensive patients with treatment-induced reduction in 24-hour PP above (broken line) or below (continuous line) the median value. Source: Schillaci *et al.* (2002).

In the baseline Cox model, age, diabetes and pre-treatment 24-hour PP and MAP all independently predicted an increased risk for subsequent cardiovascular events. However, when treatment-induced changes in SBP, DBP, MAP and PP were added one at a time to the multivariate event-free survival analysis (Cox proportional-hazards model), the reduction in 24-hour SBP, DBP and MAP was associated with a lower rate of future events, whereas changes in 24-hour PP had no prognostic impact. For every 1 SD decrease in 24-hour MAP (11 mmHg), there was an independent 39% reduction in the risk of future cardiovascular events (P <0.001), whereas for every 1 SD reduction in 24-hour PP (9 mmHg), there was a non-significant 9% reduction in events (P = NS). Risk reduction was 32% (P <0.01) for a 1 SD reduction in 24-hour SBP (14 mmHg), and 44% (P <0.001) for a 1 SD reduction in 24-hour DBP (10 mmHg).

The authors reported that pre-treatment steady and pulsatile components of BP (i.e. MAP and PP) are both independent predictors of cardiovascular events in hypertension. In addition, treatment-induced reductions in average 24-hour steady BP components, namely, SBP, DBP and MAP, are associated with a significantly lower rate of future cardiovascular events, whereas treatment-induced reduction in 24-hour PP does not appear to confer any significant prognostic benefit.

It is of note that the subjects in the present study are relatively young (mean age 48 years), and as the predictive value of PP for cardiovascular events increases with age, particularly in those >60 years of age, its prognostic value becomes more important compared with other BP components. Thus, the conclusion drawn from this study cannot be extrapolated to an older age group.

Quite rightly, as proposed by the authors, there is a need for larger, prospective, controlled studies designed to address the question of the relative importance of treatment-induced changes in the various BP components. Until the results of those studies are available, it is premature to establish PP reduction as a new target for antihypertensive therapy.

Ambulatory pulse pressure as predictor of outcome in older patients with systolic hypertension.

Staessen JA, Thijs L, O'Brien ET, Bulpitt CJ, et al. Am J Hypertens 2002; **15**(10 Pt 1): 835–43.

B A C K G R O U N D. Observational studies and recent overviews, all based on the calculation of PP and mean pressure from conventional BP readings, suggested that in middle-aged and older subjects cardiovascular prognosis gets worse with higher PP, not mean pressure. Until now, few studies addressed the question whether the use of ambulatory PP or ambulatory mean pressure may further enhance the risk stratification of hypertensive patients.

I N T E R P R E T A T I O N. In older patients with ISH higher PP estimated by 24-hour ambulatory monitoring was a better predictor of adverse outcomes than conventional PP, whereas conventional and ambulatory mean pressures were not correlated with a worse outcome.

Comment

In this study, the authors used the ambulatory BP recordings obtained in the Systolic Hypertension in Europe (Syst-Eur) Trial to investigate whether ambulatory PP is a better predictor of outcome than ambulatory mean pressure or than PP or mean pressure calculated from conventional BP readings. They studied 808 older patients with ISH (160–219/71 <95 mmHg) age ≥60 years who were randomized to nitrendipine with the possible addition of enalapril or hydrochlorothiazide (12.5–25 mg/day) or to matching placebos. At baseline, PP and mean pressure were determined from six conventional BP readings and from 24-hour ambulatory recordings.

The data showed that in untreated older patients with systolic hypertension, higher ambulatory PP consistently predicted total and cardiovascular mortality and that of cardiovascular complications. The hazard rates for 10 mmHg increases in PP ranged from 1.25 to 1.68. On the other hand, conventionally measured PP predicted only cardiovascular mortality with a hazard rate of 1.35. The 24-hour and night-time ambulatory PPs predicted cardiovascular outcome over and beyond PP calculated from conventional BP readings. Extrapolation from the Cox regression model showed that at any given level of 24-hour SBP, the cardiovascular risk increased with lower 24-hour DBP and hence with higher PP. In contrast, mean pressure determined from ambulatory or conventional BP measurements was not associated with poorer prognosis.

According to the authors, the greater number of measurements, the absence of digit preference and observer bias, and the minimization of the white-coat effect probably contributed to the predictive superiority of ambulatory over conventional PP. But, the data also in keeping with established haemodynamic concepts, as ambulatory BP measurements may more accurately reflect the dynamic interaction between the heart and the large arteries.

It is important to note, however, that in the active treatment group compared with the placebo patients, the relation between outcome and ambulatory PP was attenuated to a non-significant level. According to the authors, the point estimates of the relative hazard rates were of the same order of magnitude as those in the placebo group, but because of the smaller number of events the CIs were wider and included unity. They went on and explained that any antihypertensive drug that reduces arteriolar tone may decrease PP through a passive increase in arterial compliance. Furthermore, a reduction of the ventricular ejection rate or active relaxation of vascular smooth muscle cells may specifically reduce SBP and PP. Nearly 90% of the patients on active treatment consisted of nitrendipine given alone or in combination with other study medications, and these lowered conventional and ambulatory PPs by 4–6 mmHg. They gave evidence that nitrendipine has a high selectivity for the vasculature and increases the elasticity of the large arteries over and beyond what can be expected on the basis of BP lowering alone.

There is so far no evidence to suggest that conventional antihypertensive medications can influence outcome through altering PP. Furthermore, whether different classes of pharmacotherapy will have different effects on event reduction according to different effect on lowering PP remains speculative. A causal or reversible relationship also remains to be established.

Pulse pressure and risk of cardiovascular events in the systolic hypertension in the elderly program (SHEP).
Vaccarino V, Berger AK, Abramson J, *et al. Am J Cardiol* 2001; **88**(9): 980–6.

BACKGROUND. PP has been related to higher risk of cardiovascular events in older persons. ISH is common among the elderly and is accompanied by elevated PP. Treatment of ISH may further increase PP if DBP is lowered to a greater extent than SBP. Little is known regarding PP as a predictor of cardiovascular outcomes in elderly persons with ISH, and the influence of treatment on the PP effect.

INTERPRETATION. These results suggest that PP is a useful marker of risk for heart failure (HF) and stroke among older adults being treated for ISH.

Comment

The present study is unique in the sense that it examined the changing values of PP over time, as well as the baseline values, in the treatment and placebo groups separately. Previously published reports on the relationship of PP with cardiovascular events examined the placebo and treatment groups combined, which might not be entirely justified in the Systolic Hypertension in the Elderly Program (SHEP) given the remarkable differences in outcome in these two groups.

The results showed that in the treatment arm but not in the placebo arm, a higher PP was an independent predictor (after accounting for SBP and DBP) of HF and stroke, and was actually more strongly related to cardiovascular outcomes than SBP and DBP. However, the association between PP and CHD risk was not significant in both groups. Although the results may not be generalizable to other populations, these results do suggest that PP could provide useful prognostic information among older adults during treatment for ISH and may help optimize treatment regimens. Decreasing PP in addition to SBP may offer additional benefits to these patients.

The prognostic benefits of treatment-induced PP reduction compared with the reduction in steady BP components (SBP, DBP and MAP) remain to be determined in prospective outcome studies.

Association of increased pulse pressure with the development of heart failure in SHEP. Systolic Hypertension in the Elderly (SHEP) Cooperative Research Group.

Kostis JB, Lawrence-Nelson J, Ranjan R, Wilson AC, Kostis WJ, Lacy CR.
Am J Hypertens 2001; **14**(8 Pt 1): 798–803.

B A C K G R O U N D . Patients with ISH have increased PP and greater risk for cardiovascular events, including stroke, myocardial infarction (MI) and HF. Although the decreased DBP linked to high PP may trigger thrombotic events, ouch as stroke and MI, it cannot fully explain the relationohip between PP and HF without an intervening MI.

I N T E R P R E T A T I O N . In older persons with ISH, high PP is associated with increased risk of HF independently of MAP and of the occurrence of acute MI during follow-up.

Comment

This report presents observations on the relationship of PP to the development of HF among 4736 men and women aged ≥60 years with ISH (MAP 170/77 mmHg and mean PP 93 mmHg) who participated in the SHEP study. The main outcome measures were fatal and non-fatal HF. During 4.5 years average follow-up, fatal or non-fatal HF occurred in 160 of 4736 patients. The SBP, PP and MAP were strong predictors of the development of HF. HF was found to be inversely related to DBP but was directly related to PP. Results remained unchanged even when patients who developed MI during follow up were excluded. The mechanisms underlying the increased risk of HF in patients with high PP remains unclear. It may be explained by the association of decreased arterial compliance with both PP and increased afterload. High PP has also been associated with LVH and impaired diastolic LV relaxation, especially in elderly patients.

Pulse pressure compared with other blood pressure indexes in the prediction of 25-year cardiovascular and all-cause mortality rates: The Chicago Heart Association Detection Project in Industry Study.

Miura K, Dyer AR, Greenland P, *et al*. Chicago Heart Association.
Hypertension 2001; **38**(2): 232–7.

B A C K G R O U N D . Because recent discussions have emphasized the importance of SBP compared with DBP7–10 and because these are strongly correlated, it is also important to assess whether DBP has any additional role in the prediction of risk independent of SBP. Such analyses are relevant to understand the meaning of PP as a cardiovascular risk factor.

INTERPRETATION. The data indicate that the long-term risk of high BP should be assessed mainly on the basis of SBP or of SBP and DBP together, not on the basis of PP, in apparently healthy adults.

Comment

Recent analysis of 10 874 men aged 18–39 at baseline who were not receiving antihypertensive drugs and showed no CHD or diabetes from the Chicago Heart Association Detection Project in Industry, young men with even high-normal BP or stage 1 hypertension according to the JNC VI criteria have higher 25-year risks for death by CHD and CVD, and all-cause mortality rate than those with normal or optimal BP |**3**|.

The present report compares the relations of four BP indexes (PP, SBP, DBP and MAP) to 25-year mortality risks from CHD, CVD and all causes in five population cohorts (total, 28 360 men and women) classified by age and gender using data from a long-term prospective epidemiological study of employed persons who were screened between 1967 and 1973, and who were not receiving antihypertensive treatment, had no history of CHD, and did not have diabetes. A single supine BP measurement was obtained at baseline. Vital status was determined through 1995.

They found that the relations of PP were less strong than were those of SBP for all end-points in all age/gender groups. SBP or MAP showed the strongest relations to all end-points in all age/gender groups (hazard ratio, 1.17–1.36). The relations of SBP to death were stronger than were those of DBP, except for middle-aged men and for CVD in women. Finally, DBP showed significant positive associations with death, after control for SBP, in middle-aged participants.

Given the consistency of data from several other population studies supporting the superiority of PP, especially in persons over the age of 60, in predicting cardio-vascular morbidity and mortality, the results from this present report seems contradictory. Based on their data, the authors affirm a continued emphasis on SBP, particularly for younger men and older persons (age 60–74) of each gender. They suggested that DBP should be given concomitant careful consideration in middle-aged persons age 40–59 years because of its strong independent relation to death, and the severity of diastolic hypertension should be carefully assessed in middle-aged persons. In addition, in younger and middle-aged persons, an emphasis on PP should be avoided, as PP is likely to underestimate the true risks in these age groups. Their data also did not support the use of PP as risk predictor in men and women between the ages of 60 and 74. In fact, MAP could even turn out to be a stronger risk predictor than SBP. But use of MAP may not be practical as no guidelines for hypertension diagnosis and management using MAP. Thus, detection and evaluation of hypertension based mainly on SBP remain the most practical and easy approach in the general population. Regarding the role of PP for prognosis in considerably older 'healthy' populations, other studies are required.

Few reasons may explain the discrepancies between the Miura *et al.* study |**3**| and the majority of other studies in the older age group. The presence of a healthy cohort effect in the Miura *et al.* study |3| could well be the most important factor. The mean age of their population was only 63 years. The use of supine BPs instead of the more conventional sitting position also may have influenced results. Single BP recordings in the Miura *et al.* study |3| undoubtedly reduced precision.

In general, in patients <50 years of age, DBP is the strongest predictor. The age period 50–59 years could be seen as a transition period when all three BP indices are comparable predictors, and from 60 years of age on, DBP is negatively related to CHD risk so that PP become superior to SBP. None the less, SBP is the best single predictor for the majority of persons with hypertension. However, for older persons, the best clinical strategy for estimation of cardiovascular risk is, first, to determine the level of SBP elevation and then adjust the overall risk upward if there is wide PP, i e. discordantly low DBP.

Pulsatile BP component as predictor of mortality in hypertension: a meta-analysis of clinical trial control groups.
Gasowski J, Fagard RH, Staessen JA, *et al. J Hypertens* 2002; **20**: 145–51.

BACKGROUND. Although current guidelines rest exclusively on the measurement of SBP and DBP, the arterial pressure wave is more precisely described as consisting of a pulsatile (PP) and a steady (mean pressure) component. This study explored the independent roles of PP and mean pressure as predictors of mortality in a wide range of patients with hypertension.

INTERPRETATION. In hypertensive patients PP, not MAP, is associated with an increased risk of fatal events. This appears to be true in a broad range of patients with hypertension.

Comment
Several observational studies have showed that PP may be an independent predictor of cardiovascular risk in a wide range of individuals: in the general population, in hypertensive subjects, in survivors of MI, and patients with LV dysfunction. The collaboration of the INDANA (Individual Data Analysis of Antihypertensive Intervention Trials) project has combined results from the control groups of seven randomized clinical trials conducted in patients with systolo-diastolic or ISH and thus allowed meta-analysis in a much wider age and BP range than previous studies that included mainly older hypertensives with ISH.

In this study the relative hazard rates associated with PP and mean pressure were calculated using Cox's proportional hazard regression models with stratification for the seven trials and with adjustment for sex, age, smoking and the other pressure. The data revealed that in patients with hypertension a 10 mmHg wider PP is independently associated with an increase in risk by 6% for total mortality ($P = 0.001$), 7% for cardiovascular mortality ($P = 0.01$), and 7% for fatal coronary accidents ($P = 0.03$). The corresponding increase in risk of fatal stroke was similar (+6%,

$P = 0.27$) but there were too few strokes to reach statistical significance. These risks were consistent throughout a large pool of patients enrolled as controls and assigned to placebo or no medication in seven randomized clinical trials. In similar analyses, mean pressure was not identified as an independent predictor of these outcomes. Furthermore, significant interactions of PP or mean pressure with age suggested that the prognostic power of PP for fatal stroke was more important at higher age ($P = 0.04$), whereas the prognostic power of mean pressure for coronary mortality was greatest in the young ($P = 0.01$).

Thus, the study's results confirm and expand the previously reported findings that PP, rather than MAP, is the major risk factor of adverse cardiovascular complications. It is of note that early reports from the Framingham Heart Study emphasized that SBP was a better independent predictor of cardiovascular risk than DBP, especially in subjects over the age of 50. Increasing evidence now points towards PP as a better predictor of cardiovascular risk than SBP or DBP. However, the present study does not imply a causal relationship. A well designed clinical study is needed to clarify the issue of whether or not lowering of PP would decrease cardiovascular morbidity and mortality.

Relative role of systolic, diastolic and pulse pressure as risk factors for cardiovascular events in the Brisighella Heart Study.

Borghi C, Dormi A, Ambrosioni E, Gaddi A, On behalf of the Brisighella Heart Study Working Party. *J Hypertens* 2002; **20**(9): 1737–42.

BACKGROUND. Recent published data from the Framingham Heart Study, and other investigations have provided substantial evidence that SBP and PP may be more important predictors of cardiovascular outcomes than DBP.

INTERPRETATION. This study demonstrates that SBP is a stronger predictor of cardiovascular events than DBP in the Brisighella population. The added prognostic significance of PP is also demonstrated, particularly if PP exceeds 67 mmHg.

Comment

The Brisighella Heart Study is a prospective, population-based longitudinal epidemiological cohort, which is similar in design and duration to Framingham, provides a unique opportunity to investigate the long-term prognostic significance of BP parameters in a non-US population in Italy. The Brisighella Heart Study involved 2939 randomly selected residents of Brisighella, Italy aged 14–84 years, free of CVD at enrolment and followed since 1972. Subjects were clinically evaluated at baseline and every 4 years following enrolment when extensive clinical and laboratory data were obtained in addition to the assessment of morbidity and mortality. The objective of the present analysis was to determine the relative contribution of BP variables to the long-term incidence of cardiovascular events. For the current analysis, the period

Table 3.2 Relative risk of systolic, diastolic and pulse pressure as risk factors for cardiovascular events

SBP categories (mmHg)	Adjusted hazard ratios*	P-value (95% CI)
120–139	1.45	0.035
140–159	1.88	0.0008
>159	2.31	0.0001
DBP ranges		
70–79	0.91	0.677
80–89	1.33	0.169
>80	1.65	0.029
PP ranges		
54–67	1.23	0.149
>67	1.38	0.030

* Adjusted hazard ratios for combined CHD + CVD. Similar results were seen for CVD and CHD as separate end-points. CHD, coronary heart disease; CVD, cardiovascular disease; SBP, systolic BP; DBP, diastolic BP; PP, pulse pressure.
Source: Borghi et al. (2002).

of follow-up was from 1973 to 1996. The Cox regression analysis for CVD was used to determine the independent prognostic significance of SBP, DBP and PP. Models were adjusted for age, sex body mass index (BMI), smoking habit, presence of diabetes and plasma cholesterol.

Although variation in absolute risk may be seen from one region of Europe to the next, this study has demonstrated that the important prognostic value of SBP and to a lesser extent PP, is evident in these populations as well. DBP is a weaker indicator than SBP, particularly with increasing age. They pointed out that the U-shaped relationship between cardiovascular risk and DBP levels demonstrated in previous studies might be due to the fact that low DBP associated with increased PP resulting from loss of arterial distensibility with age. Thus, low DBP in turn may contribute to myocardial or cerebral ischaemia and accelerate the onset of cardiovascular events.

Superiority for either SBP and PP has been difficult to establish, most likely because of their high degree of correlation and the marked interaction with age. What is clear is that SBP continues to rise with age, and is associated with stiffening of the large arteries and enhanced PWV, leading to peripheral vascular damage and cardiac hypertrophy.

However, it is an incomplete basis for the unmodified use of Framingham multifactor risk estimates as a guide for public policy or personal encounter clinical practice. Several studies have evaluated the extent to which Framingham models predicted risk of CHD in more relevant local cohorts, have generally found that the Framingham risk function overestimated the absolute risk of CHD events in populations that have a low CHD risk, and may have underestimated such risk in a higher-risk group. What is still required is an accurate knowledge of the actual incidence of the disease. This could then be used to establish absolute or multifactor cardiovascular risk estimates that are appropriate to populations similar to those studied at Brisighella and, consequently, guide therapeutic interventions for those individuals and groups.

The relationship between body mass index and pulse pressure in older adults with isolated systolic hypertension.

Martins D, Tareen N, Pan D, Norris K. *Am J Hypertens* 2002; **15**(6): 538–43.

BACKGROUND. **Many longitudinal studies have reported excess cardiovascular mortality among lean hypertensive subjects, suggesting that obesity may mitigate the cardiovascular risk of hypertension. Available evidence also suggests that in middle-aged and older hypertensive subjects, PP may be a better predictor of cardiovascular complications. However, there are limited data on the relationship between BMI and PP.**

INTERPRETATION. The inverse relation between BMI and PP observed here may help to explain previous reports of increased cardiovascular risk among lean vs obese subjects with ISH.

Comment

Several studies that have examined the relationship between body weight and cardiovascular mortality report a curvilinear relationship with increased risk of mortality among the very lean and very overweight. The correlation between BP and body weight decreases significantly after age 60 years in most of these prospective studies. The relationship between BMI and PP is unclear. An understanding of the relationship between BMI and PP in older adults with ISH will be valuable to clarify further the effect of obesity on cardiovascular risk.

Using data from the Third National Health and Nutrition Examination Survey (NHANES III) the convergence validity of PP as a predictor of cardiovascular complications was assessed. The relationship between BMI and PP was also examined. The study included 1192 older adults with untreated ISH. Of note, the NHANES III data derives from a representative sample of the US population and provides some of the best available estimates of the prevalence and treatment of hypertension in the USA. The exclusion of participants on antihypertensive drugs from this study removes any confounding effect of drugs on the selection of participants with ISH.

Expectedly, the results showed a good concordance between high PP and most of the selected cardiovascular risk factors with the exception of smoking. The higher PP observed among non-smokers in this study may be attributed, in part, to a higher prevalence of smoking among the younger subset of participants, as well as to the tendency for PP to increase with advancing age.

Interestingly, both BP and PP decreased with increasing BMI. PP is higher in the lean (BMI <25) than in the overweight (BMI 25; 79 mmHg vs 74 mmHg, $P <0.001$)

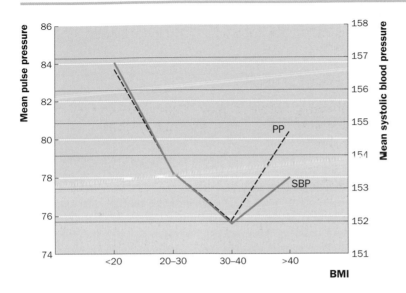

Fig. 3.3 Relationship between SBP, PP and BMI in study subjects. Source: Martins *et al.* (2002).

and decreases significantly from 82 mmHg in the first BMI quintile to 76 mmHg in the fifth BMI quintile. The negative correlation persists even after adjustment for age, sex, diabetes mellitus and hypercholesterolaemia. However, this decrease slowed when BMI was >25 and reversed when BMI was >30.1. According to the authors, the positive correlation between BMI and diabetes mellitus and the association of diabetes mellitus with arterial stiffening may account for the higher PP observed in participants with BMI >30.1.

Overall, PP was higher in women than in men among the lean and overweight participants, but there were noteworthy differences in the relationship between BMI and PP among men and women. The difference in PP between lean male and female participants was not statistically significant ($P = 0.07$), but between overweight male and female participants was statistically significant ($P = 0.001$). Also, the difference in PP between lean and overweight male participants was statistically significant ($P < 0.001$), but between lean and overweight female participants was not ($P = 0.15$). The authors, however, made no attempt to explain possible reasons for these differences observed between male and female. They pointed out that the effect of sex on morbidity associated with obesity is difficult to establish.

It is also noteworthy that the NHANES III was a cross-sectional data set from which a causal inference cannot be drawn. Therefore, more prospective studies in older patients over a wider range of BMI are needed to define better the level at which obesity assumes morbid and prognostic significance, particularly in the elderly.

Hypertension research...the focus is on arterial haemodynamics

From theory into practice: arterial haemodynamics in clinical hypertension.
O'Rourke MF. *J Hypertens* 2002; **20**(10): 1901–15.

BACKGROUND. 'My address will take you from the peripheral resistance vessels to that system which links the heart to peripheral vessels, and whose roles are to act as a conduit and as a cushion, accepting pulsatile flow at input and delivering this in a steady stream to peripheral vessels. The arterial system can be conceived as a simple tube of very low resistance, terminating in vessels with very high resistance...There are some of the issues we must consider. While the arterial system can be represented as a simple tube, the real system is far more complex. Yet it can be approximated by a simple tube.'

INTERPRETATION. The author tries in this lecture to show how theoretic and basic physiological principles can be useful: (i) in hypertension research; (ii) in the management of individual patients; and (iii) in the interpretation of clinical trials and epidemiological studies the information that the pulse affords is of so great importance and so often consulted, surely it must be to our advantage to appreciate fully all it tells us and to draw from it all that it is capable of imparting.

Comment

This was the 'Björn Folkow Lecture' given by the author during the 11th Meeting of the European Society of Hypertension, Göteborg, Sweden, June 2000. This paper is not only fun to read but also very informative. From history to theory, theory to complex physiology of haemodynamics, and from these to the clinical applications in hypertension studies—all very well connected.

Prognostic application of arterial stiffness: task forces.
London GM, Cohn JN. *Am J Hypertens* 2002; **15**(8): 754–8.

BACKGROUND. Epidemiological and clinical studies have shown that increased PP is an independent cardiovascular risk factor in the general population. PP is determined by combined effects of cardiac factors (stroke volume) and arterial stiffness. Arterial stiffness can be more directly evaluated by several measurements including that of PWV. Aortic PWV, a marker of aortic stiffness, has been shown to be a strong independent predictor of cardiovascular and all-cause mortality in patients with ESRD on haemodialysis as well as in patients with EH and older subjects over 80 years.

INTERPRETATION. Aortic stiffness measurements could serve as an important tool in identifying ESRD patients at higher risk of CVD. The ability to identify these patients would lead to better risk stratification and earlier and more cost-effective preventive therapy.

Comment

This article reviews recent clinical evidence of arterial stiffness as an independent prognostic marker of increased cardiovascular risk.

Methods and devices for measuring arterial compliance in humans.

Pannier BM, Avolio AP, Hoeks A, Mancia G, Takazawa K. *Am J Hypertens* 2002; **15**(8): 743–53.

BACKGROUND. **This review analyses methods and devices used world-wide to evaluate arterial stiffness. Three main methodologies are based upon analysis of pulse transit time, of wave contour of the arterial pulse, and of direct measurement of arterial geometry and pressure, corresponding to regional, systemic and local determination of stiffness. They are used in the clinical laboratory and/or in clinical departments. Particular attention is given to the reproducible data in the literature for each device.**

INTERPRETATION. There are two global different concepts: either systemic arterial stiffness is evaluated by adapting an electrical model to calculate a single index from one peripheral measurement of arterial BP curve, or arterial stiffness is evaluated from a direct measure of a surrogate parameter of stiffness. It is not clear whether each of these technical principles reveal the same information for any purpose such as epidemiological, comprehensive mechanical or pharmacological studies. The most widely used devices are accurate and reproducible enough to allow scientific researchers or clinicians to deepen their understanding of arterial mechanics and arterial physiopathology. At each step, validation and reproducibility procedures should be as rigorous as possible and should be conducted independently in different laboratories world-wide.

Comment

The clinical relevance of arterial stiffness is due to its fundamental role in pulsatile haemodynamics. Invasive measurement of arterial blood flow, pressure, and diameter changes have provided the basis for the measurement and interpretation of data derived from non-invasive methods, which is more suitable for clinical use. Non-invasive measurements of arterial stiffness entail measurement of surrogate parameters that are related to the functional effects of arterial stiffness, and these can be used to quantify changes, either globally, regionally or locally by a number of computerized devices. Depending on their make these methods/devices derive data based on three main methodologies: (i) pulse transit time; or (ii) analysis of the arterial

Table 3.3 Devices and methods based on measurement of pulse transit time

Device	Arterial measurement	Bland and Altman repeatability	Number of operators	Direct/ systemic measure
Complior system	Dedicated mechanotransducer; simultaneous; superficial arteries	Yes	Single	Direct
Sphygmocor system	Tonometer (Millar); not simultaneous; superficial arteries	Yes	Single	Direct
Automated ultrasound recording of PWV	Continuous ultrasound probe; aorta	No	Two	Direct
Wall Track System	Ultrasound echotracking; superficial arteries	No	±	Direct
QKd system	Brachial pressure cuff	No	Single	Direct

Source: Pannier *et al.* (2002).

Table 3.4 Devices and methods based on analysis of the arterial pressure pulse

Device	Arterial measurement	BP measurement	Bland and Altman repeatability	Direct/ systemic measure
Subclavian pulse tracing	Mechanical air transmission; subclavian artery	Brachial oscillometric device (Dinamap)	Yes	Systemic
Doppler-echocardiography Proximal and distal compliance from a modified Windkessel model	Wrist automatic tonometer	Dedicated brachial oscillometric device	Yes	Systemic
Second derivative of the finger plethysmogram	Finger photoplethysmography	Not applicable	Yes	Systemic
Sphygmocor system (AIx variable)	Hand-held tonometer (Millar) superficial arteries	Brachial sphygmomanometric method	Yes	Systemic

Source: Pannier *et al.* (2002).

pressure pulse and its wave contour; and (iii) direct stiffness estimation using measurements of diameter and distending pressure. The authors focused on the main specific devices developed and used in different experimental and clinical laboratories world-wide.

Systemic determination of arterial stiffness is based on numerous theoretical approximations. In general it requires the direct measurement of a single peripheral, and often distal, parameter: the pressure curve. On the other hand, regional, and furthermore, local, evaluations are based on direct measurements of parameters strongly linked to wall stiffness. Regional evaluation is mostly based on the principle of PWV recording that involves measurement of two quantities: transit time of the arterial pulse along the analysed arterial segment, and distance on the skin between both recording sites.

Local determination of arterial stiffness involves measurement of cross-sectional arterial distensibility. Systems are based on a vascular echotracking device using the Doppler shift principle or on echo imaging.

The authors emphasized the importance of validation/reproducibility of all the measurement techniques. There are, however, large differences in validation procedures and reproducibility evaluation of all these techniques. Indeed, there is no gold standard method for local or regional *in vivo* measurement of arterial stiffness. At present, the British Standard Institution recommended well-accepted statistical procedures to validate techniques. Particularly, Bland and Altman suggested the analysis of agreement between two methods and of reproducibility by means of the

Table 3.5 Devices and methods based on direct stiffness calculation using measurements of diameter

Device	Arterial measurement
Beta index model	*Ultrasonic phase-locked echotracking device; superficial arteries*
Suprasternal view echocardiography	*Standard B-mode echocardiography of ascending aorta*
NIUS 2	*High resolution ultrasonic echotracking; radial artery*
Wall Track System	*High resolution ultrasonic echotracking; superficial arteries*
Brachial artery transmural pressure modulation device	*High resolution ultrasonic echotracking; B mode ultrasound*
Transesophageal echocardiography	*B mode ultrasound; aorta*
Vascular echography frame grabber processing (Devereux group)	*B mode ultrasound; local reading; carotid artery*
Vascular echography frame grabber processing (ARIC study)	*B mode ultrasound; centralized reading; carotid artery*

NIUS = non-invasive ultrasound system; ARIC = the Atherosclerosis Risk in Communities study.
Source: Pannier *et al.* (2002).

repeatability coefficient, i.e. the standard deviation of the difference between measurements.

The selection of device use depends on type of research study. Physiological and physiopathological studies, particularly in specialized laboratories, require accurate and reproducible systems. The most suitable devices are those with direct calculation of surrogate measures of arterial stiffness, such as PWV, arterial compliance, or distensibility, followed by systems with off-line calculation after data acquisition. On the other hand, clinical, epidemiological or pharmacological studies may require a device that is easy to use for a technician or nurse in clinical departments and that incorporates patient data management.

Clinical applications of arterial stiffness, Task Force III: recommendations for user procedures.
Van Bortel LM, Duprez D, Starmans-Kool MJ, *et al. Am J Hypertens* 2002; **15**(5): 445–52.

BACKGROUND. *In vivo* arterial stiffness is a dynamic property based on vascular function and structure. It is influenced by confounding factors such as BP, age, gender, BMI, heart rate (HR) and treatment. As a consequence, standardization of the measurement conditions is imperative.

INTERPRETATION. The subject's conditions should be standardized before starting measurements. As it is not feasible to discuss all methods or devices measuring arterial stiffness in one article, more attention is given to user procedures of commercially available devices, because these devices are of interest for a wider group of investigators. User procedures of methods/devices are discussed according to the nature of arterial stiffness measured: systemic, regional or local arterial stiffness.

Comment

PP is an indirect index of arterial stiffening. Various methods have been developed to measure arterial stiffness in a more direct way. Indeed, increased aortic stiffness measured by PWV has been associated with all-cause and cardiovascular mortality, and recently in a longitudinal study, it has been shown to be an independent predictor of primary coronary events (fatal and non-fatal MI, coronary revascularization and angina pectoris) in patients with EH |**4,5**|. PWV appeared to predict subsequent CHD events, not only in patients with pre-existing CVD, but also in patients who were initially disease-free. The predictive power of PWV remained the same after adjustment for cardiovascular risk factors and PP. Hence, clinical applications of arterial stiffness measurements are of immense interest as these techniques might be carried out non-invasively at patients' bedside and thus improve their cardiovascular risk profiling.

At the present time, these techniques are increasingly used in clinical research and thus standardizations of the measurement conditions and of the various methods/devices are imperative, especially when used in comparative studies. As in

Table 3.6 Recommendations on general user procedures for clinical studies: standardize the subject condition

Subjects will be at rest for at least 10 min in a quiet room temperature. (consensus)
Prolong resting period or cancel measurements in conditions where subjects' basal conditions are substantially altered, like when outside temperature is high or immediately after strenuous exercise. (consensus)
Subjects have to refrain from smoking, eating, and drinking beverages containing caffeine for at least 3 h before assessments. (consensus)
Unless measurements are performed early in the morning, advise a light meal 3 to 4 h before assessments. (large agreement)
Subjects should refrain from drinking alcohol 10 h before measurements. (consensus)
Subjects may neither speak nor sleep during assessments. (consensus)
Investigators should mention in which position measurements have been done (supine, sitting). The supine position is preferred. (large agreement)
For repeated measures, subject measurements should be performed at the same time of the day and in the same position. (consensus)
Be aware of possible white coat arterial stiffness, and if suspected, perform repeated measurements within one visit or in additional visits to detect it. (consensus)
Be aware of possible disturbance of data due to cardiac arrhythmia. (consensus)

Level of agreement on the recommendations is mentioned within brackets.
Source: Bortel et al. (2002).

Table 3.7 Recommendations on user procedures for measuring local arterial stiffness

The investigator has to be well-trained. (consensus)
Do not use simplified formulas. (consensus)
Do not push the artery. (consensus)
The use of the Langewouters model versus the measurement of isobaric compliance in a small common pressure window has to be discussed. (large agreement)
Pulse pressure should be measured at the site of distension measurements. (consensus)
Pulse pressure in the common carotid artery is a valid surrogate for pulse pressure in the ascending aorta. This does not apply to the waveform. (large agreement)
In the hands of a large number of investigators pulse pressure data directly obtained from applanation tonometry are not reliable and if so, they should be avoided. (large agreement)
Assessment of local pulse pressure using calibrated pressure waves obtained from applanation tonometry appears a valid method. For calibration make use of a validated sphygmomanometer. (consensus)
Pulse pressure assessment using calibrated pulse pressures from an individual subject should be compared with those from a universal population-based transfer function. (consensus)

Level of agreement on the recommendation is mentioned within brackets.
Source: Bortel et al. (2002).

any other measurement techniques, intravariability and intervariability should be validated. The present paper described in detail experts' recommendations in carrying out these measurements. As the techniques are subject to various external 'influences' and intraindividual confounding factors or variations, e.g. diurnal variation, posture, etc., investigators are encouraged to follow these sets of recommendations meticulously.

Heart rate dependency of pulse pressure amplification and arterial stiffness.

Wilkinson IB, Mohammad NH, Tyrrell S, *et al. Am J Hypertens* 2002; **15**(1 Pt 1): 24–30.

B A C K G R O U N D . **PP and aortic PWV, measures of arterial stiffness, are both important determinants of cardiovascular risk. However, assessment of peripheral PP does not always provide a reliable measure of changes in central PP or arterial stiffness.**

I N T E R P R E T A T I O N . Peripheral PP does not provide an accurate assessment of changes in central haemodynamics in relation to changes in HR, and that aortic stiffness is not affected by acute changes in HR.

Comment

PP varies throughout the arterial tree, in part because of differences in vessel compliance and the phenomenon of wave reflection. The degree of PP amplification, from the aorta to the brachial artery can vary with posture, exercise and age. Thus, brachial artery PP may not provide a reliable estimate of central PP, which contains important information concerning both local and systemic arterial stiffness.

In the present study, Wilkinson *et al.* used cardiac pacing to evaluate the effect of HR on central and peripheral haemodynamics in a group of patients with normal LV function. They studied 20 subjects (aged 20–72 years) at cardiac catheterization. Pulse wave analysis was performed with the SphygmoCor apparatus for the derivation of central aortic waveforms from radial waveforms acquired by applanation tonometry. Central pressure, augmentation index (AIx), a measure of systemic arterial stiffness, and aortic PWV during right atrial pacing (80–120 beats/min) were determined. The results showed that PP amplification from the aorta to the brachial artery was positively and linearly related to HR. There was also an inverse, linear relationship between AIx and HR ($r = -0.70$, $P < 0.001$), but incremental pacing had no effect on aortic stiffness, as PWV did not change. The effect of HR on amplification and AIx was not influenced by age. These data indicate the important contribution that wave reflection makes to the central pressure waveform, and reinforces the notion that simply recording peripheral BP may not provide an accurate assessment of changes in central haemodynamics.

Heart rate: an important confounder of pulse wave velocity assessment.

Lantelme P, Mestre C, Lievre M, *et al. Hypertension* 2002; **39**: 1083–7.

BACKGROUND. Arterial stiffness is a strong determinant of cardiovascular risk. PWV is an index of arterial stiffness, and its prognostic value has been repeatedly emphasized. The purpose of the present study was to assess the effect of HR on PWV.

INTERPRETATION. This study demonstrates that HR is an important factor in the intraindividual variation of PWV in elderly subjects. This raises methodological concern about the measurement of this parameter. Standardizing PWV for HR level seems mandatory if one wants to interpret PWV changes in clinical trials or in the follow-up of patients.

Comment

The authors studied 22 elderly subjects (mean age 78 years) with permanent cardiac pacing. PWV was measured using a Complior® device. In each subject, PWV was measured at five different pacing frequencies in the same session (60, 70, 80, 90, 100 beats/min), the order of the various frequencies being randomly determined. Furthermore, to test the reproducibility, a repeat measurement of PWV was obtained in one randomly selected frequency. They found that PWV reproducibility was fairly good at the same HR level. However, there was a highly significant effect of HR on PWV estimated by a one-way, within-subjects analysis of variance ($P = 0.01$). The authors concluded that HR is an important factor in the intraindividual variation of PWV in elderly subjects, and they raised concerns for the use of PWV as an intermediate end-point in clinical trials, especially those devoted to the evaluation of the effects of antihypertensive drugs. They emphasized the need for standardizing PWV for HR level if one wishes to interpret PWV changes in clinical trials or in the follow-up of patients. Moreover, further studies are required, particularly in younger persons.

However, O'Rourke *et al.* (2002) commented that the interpretation of the study by Lantelme *et al.* about the relationship between HR and PWV could only be limited to the method they used (Complior®, an automatic device), but not to the conventional method (i.e. the manual method), nor to the long-established relationship between PWV and arterial stiffness. According to O'Rourke *et al.* (2002), in the conventional method, PWV is measured from the time delay between the foot (sharp initial systolic upstroke) of the wave at the two sites, whereas the Complior® depends on a proprietary algorithm. Furthermore, they are not aware of data similar to those presented by Lantelme *et al.*, showing any significant relationship between HR and PWV using the conventional method, nor can they conceive any theoretic basis for such. Whether carotid–femoral PWV is a marker of atherosclerosis in general requires more basic studies. In reply, Lantelme *et al.* gave previous studies that have demonstrated a relationship between HR and PWV measured using conventional methods. They felt that the conventional method (the gold standard) is tedious and time consuming, which probably precludes its application on a routine basis compared with the commercially available device. However, it is critical to determine the potential confounders of the automatic methods of PWV determination.

Clinical applications of arterial stiffness; definitions and reference values.

O'Rourke MF, Staessen JA, Vlachopoulos C, Duprez D, Plante GE. *Am J Hypertens* 2002; **15**(5): 426–44.

BACKGROUND. Arterial stiffening is the most important cause of increasing SBP and PP, and for decreasing DBP beyond 40 years of age. Stiffening affects predominantly the aorta and proximal elastic arteries, and to a lesser degree the peripheral muscular arteries.

INTERPRETATION. While conceptually a Windkessel model (oldest model of the arterial system) is the simplest way to visualize the cushioning function of arteries, this is not useful clinically under changing conditions when effects of wave reflection become prominent. Many measures have been applied to quantify stiffness, but all are approximations only, on account of the non-homogeneous structure of the arterial wall, its variability in different locations, at different levels of distending pressure, and with changes in smooth muscle tone.

Comment

This article summarizes the methods and indices used to estimate arterial stiffness, and provides values from a survey of the literature, followed by recommendations of an international group of workers in the field who attended the First Consensus Conference on Arterial Stiffness, which was held in Paris during 2000. Definition and units of the various indices of arterial stiffness and their reference values are given. This review is directed at arterial stiffness and its measurement, not at wave reflection and its implications. It helps immensely for one to understand the physiology that underlies these measured indices, and hence to understand and to interpret the data generated.

Recommendations:

- As a generic term, stiffness is preferable, especially to compliance, which is more frequently used to describe adherence with therapy or advice, or adherence to protocol.
- For regional measurements, diameter and pressure should be measured at the same point. When this cannot be done, note should be made of possible confounders, such as age, drugs or HR.

- For regional and other measurements, note should be made of distending pressure, and comparisons made at the same distending pressure. If technical correction for distending pressure is not possible, validated statistical 'adjustment' should be carried out and clearly described.

- For indices that give absolute values, absolute initial size should always be given.

- For global measures of arterial mechanics, analysis of the arterial pressure waveform is often performed. Although various techniques (and underlying models) are used, they should all take into account anterograde and reflected waves as important components of the measured waveform.

- A preference is given to pure physical measures.

- Reference values for all arterial properties must be given as a function of age.

Table 3.8 Definition and units of the various indices of arterial stiffness

Arterial distensibility	Relative diameter (or area) change for a pressure increment; the inverse of elastic modulus ($\Delta D/\Delta P \cdot D$) (mmHg^{-1})
Arterial compliance	Absolute diameter (or area) change for a given pressure step at fixed vessel length $\Delta D/\Delta P$ (cm/mmHg) or cm^2/mmHg)
Volume elastic modulus	Pressure step required for (theoretical) 100% increase in volume ($\Delta P/(\Delta V/V)$ (mmHg) $= \Delta P/(\Delta D/D)$ (mmHg) where there is no change in length
Elastic modulus	The pressure step required for (theoretical) 100% stretch from resting diameter at fixed vessel length ($\Delta P \cdot D/\Delta D$) (mmHg)
Young's modulus	Elastic modulus per unit area; the pressure step per square centimeter required for (theoretical) 100% stretch from resting length $\Delta P \cdot D/(\Delta D \cdot h)$ (mmHg/cm)
Pulse wave velocity	Speed of travel of the pulse along an arterial segment Distance/Δt (cm/s)
Pressure augmentation	Increase in aortic or carotid pressure after the peak of blood flow in the vessel (mmHg or as % of pulse pressure)
Characteristic impedance	Relationship between pressure change and flow velocity in the absence of wave reflections ($\Delta P/\Delta V$) ([mm Hg/cm]/s)
Stiffness index	Ratio of logarithm (systolic/diastolic pressures) to (relative change in diameter) $\beta = \ln (Ps/Pd) / ([Ds - Dd]/Dd)$ (non-dimensional)
'Large artery elasticity index'	Relationship between pressure fall and volume fall in the arterial tree during the exponential component of diastolic pressure decay $\Delta V/\Delta P$ (cm^3/mmHg)
Small artery elasticity index	Relationship between oscillating pressure change and oscillating volume change around the exponential pressure decay during diastole $\Delta V/\Delta P$ (cm^3/mmHg)

P = pressure; D = diameter; V = volume; H = wall thickness; T = time; S = systolic; D = diastolic.
Source: O'Rourke *et al.* (2002).

PWV using applanation tonometry. Three risk scores were used to estimate, for each individual, the absolute risk of stroke, CHD, and death within 10–12 years as a function of their cardiovascular risk factor profile. The results showed that increased PWV is significantly and positively associated with age, MAP, PP, HR and pack-years of cigarette smoking. Height and high-density lipoprotein cholesterol were inversely related to PWV. In addition, the absolute risks of stroke, CHD and death increased with increasing PWV in a linear graded manner. This study is limited by its cross-sectional design. Therefore, the contribution of measurement of arterial stiffness in predicting future disease, relative to that of other cardiovascular risk factors cannot be determined.

Impact of aortic stiffness attenuation on survival of patients in end-stage renal failure.
Guerin AP, Blacher J, Pannier B, Marchais SJ, Safar ME, London GM.
Circulation 2001; **103**: 987–92.

BACKGROUND. Aortic PWV is a predictor of mortality in patients with end-stage renal failure (ESRF). The PWV is partly dependent on BP, and a decrease in BP can attenuate the stiffness. Whether the changes in PWV in response to decreases in BP can predict mortality in ESRF patients has never been investigated.

INTERPRETATION. These results indicate that in ESRF patients, the insensitivity of PWV to decreased BP is an independent predictor of mortality and that use of ACE inhibitors has a favourable effect on survival that is independent of BP changes.

Comment
The results of this study indicated that persistence of aortic stiffness reversibility (or sensitivity) in response to BP lowering had a beneficial and BP-independent impact on the survival of ESRF patients, suggesting that the presence of more advanced vascular lesions characterized by the loss of BP reversibility of aortic stiffness is a major factor contributing to the mortality of ESRF patients. This finding emphasized the need to test other alternative therapies in ESRF patients in whom antihypertensive drugs are unable to alter aortic PWV. See Safar *et al.* below.

Central pulse pressure and mortality in end-stage renal disease.
Safar ME, Blacher J, Pannier B, *et al. Hypertension* 2002; **39**(3): 735–8.

BACKGROUND. Damage of large arteries is a major factor in the high cardiovascular morbidity and mortality of patients with ESRD. Increased aortic PWV and brachial PP are the principal arterial markers of cardiovascular mortality described in these patients. Whether central (carotid) PP and brachial–carotid PP amplification may predict all-cause (including cardiovascular) mortality has never been investigated.

INTERPRETATION. These results provide the first direct evidence that in patients with ESRD, the carotid PP level and, mostly, the disappearance of PP amplification are strong independent predictors of all-cause (including cardiovascular) mortality.

Comment

As pointed out before, aortic PWV, the major determinant of central PP, rather than brachial PP that may be considered as a better specific independent cardiovascular

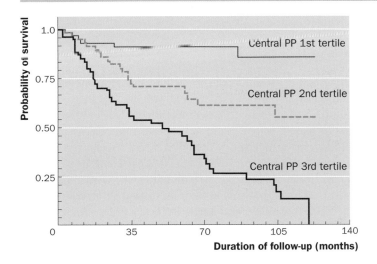

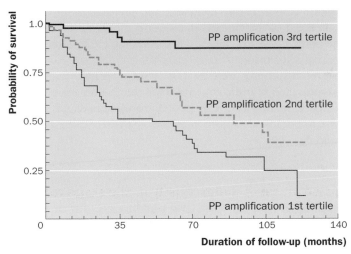

Fig. 3.4 Probabilities of survival in the study population according to the level of central PP and PP amplification divided into tertiles. Comparisons between survival curves were highly significant ($P < 0.001$ for both). Source: Safar *et al.* (2002).

Table 3.9 Predictors of all-cause mortality after adjustment of age, time on dialysis before inclusion, and previous cardiovascular events (Cox proportional hazards regression model)

Pulse pressure	Adjusted hazard ratio
Aortic	1.3 (1.0–1.7)
Carotid	1.4 (1.1–1.8)
Brachial/carotid PP	0.5 (0.3–0.8)

Source: Safar *et al.* (2002).

risk factor. Thus, it is important to determine the predictive value, in terms of cardiovascular and all-cause mortality, of central PP compared with brachial PP.

The purpose of this study was to evaluate the comparative values of brachial PP, carotid PP and carotid–brachial PP amplification in the prediction of all-cause mortality in patients with ESRD, independently of the usual cardiovascular risk factors observed in this population, such as age, previous cardiovascular events or LVH.

A cohort of 180 patients (mean age 51.5 ± 16.3) with ESRD who were undergoing haemodialysis was studied. At entry, patients underwent carotid PP measurements (pulse wave analysis), echocardiography, and aortic PWV (Doppler ultrasonography), together with standard clinical and biochemical analyses.

After about 52 months followed-up, 70 deaths occurred, including both cardiovascular and non-cardiovascular fatal events. On the basis of Cox analyses, after adjustment of age, time on dialysis before inclusion, and previous cardiovascular events, three factors emerged as predictors of all-cause mortality: carotid PP, brachial/carotid PP and aortic PWV. But, brachial BP, including PP, had no predictive value for mortality after adjustment.

The salient findings of this study were that in ESRD patients undergoing haemodialysis, the disappearance of aortic–brachial PP amplification was a significant predictor of all-cause mortality, independent of age and other standard confounding factors, and carotid PP was more powerful than brachial PP in the prediction of overall mortality.

Influence of age, risk factors, and cardiovascular and renal disease on arterial stiffness: clinical applications.

Benetos A, Waeber B, Izzo J, *et al. Am J Hypertens* 2002; **15**(12): 1101–8.

BACKGROUND. Age is the main clinical determinant of large artery stiffness. Central arteries stiffen progressively with age, whereas peripheral muscular arteries change little with age. Increase of central artery stiffness with age is responsible for earlier wave reflections and changes in pressure wave contours.

INTERPRETATION The stiffening of aorta and other central arteries is a potential risk factor for increased cardiovascular morbidity and mortality. Arterial stiffening with ageing is accompanied by an elevation in SBP and PP. Hypertension may increase arterial stiffness, especially in older subjects. Patients with HF, ESRD and those with atherosclerotic lesions often develop central artery stiffness. Decreased carotid distensibility, increased arterial thickness, and presence of calcifications and plaques often coexist in the same subject.

Comment

This is an excellent review paper written by experts in the field of 'arterial stiffness' and its clinical applications. The paper was carefully written, summarizing the latest evidence related to arterial stiffness in various 'disease states' especially hypertension, ESRD, ageing, HF and type 1 and 2 diabetes mellitus, and with risk factors includes smoking and dyslipidaemia.

Amplitude and timing of central aortic pressure wave reflections in heart transplant recipients.

Schofield RS, Schuler BT, Edwards DG, et al. Am J Hypertens 2002; **15**(9): 809–15.

BACKGROUND. Hypertension assessed by sphygmomanometer is a common finding in heart transplant recipients (HTR); however, little is known about the contribution of arterial wave reflection to central aortic pressure in these patients. The aim of this study was to measure the central aortic pressure wave in HTR on antihypertensive therapy and determine the effects of amplitude and timing of wave reflection on the various components of the wave.

INTERPRETATION. Non-invasive analysis of the central aortic pressure wave identified a subgroup of hypertensive HTR with increased arterial stiffness, increased propagation of the reflected wave, and augmented aortic SBP and PP not identified with the sphygmomanometer.

Comment

Patients who have had transplants are at a high risk for cardiovascular events as they are frequently hypertensive, diabetic, hyperlipidaemic, overweight, and have a high incidence of insulin resistance. Post-transplant hypertension is well recognized and usually requires three or more antihypertensive agents to control optimally.

The objectives of this study were to compare central aortic SBP with simultaneous brachial artery pressure, and to analyse the various components of the aortic pressure wave, pulse wave reflections and LV afterload. The central aortic pressure was measured non-invasively by radial artery applanation tonometry (and use of a generalized transfer function) at rest. The central aortic AIx, an indicator of arterial stiffness, was calculated from the aortic pressure waveform. A total of 53 stable adult HTR on antihypertensives were studied.

Despite similar brachial BP measured by standard cuff-sphygmomanometry, patients can be stratified into groups of high, medium and low degrees of arterial stiffness according to the amplitude of aortic AIx. They found that a subgroup of patients with high aortic AIx (and, to a lesser extent, patients with medium aortic AIx) was identified with highly abnormal arterial stiffness and elevated augmented SBP despite relatively controlled brachial BP. The study identified those with an increased aortic AIx also had an increased PP and a reduced travel time of the reflected pressure wave from the periphery to the heart ($\Delta t_p/2$), all of which are markers of increased LV afterload and cardiovascular risk. The authors felt that these patients with high aortic AIx are already at increased risk for cardiovascular events and should be treated more aggressively. They suggested that the goal of antihypertensive drug therapy in these patients, in addition to reducing MAP, should also be to reduce the amplitude of the reflected wave by delaying its return to the central aorta so that it occurs after peak pressure or during diastole.

The authors pointed out that radial artery applanation tonometry as applied in the present study is a non-invasive, reproducible and portable measuring tool for estimating central aortic pressure and wave reflection. They suggest that more widespread use of this simple technique (which describes the state of central arterial function and compliance more completely) as a supplement to conventional BP measurement might allow more optimal risk factor management and better monitoring of antihypertensive therapy in high-risk patients.

It is not surprising that patients in this study could be further stratified into three different risk levels according to their aortic AIx in spite of similar brachial BP. Brachial BP, when used singly as a gauge of cardiovascular risk is misleading as this ignores the value of other risk factors such as smoking, dyslipidaemia and diabetes, which also contribute to an individual absolute cardiovascular risk. This has been well established by the use of the Framingham algorithm. The study would be more informative if the authors adjusted for these baseline risk factors as covariates in multivariate analysis to see whether aortic AIx, travel time and PP are still significantly different among the patients. If there was no difference, then these indices add little value in fine-tuning the risk stratification in these patients.

Aortic pulse pressure and extent of coronary artery disease in percutaneous transluminal coronary angioplasty candidates.

Philippe F, Chemaly E, Blacher J, *et al. Am J Hypertens* 2002; **15**(8): 672–7.

BACKGROUND. PP and aortic stiffness are both predictors of CAD. Whether these parameters are directly related to coronary structural alterations has never been studied.

INTERPRETATION. Aortic PP was a significant risk factor for the extent of CAD. There was only a borderline significant association of restenosis to the steady, but not pulsatile, component of aortic BP in the stent era.

Comment

The recent analysis of data from the SHEP Study has indicated that PP derived from 24-hour ambulatory BP monitoring is a better predictor for cardiovascular events than PP derived from office BP. However, recently, there has been more emphasis on aortic rather than peripheral PP to predict cardiovascular risk. Indeed, aortic pulsatility, but not brachial pulsatility, has been shown to be independently associated to the presence of CAD in patients undergoing coronary angiography. The objectives of the present study were to investigate the relationship between the level of intra-aortic PP and the extent of CAD, and between the level of intra-aortic PP and in-stent restenosis in 99 patients who underwent percutaneous transluminal coronary angioplasty as a result of acute MI.

Philippe *et al.* demonstrated that high intra-aortic but not brachial PP was significantly associated with the extent of CAD in patients who underwent percutaneous transluminal coronary angioplasty. There was, however, no significant association observed between aortic or brachial PP and restenosis after angioplasty. According to the authors, intra-aortic PP measured during cardiac catheterization should be a better index of aortic stiffness than brachial PP. In addition it is closer to the heart, coronary vessels and carotid arteries and it allows an accurate measurement of MAP by direct integration of the BP curve. To the best of their knowledge, the present study is the first to relate an independent and significant association between aortic PP and the extent of CAD quantitatively assessed from the number of diseased coronary vessels. However, a similar finding may be observed using carotid PP instead of aortic PP as an index of central BP (see below).

The mechanisms through which PP associated with the presence and severity of CAD may be related to two factors: an increase in oxygen demand, related to the increase in SBP and the resulting increase in cardiac mass; and a reduction in oxygen supply, related to the decrease in DBP and the resulting decrease in coronary perfusion. The present study clearly indicates for the first time that structural alterations of the coronary arterial wall are also directly and quantitatively involved. However, whether this implies a causal or reversible relationship, needs to be further evaluated.

Large artery stiffness predicts ischemic threshold in patients with coronary artery disease.

Kingwell BA, Waddell TK, Medley TL, Cameron JD, Dart AM. *J Am Coll Cardiol* 2002; **40**(4): 773–9.

BACKGROUND. Large artery stiffness is an independent predictor of cardiovascular mortality and a major determinant of PP and, thus, cardiac afterload and coronary perfusion. Clinical relevance of the haemodynamic consequences of large artery stiffening has not previously been demonstrated in relation to myocardial ischaemia.

INTERPRETATION. Within a patient group with moderate CAD, large artery stiffness was a major determinant of myocardial ischaemic threshold.

Comment

Clinical studies have demonstrated a strong association between PP at baseline and future cardiovascular, including coronary, events. Elevated PP could affect coronary outcomes through increased systolic pressure and, thus, afterload and diminished coronary perfusion secondary to diastolic pressure reduction. Thus, aortic stiffening tightens the link between cardiac systolic performance and myocardial perfusion.

The main objective of this study was to determine whether large artery stiffness contributes to exercise-induced myocardial ischaemia in patients with CAD. They hypothesized that for any degree of coronary stenosis, patients with stiffer large vessels would have a lower ischaemic threshold, measured as the time to ST segment depression of 0.15 mV during a treadmill exercise test. Systemic arterial compliance, distensibility index, PWV and AIx were used to assess different aspects of large artery stiffness at rest in relation to ischaemic threshold. A total of 96 patients with angiographically confirmed CAD were studied. It is obvious that this study was carefully planned and well-thought, and possible confounders have been minimized. Intriguingly, all large artery stiffness/compliance indices were correlated with time to ischaemia ($P = 0.01–0.009$). Both carotid ($P = 0.007$) and brachial ($P = 0.001$) PP also correlated inversely with time to ischaemia. Importantly, other major risk factors plus severity of coronary stenosis did not materially change the results, i.e. indices of arterial stiffness were significant independent predictors of ischaemic threshold. Interestingly, arterial stiffness indices were felt to be stronger determinants of time to ischaemia than angiographic assessment of severity of coronary stenoses. This finding implicates large artery stiffness as a potentially important target for therapy in patients with CAD.

The authors pointed out that because aortic and coronary diseases are known to develop in parallel, it is likely that aortic atherosclerosis was a major determinant of large artery stiffness in this cohort. However, it was not possible in this study to determine the relative contribution of aortic atherosclerosis to large artery stiffness and, therefore, ischaemic threshold. It is evident, however, that atherosclerosis promotes myocardial ischaemia not only via coronary artery obstruction but also via large artery stiffening. These data highlight large artery stiffness as an ischaemic mechanism and potential therapeutic target in patients with CAD.

Aortic stiffness is an independent predictor of primary coronary events in hypertensive patients: a longitudinal study.

Boutouyrie P, Tropeano AI, Asmar R, *et al. Hypertension* 2002; **39**: 10–15.

BACKGROUND. Arterial stiffness may predict CHD beyond classic risk factors. In a longitudinal study, the predictive value of arterial stiffness on CHD in patients with EH and without known clinical CVD was assessed.

INTERPRETATION. This study provides the first direct evidence in a longitudinal study that aortic stiffness is an independent predictor of primary coronary events in patients with EH.

Comment

Recent longitudinal studies directly demonstrated that arterial stiffness, measured through PWV, carotid elastic modulus, or ratio of stroke volume to PP, was an independent predictor of all-cause and cardiovascular mortality in patients with ESRD and in essential hypertensives |6|. However, the predictive value of aortic stiffness on primary CHD events has never been established in patients with EH in a longitudinal study.

Indeed, the same group further provides data in support of their previous conclusion of the independent predictive value of aortic stiffness for cardiovascular events, and in this paper, more specifically predicting for primary coronary events (fatal and non-fatal MI, coronary revascularization and angina pectoris) in a longitudinal study. The risk assessment of CHD was made by calculating the Framingham risk score (FRS) according to the categories of gender, age, BP, cholesterol, diabetes and smoking. The cohort included 1045 essential hypertensive patients with no overt CVD or symptoms who attended the out-patient hypertension clinic between 1980 and 1996 and had a baseline measurement of arterial stiffness. Mean age at entry was 51 years, and mean follow-up was 5.7 years.

The FRS significantly predicted the occurrence of coronary and all cardiovascular events in this population ($P < 0.01$ and $P < 0.0001$, respectively). PWV remained significantly associated with the occurrence of coronary event after adjustment either of FRS (for 3.5 m/s: RR 1.345%, CI 1.01–1.79; $P = 0.039$) or classic risk factors (for 3.5 m/s: RR 1.395%, CI 1.08–1.79; $P = 0.01$), i.e. arterial stiffness measured through PWV predict CHD event in hypertensive patients beyond that which could be predicted by classic risk factors assessed through either a Framingham algorithm or a multivariate Cox model, including previous antihypertensive treatment.

It is interesting to see that the predictive value of PWV for primary CHD events was more marked for patients considered at low risk, i.e. belonging to the first and second FRS tertiles, than for patients at high risk, i.e. belonging to the third FRS tertile, indicating that this low-to-intermediate risk population benefited the most from risk assessment with PWV. However, the authors did not attempt to give explanations why this could be the case.

Overall, these results showed that measuring aortic stiffness may help to identify patients at high risk of CHD who may benefit from more aggressive management.

Bedside quantification of atherosclerosis severity for cardiovascular risk stratification: a prospective cohort study.

Hunziker PR, Imsand C, Keller D, *et al.* J Am Coll Cardiol 2002; **39**(4): 702–9.

BACKGROUND. Drug prevention of cardiovascular events is effective but costly, leading to a debate about who should receive this treatment. Patient selection is often based on surrogate markers, but quantification of atherosclerosis severity is desirable.

INTERPRETATION. Bedside measurement of specific aortic elastance allows assessment of atherosclerosis severity. It predicts the risk for future atherosclerotic events beyond conventional risk factors, promising better targeting of pharmacological prevention and improved cost-effectiveness.

Comment

The objectives of this study were to assess the ability of a new non-invasive method to quantify atherosclerosis severity and to examine its power to predict cardiovascular events.

Using conventional transthoracic echocardiography, Hunziker *et al.* attempt to quantify aortic atherosclerosis severity in a novel way by determining the specific aortic elastance based on the biomechanics of pulse wave–vessel wall interaction, i.e. pulse wave propagation. The wave front propagation time from the LV outflow tract to the common femoral artery is measured using pulsed wave Doppler. The wave front is defined as the extrapolation of the first segment of the Doppler flow profile to the baseline.

Two independent consecutive patient cohorts were prospectively studied: (i) validation study (52 patients referred for transesophageal echocardiography, and results were compared with aortic plaque burden visualized directly), and (ii) risk stratification (336 patients referred for transthoracic echocardiography were prospectively studied by monitoring atherosclerotic events at 1 year and comparing the results with conventional risk stratification).

They found that specific aortic elastance was well correlated with plaque burden ($P < 0.0001$) and largely independent of confounding variables. Specific aortic elastance also predicted the primary end-point of 'atherosclerotic death, MI or stroke' at 1 year ($P < 0.0002$). Event rate at 1 year in the lowest specific elastance tertile was 1.8% (CI 0.0–4.3%), in the middle tertile 5.4% (CI 1.1–9.7%) and in the highest tertile 12.7% (CI 6.3–19%). Specific aortic elastance, prior atherosclerotic events and LV ejection fraction were found to be independent risk predictors. In addition, specific elastance was of incremental value to clinically identified variables.

Thus, bedside quantification of atherosclerosis severity is feasible by echocardiographic determination of specific aortic elastance. The method further confirms the working hypothesis that non-invasive quantification of atherosclerosis severity might be as promising for risk prediction as are classical 'risk factors'.

Determinants of accelerated progression of arterial stiffness in normotensive subjects and in treated hypertensive subjects over a 6-year period.

Benetos A, Adamopoulos C, Bureau JM, *et al. Circulation* 2002; **105**(10): 1202–7.

BACKGROUND. Elastic artery stiffness, a result of arterial ageing, is an independent indicator of cardiovascular risk. The aim of the present longitudinal study was to compare the progression of aortic stiffness over a 6-year period in treated hypertensive subjects and normotensive subjects, and to evaluate the determinants of this progression.

INTERPRETATION. The presence of high BP, high HR and high serum creatinine were the major determinants of accelerated progression of aortic stiffness in treated hypertensives. This is the first longitudinal study to evaluate the determinants of arterial ageing over an extended period of time.

Comment

Classic cardiovascular risk factors, increase in BP, dyslipidaemia, diabetes and tobacco smoking are often associated with increased arterial stiffness. However, the impact of these risk factors with increasing age in the development of arterial stiffness is still unclear. According to the authors most of these observations are based on short-term pharmacological studies and on cross-sectional observational data.

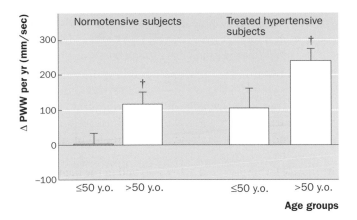

Fig. 3.5 Annual PWV progression in younger (≤50 years) and older (>50 years) normotensive (left) and treated hypertensive (right) subjects (adjusted for initial PWV and sex); †P <0.001 vs younger subjects. Source: Benetos *et al.* (2002).

In this study, the investigators followed longitudinally 187 hypertensives on treatment and 296 normotensive subjects for about 5 years. Carotid–femoral PWV was used to evaluate aortic stiffness in all at baseline and at end of follow-up. The impact of several risk factors on the annual rates of progression in PWV adjusted for age was examined. They found that the progression was higher in older subjects in both populations, while treated hypertensives had higher rates of progression than normotensives. Only treated hypertensives with well-controlled BP levels at the time of both visits had a PWV progression similar to that of normotensives. PWV progression in patients with uncontrolled BP levels at both visits was more than three times higher than in well-controlled hypertensives. In treated hypertensives, high HR and high creatinine during the first visit were associated with an accelerated progression in PWV. The type of treatment and the number of antihypertensive drugs at the time of the first and second visits had no influence on the progression of PWV.

As the increase in aortic stiffness (PWV) over a period of 6 years is more marked in treated hypertensives than in normotensives, the authors concluded that treated hypertensives have accelerated arterial ageing. Three factors were identified as being responsible for accelerated progression in PWV (i.e. to promote accelerated arterial ageing): BP elevation, increased HR and increased serum creatinine. These results reinforce recent data from the Framingham cohort showing that people with high BP are more likely to present an excessive increase in SBP and a decrease in DBP later in life, which suggests accelerated arterial ageing in subjects with high BP levels.

By contrast, there was no association between other major cardiovascular risk factors and progression in aortic stiffness found. This finding was rather surprising. However, the authors did point out that their study was limited by the small number of subjects with diabetes and severe dyslipidaemia, and thus possibly leading to a type II error, i.e. the inability to detect a possible contribution of these metabolic parameters on PWV progression because of the weak number of affected patients. It is also interesting to note that, as for HR, serum creatinine was a determinant of PWV progression in hypertensive but not in normotensive subjects. This result may suggest that hypertensives are more vulnerable than normotensive subjects to the deleterious effects of certain risk factors.

Based on their findings, the authors advocate controlling BP and lowering HR are important to reduce age-related progression of arterial stiffness.

Relations of pulse pressure and other components of blood pressure to preclinical echocardiographic abnormalities.

Celentano A, Palmieri V, Di Palma Esposito N, *et al. J Hypertens* 2002; **20**(3): 531–7.

BACKGROUND. To evaluate the extent to which PP is associated with echocardiographic abnormalities, and in particular to whether PP is related to LVH taking into account other BP components.

INTERPRETATION. Middle-aged clinically healthy hypertensives with PP >50 mmHg had twofold higher prevalence of LVH than those with PP ≤50 mmHg, which may contribute to the higher cardiovascular risk in subjects with higher PP. However, in our sample, PP was not related to LVH independently of SBP, suggesting that SBP is the explanatory link of the relation between PP and LVH.

Comment

In the MAVI Study, Verdecchia et al. |7| reported that for each 39 g increase in LV mass per m², there is a 40% increase in cardiovascular events. In a French study of normotensive and untreated hypertensive adults, the pulsatile component index of BP was associated with LVH |8|. It is therefore important to examine the relationship of components of BP to LVH and systolic dysfunction, as performed by Celentano et al. This can provide further valuable insights into the pathogenesis of this ominous sequel of hypertension and the optimal therapy required to prevent or correct it.

The objective of this cross-sectional study were to evaluate: (i) whether PP is associated with prognostically relevant LV abnormalities, such as LVH, LV geometric remodelling and systolic dysfunction, and (ii) whether relations of PP to LVH might be explained by a greater severity of arterial hypertension associated with higher SBP.

A total of 275 middle-aged adults with asymptomatic EH (mean age 47 years, range 19–69, 3% aged ≥65) were recruited from a specialized out-patient hypertension unit. Subjects were divided in two groups with PP ≤50 or PP >50 mmHg. They found that the prevalence of echocardiographically estimated LVH was twofold higher in subjects with clinic PP >50 mmHg, independent of a number of physiological and demographic confounders. Subjects with PP >50 mmHg also had higher clinic and ambulatory SBP whereas DBP did not differ between groups. PP and SBP, either clinic or ambulatory, showed similar correlation to LVH in separate logistic multivariate models. Using different methodologies, PP was also not related to LV mass index or LVH when the effect of its component SBP was taken into account. Furthermore, in separate analyses, PP was not significantly related to ejection fraction or mid-wall mechanics. Based on these findings, the authors concluded that, in relatively young asymptomatic hypertensives, the variability of PP was mostly due to SBP, and SBP is the pathophysiological link of the relation between PP and LVH. However, they felt that the relation of PP to target organ damage might differ in different age strata, and in particular in elderly individuals. Diabetes was an independent correlate of PP and may represent a significant additional pathophysiological factor in the relation between pressure overload and cardiovascular target organ damage.

From a methodological viewpoint, the concept that PP, *per se*, plays an independent role in addition to SBP, DBP and MAP is difficult to demonstrate. This is due to the fact that these BP components are highly correlated with each other, and thus making the evaluation of their relative and net impact on the LV structure and function difficult. Indeed, data presented by Celentano et al. confirms the high correlation between SBP and PP ($r = 0.9$), making dissociation of the effects extremely problematic by whatever statistical methodology is employed. The interaction of age

with these BP variables complicates interpretations further, such that with age there
is a trend of declining importance of DBP and a corresponding increase in SBP as
predictors of CHD. A recent Framingham Study investigation reported that there
was a gradual shift from DBP to SBP and then to PP as predictors of CHD risk. From
the age of 60 years onward, DBP is negatively related to CHD so that PP becomes
superior to SBP |4,5,9|. The relative young age (mean 47 years) in the study by Celen-
tano *et al.* may explain why this study fails to agree on the relative importance of SBP
and PP on changes in LV function and structure. Furthermore, brachial SBP tends to
overestimate central BP in young subjects, and the difference between central and
brachial BP decreases with age, and patients with PP ≤50 mmHg were younger than
those with elevated PP. Another possible problem is the fact that the data reported by
Celentano *et al.* are derived from cross-sectional rather than prospective population-
based data and thus are subject to selection bias. As pointed out, their study requires
confirmation in a longitudinal prospective population-based investigation.

Correlates of pulse pressure reduction during antihypertensive treatment (losartan or atenolol) in hypertensive patients with electrocardiographic left ventricular hypertrophy (the LIFE study).

Gerdts E, Papademetriou V, Palmieri V, *et al. Am J Cardiol* 2002; **89**(4):
399–402.

BACKGROUND. In hypertensive patients, PP has been related to hypertension-induced
target organ damage and risk of cardiovascular events. However, correlates of PP
reduction during antihypertensive treatment have been less extensively investigated.

INTERPRETATION. In hypertensive patients with electrocardiographic left ventricular
hypertrophy, older age, less reduction in MAP, concomitant diabetes mellitus and shorter
stature are associated with attenuated PP reduction during antihypertensive treatment.

Comment

Previous outcome studies in hypertensive patients have demonstrated PP to be a predictor of cardiovascular morbidity and mortality, but less is known about factors
associated with PP reduction during antihypertensive treatment. Of note, the reduction in PP during antihypertensive treatment does not necessarily parallel that of SBP
and DBP. Thus, to describe further factors associated with PP reduction during antihypertensive treatment, 767 patients aged 55–80 years in the LIFE Study were evaluated. The study found that over 2 years of treatment, BP and PP were reduced from
173/98 to 147/84 mmHg and from 75 to 63 mmHg, respectively, both P <0.001.
When dividing the study population into two groups using a prognostically validated
partition for PP, patients with PP greater or equal 63 mmHg after 2 years of antihypertensive treatment ($n = 349$), they identified four clinical variables, besides initial
PP, as independent correlates of an attenuated PP reduction: older age, shorter

stature, concomitant diabetes mellitus and less reduction in MAP. It would be interesting to see further analyses on unblinded study treatment (atenolol vs losartan) on PP in relation to outcomes.

Effect of angiotensin II on pulse wave velocity in humans is mediated through angiotensin II type 1 (AT1) receptors.

Rehman A, Rahman AR, Rasool AH. *J Hum Hypertens* 2002; **16**(4): 261–6.

BACKGROUND. The objective of this study was to examine the effect of Ang II and Ang II type 1 (AT1) receptor blockade on PWV in healthy humans.

INTERPRETATION. Valsartan completely blocks the effect of Ang II on PWV. The effect of Ang II on PWV is mediated through AT1 receptors. Reduction in PWV by Ang II antagonist is not fully explained by its pressure lowering effect of Ang II and may be partially independent of its effect on BP.

Comment

The authors have previously shown in another clinical study that intravenous Ang II increases PWV in young healthy male volunteers, only when given in doses that significantly increase BP. Interestingly, only less than 30% of the total Ang II-induced rise in PWV was explained by the Ang II-induced rise in BP. The present paper described an extension of this work with the objective to investigate if the effect of Ang II on arterial stiffness (measured as PWV) could be influenced by AT1 receptor blockade.

Again, nine young male volunteers were studied in a double-blind randomized cross-over design. Subjects were previously treated for 3 days with once-daily dose of either a placebo or valsartan 80 mg. On the third day, they were infused with either placebo or 5 ng/kg per min of Ang II over 30 min. Carotid–femoral PWV was measured by using a Complior® machine. Healthy male volunteers were chosen to exclude the confounding effects of age, gender and disease states.

Results from the study showed that Ang II, at the given dose, increased BP (SBP, DBP and MAP) and PWV significantly. Rises in BP were similar to those seen in their previous study. Increase in BP was in the range of 15–20 mmHg systolic and diastolic. Interestingly, such Ang II-induced rises in BP and PWV were completely blocked by 3 days treatment with valsartan. This observation implied that the effect of Ang II on BP and PWV is mediated via AT1 receptors. Again, multiple linear regression analysis of the data in present study also suggested that not all of the Ang II-induced rise in PWV could be explained by the Ang II-induced rise in BP. The analysis also revealed that less than 30% of the total effect of valsartan on PWV could be explained by the effect of valsartan on BP. The authors suggested that the remaining effect of valsartan on PWV was probably due to an independent effect of the drug on the arterial wall that may include not only blockade of the effects of Ang II mediated through AT1 but also enhancing those mediated via AT2 (Ang II type 2 receptors). The authors pointed out that these observations are not novel as Asmar *et al.* |**10**| have demonstrated that long-term (6 months) treatment of perindopril reduced BP and PWV in these patients but less than 10% of the total reduction in PWV could be explained by the reduction in BP. However, the present study was the first one to investigate the effect of prior blockade of AT1 receptors on the Ang II-induced rise in PWV in humans.

The authors did acknowledge that the main limitation of their study was the lack of plasma levels measurements of valsartan and hormones, including Ang II, endothelin-1, atrial natriuretic peptide and antidiuretic hormone at the time of PWV measurements so as to correlate the prevailing plasma levels with the results. However, they pointed out that a concomitant rise in BP suggested the presence of circulating Ang II, and the prevention in the rise in BP when Ang II was infused after prior treatment with valsartan suggests an adequate drug effect.

As Ang II may be formed by non-ACE chymase pathway as well, the authors suggested that more specific blockade of Ang II with the combination of ACE inhibitor and AT1 receptor blocker can be used to investigate further their effects on PWV and to explore the role of bradykinin and alternative pathways of Ang II formation in arterial compliance.

Reduction in arterial stiffness with angiotensin II antagonist is comparable with and additive to ACE inhibition.
Mahmud A, Feely J. *Am J Hypertens* 2002a; **15**: 321–5.

BACKGROUND. In poorly controlled hypertension, an Ang II receptor antagonist added to a regimen of more than three antihypertensive agents, including an ACE inhibitor, has a beneficial effect on arterial wave reflection and PP amplification. The effect of monotherapy with an Ang II receptor antagonist on large artery function, however, has not been described. Furthermore, although both Ang II receptor antagonists and ACE inhibitors target the same pressor system, because of their different sites of action they may have additive or synergistic effects.

INTERPRETATION. Angiotensin receptor antagonists reduce arterial stiffness in hypertension comparable with and possibly additive to ACE inhibition.

Comment

ACE inhibitors lower BP and decrease arterial stiffness both in humans and in experimental animals beyond that expected from the reduction in BP alone. The study by Guerin *et al.* (2001) (see above) have indicated that, in patients with ESRD, a reduction in PWV was of greater prognostic significance than a reduction in BP alone, i.e. independent of BP changes, survival was substantially better for those subjects whose aortic PWV declined in response to decreased BP. In addition, the use of ACE inhibitors has a favourable effect on survival that is independent of BP changes. As discussed above, Rehman *et al.* (2002) demonstrated that infusion of Ang II in young healthy subjects increased BP and PWV, but these effects were completely blocked by valsartan, an ARB, and thus suggested that the effect of Ang II on PWV is mediated through AT1 receptors. However, only 30% of the reduction in PWV can be attributed to BP lowering by valsartan, i.e. valsartan decrease PWV (arterial stiffness) beyond its effect on BP, i.e. independent of BP.

Mahmud and Feely (2002a) take a step further and this study was to explore the effects of valsartan on large artery properties, particularly arterial stiffness, in comparison and in combination with an ACE inhibitor, captopril.

They measured the effects of Ang II blockade on arterial stiffness, AIx, PWV and BP in 12 untreated hypertensive patients (mean 49 ± 11 years) in a 4-week, randomized, cross-over study comparing valsartan 160 mg/day with captopril 100 mg/day, with a 2-week washout period. Subsequently both therapies were combined. The results showed that valsartan reduced PWV and AIx similar to captopril. The reductions in PWV and AIx remained significant when corrected for BP. Interestingly, combined therapy reduced PWV and AIx more than monotherapy, even when corrected for BP.

The novel finding in this study is that ARB significantly reduces AIx and PWV in hypertensive subjects and is as effective as ACE inhibitor. As the relationship between BP and arterial stiffness is non-linear, the authors also analysed the changes in AIx and PWV corrected for BP. After correcting for BP reduction and baseline PWV, the reduction in PWV and AIx still remains significant. This suggests that ACE inhibitor and ARB decrease arterial stiffness independent of BP lowering and thus suggests that these drugs (by blocking Ang II) have a direct effect on vascular wall beyond BP reduction. Furthermore, there may be an additive effect of the ARB and ACE inhibitor in combination, not only on BP but also on arterial stiffness. Long-term study is required to separate the likely functional and structural mechanisms underlying the changes in arterial stiffness. Finally, these data do suggest an important role for the renin–angiotensin system in the control of large arterial function.

Effect of angiotensin II receptor blockade on arterial stiffness: beyond blood pressure reduction.

Mahmud A, Feely J. *Am J Hypertens* 2002b; **15**(12): 1092–5.

BACKGROUND. For the same BP reduction, antihypertensive drugs do not cause the same arterial changes in hypertensive patients. ACE inhibitors, calcium channel blockers and some beta-blockers decrease arterial stiffness, but not the diuretic compound, hydrochlorthiazide. Valsartan has been shown to reduce arterial stiffness to a similar extent as an ACE inhibitor in EH.

INTERPRETATION. The results suggest that an AT1 receptor antagonist losartan induces a BP-independent decrease in aortic stiffness and arterial wave reflection.

Comment

To explore further a BP independent effect, Mahmud and Feely (2002b) hypothe-sized that if an AT1 receptor antagonist reduced arterial stiffness, in addition to low-ering BP of a magnitude similar to that seen with a diuretic (e.g. hydrochlorthiazide, which is known not to affect arterial stiffness), a direct arterial effect of the AT1 receptor antagonist may be implied (also see paper by Rehman *et al.* 2002 above).

In this study, they compared the effect of losartan (50 mg/day) with hydrochlor-thiazide (12.5 mg/day) on BP and arterial stiffness in 11 untreated hypertensive patients (five men) aged 47–69 years in a 4-week single blind randomized cross-over study with an intervening 4-week washout period. Carotid–femoral PWV was deter-mined by the foot-to-foot method using the Complior® device. The results showed that both drugs produced a significant ($P < 0.001$) and similar decrease in brachial BP. But, only losartan induced a significant decrease in arterial wave reflection ($P < 0.0001$), with a preferential reduction in aortic ($P < 0.001$) compared with brachial PP. Losartan also significantly increased PP amplification and reduced PWV.

These findings suggest that losartan, an AT1 receptor antagonist, has a BP-inde-pendent effect on the vasculature, i.e. for the same BP reduction as hydrochlorthi-azide, losartan induced a significant reduction in the magnitude of wave reflection (AIx) in the ascending aorta with a greater reduction in aortic PP than brachial PP, favourably modifying PP amplification. Furthermore, hydrochlorthiazide had no effect on PWV, whereas losartan significantly decreased PWV, i.e. reduced aortic stiffness. This implies a BP independent effect of losartan on arterial stiffness and wave reflection in the ascending aorta, afforded by blocking the AT1 receptor.

Prolonged treatment with the AT(1) receptor blocker, valsartan, increases small and large artery compliance in uncomplicated essential hypertension.

Shargorodsky M, Leibovitz E, Lubimov L, Gavish D, Zimlichman R. *Am J Hypertens* 2002; **15**(12): 1087–91.

BACKGROUND. Decreased arterial compliance is considered an early marker of vascular wall damage. Hypertension gradually decreases arterial compliance. The aim of this study was to investigate whether treatment with the AT1 antagonist valsartan will affect arterial compliance in patients with EH.

INTERPRETATION. Treatment with valsartan in patients with EH improves small and large arterial compliance. The improvement in arterial compliance was significant only after 3 months of treatment, whereas SBP, DBP and systemic vascular resistance decreased earlier. The AT1 receptor blockade with valsartan seems to be an effective means of not only lowering BP but of reversal of vascular wall damage, which predisposes to cardiovascular events.

Comment

Structural changes within the arterial wall and atherosclerotic plaques reduce the compliance of the arterial wall. Determination of arterial compliance may allow us to estimate the extent of vascular damage and the probability of the development of cardiovascular events, as well as to estimate the efficacy of therapeutic intervention. Ang II plays a major part in the development of elevated BP and vascular damage and its blockade may improve remodelling of the vascular wall by reversing damage in patients with EH. The purpose of this study was to determine whether antihypertensive treatment with the AT1 receptor blocker valsartan will improve arterial elasticity in addition to its BP-lowering effect.

The study included 22 patients with EH (six men, mean age 59 ± 4 years), without overt target organ damage. Antihypertensive medications were withdrawn for 3 weeks, and valsartan was given at 80 mg. If BP remained above the target level (below 135/85 mmHg) the dose was increased to 160 mg. Large (C1) and small (C2) arterial compliance were derived from radial artery waveforms, obtained using a calibrated tonometer (model CR-2000). The arterial compliance, BP, blood and urine were measured monthly. Systemic vascular resistance was also determined. The decrease in SBP and DBP was significant within 1 month and improved further on at 3 months. Both C1 and C2 also increased but reached statistical significance only after 3 months. The C1 increased by 22%, and C2 by 35%. Systemic vascular resistance decreased by 15% at 3 months.

Based on the dissociation in time of improvement of BP from the change in arterial properties (C1 and C2), the authors believe Ang II blockade provides a real beneficial remodelling of the arterial wall in addition to its effect on BP lowering. While significant changes in BP occur early at first month of treatment, arterial remodelling is a lengthy process that needs longer periods to occur. They concluded that the increase in arterial compliance seen in their patients is therefore the result of improvement in arterial properties, rather than BP reduction *per se*. However, presence of a technical component of BP effect on the calculated value cannot be totally excluded.

Indeed, this study merely observed the different time course of changes in BP and arterial compliance of both large and small arteries estimated by analysis of the radial arterial pressure pulse. Quite rightly, the authors are probably only 'seeing' a 'valsartan-related effect' on BP and arterial compliance changes at different times. However, the dissociation in time of these changes cannot be taken as evidence of an 'additional' effect of angiotensin blockade. A multivariate analysis on changes in C1 and C2 corrected for changes in BP between baseline and at 3 months should clarify the matter further. Therefore, the main question of whether the observed changes in arterial compliance afforded by angiotensin blockade is 'unrelated to' or 'independent of' or 'beyond' or 'in addition to' its effect on BP changes remains to be answered.

Unlike the present study, Mahmud and Feely (2002a) evaluated the effect of Ang II blockade using valsartan and captopril on arterial stiffness, AIx, PWV and BP in a cross-over study. Using a different method of estimation of arterial stiffness, this study shows also improvement in arterial properties upon blockade of the renin–angiotensin system. The improvement remains significant after adjustment for BP, i.e. a BP-independent effect.

From breaking to inhibiting the 'advanced glycation end-products products'…is the only answer to reverse arterial stiffness?

 Inhibitor for advanced glycation end products formation attenuates hypertension and oxidative damage in genetic hypertensive rats.
Mizutani K, Ikeda K, Tsuda K, Yamori Y. *J Hypertens* 2002; **20**(8): 1607–14.

B ACKGROUND. A recent study demonstrated that free radicals were involved in the maintenance of hypertension in SHRSP. AGEs accumulate progressively in the vasculature with ageing, and have been identified to be relevant mediators for various vascular complications.

I NTERPRETATION. Because long-term administration of an AGEs inhibitor reduces BP and oxidative damage in SHRSP, this study suggests a role for AGEs in the progression or maintenance of hypertension and related diseases in genetic hypertension.

Comment

Non-enzymatic glycation, in which reducing sugars are covalently attached to free amino groups and cross-link to other proteins and form complexes that ultimately form AGEs, which has been found to occur during normal ageing and at an accelerated rate in disease states such as diabetes mellitus. AGE formation and protein cross-linking are irreversible processes that alter the structural and functional properties of proteins, lipid components and nucleic acids. AGEs elicit a wide range of cell-mediated responses that might contribute to the pathogenesis of diabetic complications, vascular and renal disease and Alzheimer's disease.

As parts of the ageing process, collagen and elastin (which maintain cardiovascular elasticity) are prone to the formation of AGE cross-links, leading to stiffening of the blood vessels, including the large arteries. This loss of flexibility in the vasculature may account for the increase in the arterial PP and the development of ISH, which substantially increases the risk of CVD and death. Substances that inhibit AGE formation, reduce oxidative stress or destroy already formed cross-links may limit the progression of disease and may offer new tools for therapeutic interventions in the therapy of AGE-mediated disease.

Indeed, ALT-711, is one of the novel non-enzymatic breakers of AGE cross-links, and has been shown in a randomized, double-blind, placebo-controlled study (performed in nine US centres) to improve selectively total arterial compliance (15% increase in ALT-711 treated-subjects) and lowers PP in older individuals with vascular stiffening, but does not alter cardiac output or systolic vascular resistance |11|.

Unlike ALT-117, OPB-9195 is a novel compound designed to inhibit the formation of AGEs, rather than breaking them. To elucidate the role of AGEs in genetic hypertension, the authors of the present paper investigated the effect of OPB-9195 treatment on hypertension and oxidative damage in SHRSP rats. They hypothesized that increased deposition or circulating AGEs in genetic hypertensive rats would affect nitric oxide (NO) synthase/nitric oxide pathway or oxidative stress, which leads to the progression or maintenance of hypertension.

They found that the plasma of OPB-9195-treated SHRSP had lower levels of glycated albumin as compared with that of control SHRSP. The treated rats also had a reduced SBP, as well as a decreased oxidative state and an increased urinary NO release. They also observed an increase in endothelial NO synthase activity and endothelial NO gene expression in the aorta, which might explain the higher levels of NO production. In addition, they also confirmed that the expression of glutathione peroxidase in the aorta was significantly increased in OPB-9195-treated SHRSP.

Although the real mechanisms through which these novel compounds, AGE inhibitors or breakers, affect physiological changes and hence lead to vascular benefits are unclear, these molecules are effective at different levels in cardiac and vascular cells, and the development of their therapeutic use appears to be highly promising.

Conclusion

In general, in patients 50 years of age, DBP is the strongest predictor. The age period 50–59 years could be seen as a transition period when all three BP indices are comparable predictors; from 60 years of age on, DBP is negatively related to CHD risk so that PP becomes superior to SBP. None the less, SBP is the best single predictor for the majority of persons with hypertension |4|. However, for older persons, the best clinical strategy for the estimation of cardiovascular risk is, first, to determine the level of SBP elevation and then adjust the overall risk upward if there is wide PP, i.e. discordantly low DBP.

Hardening of the pulse, i.e. arterial stiffness, was perhaps first described thousands of years ago by Chinese healers, as an adverse prognostic sign. In 1872, the young medical student Frederick Mahomed at Guy's Hospital, London described elevated arterial pressure on the basis of pulse wave contour measured with the sphygmograph, many years before clinical acceptance of the cuff sphygmomanometer. In Western medicine, the importance of arterial stiffness in hypertension and vascular disease is only receiving more attention until recently. The few task forces articles published in the May and August 2002 issues of the *American Journal of Hypertension* above have reflected this. Indeed, as stated by O'Rourke (2002) in his review paper:

'the information that the pulse affords is of so great importance and so often consulted, surely it must be to our advantage to appreciate fully all it tells us and to draw from it all that it is capable of imparting.'

Such improved clinical recognition of the prognostic value of age-related vascular stiffening will lead to better therapy and improved outcomes for patients with hypertension. ACE inhibitors and ARBs that block the Ang II seem promising. Ultimately, however, newer compounds such as ALT-117 and OPB-9195 that inhibit the formation of AGEs may alter the adverse consequences of age-related arterial stiffness.

References

1. Franklin SS, Khan SA, Wong ND, Larson MG, Levy D. The relation of blood pressure to coronary heart disease risk as a function of age: The Framingham Heart Study. *J Am Coll Cardiol* 2000; **35** (Suppl. A): 291.

2. Verdecchia P, Schillaci G, Borgioni C, Ciucci A, Pede S, Porcellati C. Ambulatory pulse pressure: a potent predictor of total cardiovascular risk in hypertension. *Hypertension* 1998; **32**: 983–8.

3. Miura K, Daviglus ML, Dyer AR, Liu K, Garside DB, Stamler J, Greenland P. Relationship of blood pressure to 25-year mortality due to coronary heart disease, cardiovascular diseases, and all causes in young adult men. The Chicago Heart Association Detection Project in Industry. *Arch Intern Med* 2001; **161**: 1501–8.

4. Franklin SS, Wong ND, Larson MG, Kannel WB, Levy D. How important is pulse pressure as a predictor of cardiovascular risk? *Hypertension* 2002; **39**(2): E12–13.

5. Boutouyrie P, Tropeano AI, Asmar R, Gautier I, Benetos A, Lacolley P, Laurent S. Aortic stiffness is an independent predictor of primary coronary events in hypertensive patients: a longitudinal study. *Hypertension* 2002; **39**: 10–15.

6. Laurent S, Boutouyrie P, Asmar R, Gautier I, Laloux X, Guize L, Ducimetière P, Benetos A. Aortic stiffness is an independent predictor of all-cause and cardiovascular mortality in hypertensive patients. *Hypertension* 2001; **37**: 1236–41.

7. Verdecchia P, Carini G, Circo A, Dovellini E, Giovanni E, Lombardo M *et al.* Left ventricular mass in essential hypertension. The MAVI Study. *J Amer Coll Cardiol* 2001; **38**: 1829–35

8. Darne B, Girerd X, Safar M, Cambien F, Guize L. Pulsatile versus steady component of blood pressure: a cross-sectional and a prospective analysis on cardiovascular mortality. *Hypertension* 1989; **13**: 392–400.

9. Franklin SS, Larson MG, Kahn SA, Wong ND, Leip EP, Kannel WB, Levy D. Does the relation of blood pressure to coronary heart disease change with aging? The Framingham Study. *Circulation* 2001; **103**: 1245–9.

10. Asmar RG, Pannier B, Santoni JP, Laurent S, London GM, Levy BI, Safar ME. Reversion of cardiac hypertrophy and reduced arterial compliance after converting enzyme inhibition in essential hypertension. *Circulation* 1988; **78**: 941–50.

11. Kass DA, Shapiro EP, Kawaguchi M, Capriotti AR, Scuteri A, deGroof RC *et al.* Improved arterial compliance by a novel advanced glycation end-product crosslink breaker. *Circulation* 2001; **104**: 1464–70.

4

Genes in hypertension: some insights

Introduction

The origin of hypertension is not well understood. In Western societies it has been estimated that about 40% of the variation of blood pressure (BP) is attributable to genetic factors while the remaining can be traced back to environmental exposure. A number of common variants in different genes have been identified, each of which may have a moderate effect on BP. The genetic component of the development of high BP may not itself necessarily cause hypertension. Rather there may be a genetic predisposition to develop raised pressure when exposed to various environmental factors. Recently, a number of rare salt sensitive monogenic defects that leads to increased reabsorption of sodium in the renal tubules have been identified. Such discoveries have highlighted the clinical needs to search for other hypertensive genes as they allowed early diagnosis, prevention, pharmacological treatment or even enable the design of target gene therapy. The identifications of hypertension susceptibility genes are increasingly reported, thanks to the enormous development of molecular genetics and genetic statistics. As more genes are being researched and with the ever increasing demand for better therapy to prevent or treat hypertension, effective and specific drugs can be chosen according to the nature of the genetic defect, and with time, more clinical trials will be carried out on possible gene therapy. However, it should be borne in mind that the development of hypertension is a multifactorial and polygenic complex disorder. It makes sense that several genes have to be targeted, which may not be technically feasible in large-scale clinical trials. The dissection of the genetics of primary hypertension has just begun, but genome-wide scans have the potential of localizing any gene in the entire genome relevant to hypertension and hence, facilitating our understanding and identification of previously unknown genes and pathophysiological pathways that are of importance to the development of hypertension. This will certainly require a tight collaboration between clinicians and molecular geneticists.

The FBPP investigators multi-center genetic study of hypertension.

Multi-center genetic study of hypertension: The Family Blood Pressure Program (FBPP). *Hypertension* 2002 Jan; **39**(1): 3–9.

B A C K G R O U N D. The Family Blood Pressure Program (FBPP) consists of four independently established multi-centre networks of investigators who have complementary approaches to the genetics of BP levels and hypertension. The programme has recruited participants from the African American, Mexican American, Asian and non-Hispanic white populations. Each network utilized study designs, laboratory measurements and analytic methods that made efficient use of the unique characteristics of their populations and the investigators' expertise. The individual networks subsequently unified core study components into a single cohesive programme. The unified FBPP includes: (i) standardized clinic and laboratory protocols for core variables to facilitate direct comparison of results among networks; (ii) co-ordination among laboratories to avoid unnecessary duplication of effort; (iii) utilization of a single laboratory for genome-wide marker typing; and (iv) a pooled data set containing phenotype and genotype information from >11 000 individuals.

I N T E R P R E T A T I O N. Identifying functional variation in genes contributing to interindividual differences in BP levels and hypertension status will suggest improved interventions to reduce the risk and improve treatment of hypertension in several ways: (i) more accurate and earlier identification of those individuals at increased risk to develop hypertension; (ii) improved understanding of the aetiology and pathophysiology of hypertension; (iii) development of new, more efficacious treatments, and tailoring of particular treatments to patients who are most likely to respond; and (iv) a better understanding of the factors contributing to differences in the prevalence of hypertension among populations.

Comment

Family studies have demonstrated a significant genetic component underlying inter-individual variation in BP levels and the occurrence of hypertension, but the identity of the individual genes remains uncertain. BP control involves a redundancy of traits with balancing pressor and depressor roles, and therefore, the impact of any one gene will likely be reduced as its effect is transmitted across intervening levels of a biological hierarchy. This type of variation is difficult to elucidate, but advances in both laboratory and analytical approaches continue to facilitate progress. FBPP was established by the National Heart, Lung, and Blood Institute (NHLBI) to localize and identify genes influencing interindividual BP variation and the occurrence of hypertension in the population-at-large.

Four separate 'genetic determinants of high BP' networks were established in 1995 under collaborative agreements with the NHLBI. Each network had multiple field sites collecting data on multiple racial or ethnic groups. In addition, each network included components for biochemical measurements, genotyping, data management and statistical analyses. Each network had, and continues to have, unique areas of expertise and interests that are reflected in a diversity of study designs. All networks ascertained families having individuals with elevated BP. Most networks ascertained families having individuals with a clinical diagnosis of hypertension, whereas others focused on younger individuals who were in the upper portion of the BP distribution for their age and gender but would not be classified as having overt hypertension.

GenNet sought to address BP as a continuously distributed quantitative pheno-type. Non-Hispanic white subjects were recruited from Tecumseh, MI and African American subjects were recruited from Maywood, Illinois. Probands were defined as individuals age 18–50 years with BPs in the upper 20–25% of the age/gender-specific BP distribution. Once the proband was identified, an attempt was made to enrol all siblings and parents of the proband, irrespective of their BP or hypertension treat-ment status. Biochemical measurements included plasma renin activity, serum angio-tensinogen concentration, angiotensin-converting enzyme (ACE) activity, red blood cell lithium–sodium countertransport, and urinary fractional lithium clearance. In addition, GenNet included an animal project in which inbred hypertensive rat strains were used to identify genetic regions to be compared with human orthologs iden-tified from genetic linkage studies to target regions of the human genome for further study.

GENOA (Genetic Epidemiology Network of Atherosclerosis) includes three field centres: the field centre in Jackson, MI, recruited African Americans; the field centre in Starr County, TX, recruited Mexican Americans; and the field centre in Rochester, MN, recruited non-Hispanic white subjects. The field centres in Jackson, MI, and Rochester, MN, recruited sibships containing at least two individuals with hypertension diagnosed before age 60. Because of the high prevalence of non-insulin-dependent diabetes in the Mexican American population, and the resulting confounding that this would create, the field centre in Starr County recruited sib-ships containing at least two individuals with adult onset diabetes. All available full biological siblings of the index sibling pairs were invited to participate in interviews, physical examinations and phlebotomy.

HyperGEN (Hypertension Genetic Epidemiology Network) has field centres in: Birmingham, AL; Forsyth County, NC; Framingham, MA; Minneapolis, MI; and Salt Lake City, UT. African American and non-Hispanic white hypertensive siblings and their parents (when available) and one untreated adult offspring of some of the siblings were recruited. Preference in ascertainment and recruitment was given to hypertensive sibships in which at least one of the subjects was classified as having severe hypertension. In addition to the core examination, stressed BPs and a variety of hypertension-related intermediate traits (e.g. urinary aldosterone and catechola-mines) were also measured.

SAPPHIRe (Stanford Asian Pacific Program in Hypertension and Insulin Resist-ance) focused its investigation on Asian Pacific populations of Chinese and Japanese origin residing in Taiwan, Hawaii and California. Two types of sibling pairs were recruited: those concordant for hypertension (both siblings with hypertension) and those with one hypertensive individual and one individual with low BP. In addition

to the core examination, all SAPPHIRe participants underwent an oral glucose toler-
ance test.

Genes for hypertension and hyperlipidaemia

Genome scan for BP in Dutch dyslipidaemic families reveals linkage to a locus on chromosome 4p.
Allayee H, de Bruin TW, Michelle Dominguez K, *et al. Hypertension* 2001;
38(4): 773–8.

BACKGROUND. Genes contributing to common forms of hypertension are largely
unknown. A number of studies in humans and in animal models have revealed
associations between insulin resistance (IR), dyslipidaemia and elevated hypertension.
To identify genes contributing to BP variation associated with insulin-resistant
dyslipidaemia, a genome-wide scan for BP was carried out in a set of 18 Dutch families
exhibiting the common lipid disorder familial combined hyperlipidaemia.

INTERPRETATION. The genome scan results support the existence of multiple genetic
factors that can influence both BP and plasma lipid parameters.

Comment

A number of studies have revealed associations between hyperlipidaemia, IR and elevated BP leading to the definition of a condition similar to the metabolic syndrome
termed familial dyslipidaemic hypertension, involving a clustering of traits, including central obesity, lipid abnormalities, hypertension and elevated fasting insulin
levels. Several studies have demonstrated a high degree of heritability of this trait,
which occurs in approximately 1% of the general population but in approximately
12% of patients with essential hypertension.

   The study by Allayee *et al.* supports the existence of multiple genetic factors that
can influence both BP and plasma lipid parameters. They applied a genomic scan to
the common lipid disorder familial combined hyperlipidaemia, which is characterized by IR and dyslipidaemia and is present in 10–20% of patients with premature
coronary artery disease (CAD). Sibpair linkage analysis of the data by both two-point
and multipoint approaches revealed strong evidence for linkage of SBP (systolic BP)
to a locus on the short arm of chromosome 4.

Angiotensin genes

Relationship between angiotensin-converting enzyme gene polymorphism and insulin resistance in never-treated hypertensive patients.
Perticone F, Ceravolo R, Iacopino S, *et al. J Clin Endocrinol Metab* 2001; **86**: 172–8.

BACKGROUND. The association between ACE gene polymorphism and IR in hypertensive subjects remains controversial. Thus, this study evaluated the possible association between IR and ACE gene polymorphism in a group of hypertensive, never-treated patients compared with that in a normotensive control group.

INTERPRETATION. The results extended previous data regarding the relationship of hypertension and IR by demonstrating a dependence of this relationship upon the ACE gene polymorphism.

Comment

IR has been regarded as part of the metabolic syndrome, with associated abnormalities of hypertension, hyperlipidaemia, etc., leading to a high cardiovascular risk.

ACE plays a key part in regulating BP as well as fluid and electrolyte balance. ACE has several functions related to the renin–angiotensin system, including the proteolytic activation of angiotensin II (Ang II), a potent vasopressor and aldosterone-stimulating peptide, and not related to the renin–angiotensin system, such as the degradation of kinins. The cloning of the ACE gene has made it possible to identify an insertion (I)/deletion (D) polymorphism in intron 16 that appears to be associated with different levels of serum ACE activity.

Subjects homozygous for the short allele (DD) have serum ACE levels about twofold higher than II subjects. In clinical epidemiological studies, the DD genotype has been identified as a novel risk factor for CAD and myocardial infarction.

In addition, ACE gene polymorphism could be related to the development of IR and the pathogenesis of hypertensive status and CAD in type II diabetic patients.

Essential hypertension is frequently associated with IR and hyperinsulinaemia, such as the compensatory response to decreased sensitivity to insulin-stimulated glucose uptake in peripheral tissues, particularly skeletal muscle. Nevertheless, the mechanism responsible for the development of IR in hypertension and other common IR states remains unknown. Moreover, the fact that IR is found among normotensive relatives of hypertensive patients implies that the predisposition to IR might be inherited.

Furthermore, ACE inhibitors improve the insulin sensitivity in normal subjects, non-insulin-dependent diabetes patients, and non-diabetic hypertensive patients.

The effect of treatment with ACE inhibitors on insulin sensitivity suggests the possibility of a relationship between the renin–angiotensin system, the system of bradykinins, and insulin action, making the gene coding for ACE a candidate for the genetic basis of IR. These findings support the idea that the ACE gene is related to a predisposition to IR, and Perticone *et al.* investigate this relationship of hypertension and IR—clearly demonstrating a dependence of this relationship upon the ACE gene polymorphism.

Angiotensinogen gene core promoter variants and non-modulating hypertension.

Hilgers KF, Delles C, Veelken R, Schmieder RE. *Hypertension* 2001 Dec 1; **38**(6): 1250–4.

B A C K G R O U N D . **Non-modulation has been suggested as a possible intermediate phenotype defining a subgroup of genetic hypertension. The trait is characterized by an attenuated response of renal blood flow and/or aldosterone to Ang II. This study tested the hypothesis that functional polymorphisms of the core promoter of the angiotensinogen gene are associated with non-modulation.**

I N T E R P R E T A T I O N . The −20C variant or the −20C/−6A haplotype of the angiotensinogen core promoter is associated with a blunted aldosterone response to Ang II and may thus contribute to the non-modulating phenotype.

Comment

Non-modulation has been described as an abnormal response of aldosterone release or renal blood flow to Ang II or to sodium restriction, occurring in a subset of hypertensive patients. Somewhat different definitions have been used, emphasizing either renal blood flow or aldosterone responses and sometimes substituting sodium restriction for Ang II infusion. Non-modulating hypertension has been described as a heritable intermediate phenotype that may precede the development of hypertension.

The molecular genetic basis of non-modulating hypertension is not fully understood, but an association with the M235T polymorphism of the angiotensinogen gene has been suggested, being associated with hypertension and elevated plasma angiotensinogen in several populations. The elevation of plasma angiotensinogen is not due to the M235T substitution itself but a linked A for G substitution at position −6 in the core promoter of the gene. The −6A variant was reported to be associated with elevated angiotensinogen gene transcription, increased angiotensinogen gene expression in uterine spiral arteries, elevated plasma angiotensinogen levels and hypertension.

In addition, two other polymorphisms of the angiotensinogen gene core promoter that may cause altered gene transcription have been described: C for A substitution at position −20 leads to increased angiotensinogen transcription *in vitro* and is associated with hypertension and elevated plasma angiotensinogen. The C/T polymorphism at position −18 may affect transcription factor binding *in vitro*, and the C allele was associated with hypertension.

This paper by Hilgers *et al.* reports that the −20C variant or the −20C/−6A haplotype of the angiotensinogen core promoter is associated with a blunted aldosterone response to Ang II and may thus contribute to the non-modulating phenotype.

Molecular basis of salt sensitivity in human hypertension evaluation of renin–angiotensin–aldosterone system gene polymorphisms.

Poch E, González D, Giner V, *et al. Hypertension* 2001 Nov; **38**(5): 1204–9.

B A C K G R O U N D . **This study designed to analyse the association between salt sensitivity in essential hypertension and eight genetic polymorphisms in six genes of the renin–angiotensin–aldosterone system (RAAS).**

I N T E R P R E T A T I O N . The I allele of ACE I/D polymorphism is significantly associated to salt-sensitive hypertension. The BP response to high salt intake was different among genotypes of ACE I/D and 11β-hydroxysteroid dehydrogenase (11β-HSD) G534A, suggesting that these polymorphisms may be potentially useful genetic markers of salt sensitivity.

Comment

Although many factors influence the BP response to a high-salt diet, the RAAS has been demonstrated to play a central part. Low-renin hypertensives show an increased BP response to salt load, and salt-sensitive individuals exhibit a blunted response of the RAAS when switching from low to high salt intakes, compared with that of salt-resistant subjects.

Polymorphisms in candidate genes of this system have been extensively tested as genetic determinants of essential hypertension in the past several years. Some of the polymorphisms that have been associated with hypertension are the ACE I/D (D allele, only in males), the angiotensinogen M235T (T allele), and the aldosterone synthase C-344T (T allele). In addition, these apolymorphisms determine part of the variations in plasma levels of ACE, angiotensinogen, and aldosterone, respectively.

The mineralocorticoid receptor gene (MLR) and the 11β-HSD2 gene have also been considered as candidate genes for essential hypertension because they play a causative role in rare forms of monogenic hypertension or hypotension. Mutations in the former gene cause pseudohypoaldosteronism type I, a monogenic syndrome of hypotension and salt wasting and a rare form of hypertension, whereas mutations in the latter cause the apparent mineralocorticoid excess, a form of salt-sensitive monogenic hypertension.

Essential hypertension, as well as the target organ damage and other associated phenotypes, such as salt sensitivity, appear to be polygenic in nature. Poch *et al.*

previously reported |1| an association between the ACE I/D polymorphism and the molecular genetic analysis of salt sensitivity in a sample of patients with essential hypertension. This has been extended in the present study, to eight polymorphisms of six genes of the RAAS: the ACE I/D, the angiotensinogen M235T, the angiotensin II receptor type 1 (AT1) A1166C, the aldosterone synthase C344T and intron 2 conversion, the MLR G3524C and A4582C, and the 11βHSD2 G534A in an extended sample of patients with essential hypertension. They found that the BP response to high salt intake was different among genotypes of ACE I/D and 11β-HSD G534A, suggesting that these polymorphisms may be potentially useful genetic markers of salt sensitivity.

T+31C Polymorphism of angiotensinogen gene and essential hypertension.

Ishikawa K, Baba S, Katsuya T, *et al. Hypertension* 2001 Feb; **37**(2): 281–5.

BACKGROUND. A common variant at codon 235 of the angiotensinogen gene (AGT) with methionine to threonine amino acid substitution (AGT M235T) has been reported as a genetic risk for essential hypertension. However, the frequency of AGT T235 was heterogeneous among races, and a positive association between AGT M235T and hypertension was not settled. To examine the association in a general population of Japanese ($n = 4013$), we introduced the TaqMan polymerase chain reaction method and examined the relation between hypertension and T+31C polymorphism, which was in absolute linkage disequilibrium with AGT M235T.

INTERPRETATION. The C+31 allele of AGT was significantly associated with the positive family history of hypertension but not with the presence of hypertension or BP. The subjects with CC tended to have hypertensive relatives, especially a hypertensive father or siblings, and its statistical significance was stronger in men. Adjustment of confounding factor did not alter the results of simple association study, suggesting that this positive association with positive family history of hypertension (FH) is independent and significant. These findings revealed that the TaqMan polymerase chain reaction method is a powerful tool for genetic association study with a large number of subjects and that AGT T+31C is significantly associated with paternal FH.

Comment

In 1992, the AGT polymorphism AGT M235T was reported to be associated with essential hypertension and increased concentration of plasma angiotensinogen in white subjects. A common variant of AGT G-6A in the proximal promoter, which is in almost complete linkage disequilibrium with M235T, leads to a higher basal transcription rate of the AGT gene. In regard to the association between T235 or the A-6 allele and hypertension; however, the results obtained from many case–control studies or affected sib-pair methods are still inconsistent. Ishikawa *et al.* examine the effect of the AGT allele for hypertension by studying a large general population of randomly selected urban residents and using the TaqMan polymerase chain reaction (a powerful tool for genetic association study) conclude that AGT T+31C is significantly associated with paternal FH.

Genes and response to antihypertensive therapy

C825T Polymorphism of the G protein β3-subunit and antihypertensive response to a thiazide diuretic.

Turner ST, Schwartz GL, Chapman AB, Boerwinkle E. *Hypertension* 2001 Feb; **37**(2 Part 2): 739–43.

BACKGROUND. The T allele of the C825T polymorphism of the gene encoding the β3-subunit of G proteins has been associated with increased sodium-hydrogen exchange and low renin in patients with essential hypertension. To assess its association with BP response to diuretic therapy, we measured the C825T polymorphism in 197 black people (134 men, 63 women) and 190 non-Hispanic white people (76 men, 114 women) with essential hypertension, who underwent monotherapy with hydrochlorothiazide for 4 weeks.

INTERPRETATION. The C825T polymorphism of the G protein β3-subunit may help identify patients with essential hypertension who are more responsive to diuretic therapy.

Antihypertensive pharmacogenetics: getting the right drug into the right patient.

Turner ST, Schwartz GL, Chapman AB, Hall WD, Boerwinkle E. *J Hypertens* 2001 Jan; **19**(1): 1–11. Review.

BACKGROUND. Pharmacogenetic investigation seeks to identify genetic factors that contribute to interpatient and interdrug variation in responses to antihypertensive drug therapy. Classical studies have characterized single gene polymorphisms of drug metabolizing enzymes that are responsible for large interindividual differences in pharmacokinetic responses to several antihypertensive drugs. Progress is being made using candidate gene and genome scanning approaches to identify and characterize many additional genes influencing pharmacodynamic mechanisms that contribute to interindividual differences in responses to antihypertensive drug therapy.

INTERPRETATION. Knowledge of polymorphic variation in these genes will help to predict individual patients' BP responses to antihypertensive drug therapy and may also provide new insights into molecular mechanisms responsible for the elevation of BP.

Comment

Within each class of antihypertensive drugs, BP responses vary considerably among patients, with a range of response that is several times greater than the mean response. This interindividual variation in response is primarily due to pharmacodynamic, not pharmacokinetic, differences and likely reflects variation in pathophysiological mechanisms that contribute to hypertension in individual patients.

It has long been suspected that interindividual variation in drug responses may be influenced by genetic factors. Recently, a polymorphism (C825T) was described in exon 10 of the gene encoding the β3-subunit of G proteins (GNB3), and subsequently it was found to be associated with a shortened splice variant of the Gβ3-protein that gives rise to enhanced signal transduction via pertussis toxin-sensitive G proteins. The C825T polymorphism was originally identified through

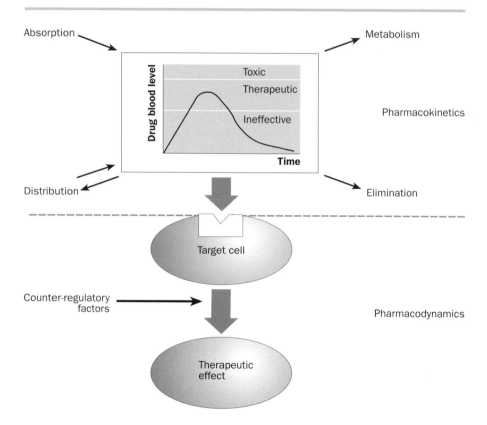

Fig. 4.1 Determinants of drug response. Genetic variation may contribute to individual differences in drug response by altering the structure, configuration or quantity of proteins involved in pharmacokinetic or pharmacodynamic mechanisms determining drug response. Source: Turner *et al.* (2001) |3|.

Table 4.1 Single gene polymorphisms with large effects on the metabolism of antihypertensive medications

Polymorphism	Gene	Antihypertensive drug	Clinical consequence	Other drugs metabolized
Debrisoquine hydroxylation	Cytochrome P450 CYP2D6 Chromosome 22	Alprenolol Bufuralol Metoprolol Propranolol Timolol	Poor metabolizers: excessive β-blockade Extensive metabolizers: loss of blood pressure control at end of dose interval	Antiarhyfimica: encainide, flecainide, maxilatine, propafenone Antidepressants: amitriptyline, domipramine, desipramine, imipramine, nortriptyline Neuroleptics, perphenazine, resperidone, thioridazine
N-acetylation	N-acetyltransferase NAT2* Chromosome 8	Hydralazine	Slow acetylators: antinuclear antibodies and systemic lupus erythematosus-like syndrome Rapid acetylators: higher dose required for blood pressure control	Antiarrhthmic: procainamide Antidepressant: phenelzine Anti-infectives: dapsone, isoniazid Anti-inflammatory: P-salicyclic acid, sulfasalazine
Catechol-O-methylation	Catechol-O-methyl transferase COMT Chromosome 22	Methyedopa	Low methylators: lower dose required for blood pressure control	Antiparkinonian: levodopa

Source: Turner et al. (2001) [3].

Table 4.2 Candidate gene studies of blood pressure response to antihypertensive drug therapy

Gene	Polymorphiam	Allele Association	Antihypertensive drug	Duration of therapy	Sample
Adducin	Gly460Trp	Trp460 allele associated with greater blood pressure reduction	D-THZ	8 weeks	Essential hypertension; $n = 143$ Caucasians
Angiotensinogen	M235T	T235 allele associated with greater blood pressure reduction	ACE-1	4 Weeks	Essential hypertension; $n = 125$ Caucasians
		None	CCB-D BRB-S ACE-1	4 weeks	Essential hypertension; $N = 63$–91 Caucasians
Angiotensin converting enzyme	Insertion/ deletion	None	CCB-D BRB-S ACE-1	4 weeks	Essential hypertension; $n = 63$–91 Caucasian
		None	ACE-1	4 weeks	Essential hypertension; $n = 125$ Caucasians
		None	ACE-1	52 weeks	Essential hypertension; $n = 60$ Japanese
		None	ACE-1	12 weeks	Proteinuric renal disease; $n = 36$ Japanese
Angiotensin II receptor type 1	A1166C	None	ACE-1	4 weeks	Essential hypertension; $n = 125$ Caucasians
G_s protein, α-subunit	FokI (+/−)	FokI (+) allele associated with greater blood pressure reduction	BRB-B	4 weeks	Essential hypertension; $n = 66$ Caucasians

Antihypertensive drugs: ACE-1, angiotensin converting enzyme inhibitor; CCB-D, calcium channel blocker, dihydropyridine; BRB-S β_1-selective andrenoceptor blocker; BRB-B, β-adrenoceptor blocker; both B_1-selective and non-selective; D-THZ, thiazide diuretic.

studies of lymphoblasts, derived from white people with essential hypertension, in which sodium-proton antiport activity was increased as a consequence of enhanced G-protein-dependent signal transduction in response to a variety of vasoactive and growth-promoting stimuli.

Turner et al. |2|. report a study in which the C825T polymorphism of the G protein β3-subunit may help identify patients with essential hypertension who are more responsive to diuretic therapy. This may have some therapeutic implications and may help us appreciate why some patients respond well to diuretics while others do not.

The review by Turner et al. |3|. takes this further by providing an overview of the data, and aims to do the following: (i) to present pharmacogenetic concepts relevant to antihypertensive drug therapy; (ii) to consider the challenge of identifying individual genetic factors that contribute to differences in responses to antihypertensive medications; (iii) to describe classical pharmacogenetic investigations successful in identifying single gene polymorphisms with large effects on the metabolism of several antihypertensive drugs; (iv) to provide examples of candidate gene and genome scanning approaches now being applied to identify genes contributing to a continuously distributed variation in BP response to antihypertensive medications; and (v) to suggest developments likely in the future to expand the role of pharmacogenetics in the evaluation, treatment and control of hypertension and its complications.

Table 4.3 Candidate gene studies of other cardiovascular responses

Gene	Polymorphism	Drug	Response phenotype	Sample description
Angiotensin converting enzyme	Insertion/ deletion	ACE-1	Cough	EHT,CHF
			Plasma ACE	NT
			Plasma ACE	EHT
			AT_1R mRNA	EHT
			Renal plasma flow	NT
			Proteinuria	PRN
			LV mass	EHT
			Diastolic filling	EHT, CRF
			Glomerular filtration	nDRD
		BRB S	Glomerular filtration	nDRD
Angiotensin II receptor, type 1	A1166C	Phenylephrine, AII	Coronary vasoconstriction	CAD
		ACE-1, CCB-D	Pulse wave velocity	EHT

Drug abbreviations are as given in Table 4.2; AII, angiotensin II; AT_1R, angiotensin II receptor, type 1; LV, left ventricular; EHT, essential hypertension; CHF congestive heart failure; NT, normotension; PRD, proteinuric renal disease; CRF, chronic renal failure; nDRD, non-diabetic renal disease; CAD, coronary artery disease.
Source: Turner et al. (2001) |3|.

Gene therapy

Gene therapy for hypertension. The preclinical data.

Phillips MI. *Hypertension* 2001 Sep; **383**(3 Pt 2): 543–8. Review.

B A C K G R O U N D . **Despite several drugs for the treatment of hypertension, there are many patients with poorly controlled high BP. This is partly because all of the available drugs are short-lasting (<24 h), have side-effects, and are not highly specific. Gene therapy offers a possibility of producing longer-lasting effects with precise specificity based on the genetic design.**

I N T E R P R E T A T I O N . There is sufficient preclinical data to give serious consideration to phase I trials for testing some of the anti-sense oligodeoxynucleotides, although testing the viral vectors needs much more work.

Comment

Preclinical studies on gene therapy for hypertension have taken two approaches. Chao J *et al.* |4| have performed extensive studies on gene transfer to increase vaso-dilator proteins. They have transferred kallikrein, atrial natriuretic peptide (ANP), adrenomedullin and endothelin nitric oxide (NO) synthase into different rat models. Their results show that BP can be lowered for 3–12 weeks with the expression of these genes. The anti-sense approach, which we began by targeting angiotensinogen and the angiotensin type 1 (AT1) receptor, has now been tested independently by several different groups in multiple models of hypertension. Other genes targeted include the β1-adrenoceptor, thyrotrophin-releasing hormone, angiotensin gene-activating elements, carboxypeptidase Y, c-*fos* and CYP4A1. There have been two methods of delivering anti-sense: one is by oligodeoxynucleotides, and the other is with full-length DNA in viral vectors. All the studies show a decrease in BP lasting several days to weeks or months. Oligodeoxynucleotides are safe and non-toxic and could be delivered orally or eventually by skin patches. Systemic delivery of recombinant adeno-associated virus with DNA anti-sense to AT1 receptors in adult rodents decreases hypertension for up to 6 months.

Gene therapy for cardiovascular disease. A case for cautious optimism.

Khurana R, Martin JF, Zachary I. *Hypertension* 2001 Nov; **38**(5): 1210–16. Review.

B A C K G R O U N D . **There is currently intense interest in the development of gene therapy for cardiovascular disease. The stimulation of therapeutic angiogenesis for ischaemic** heart disease has been one of the areas of greatest promise. Encouraging results have been obtained with the angiogenic cytokines vascular endothelial growth factor (VEGF) and basic fibroblast growth factor in animal models, leading to clinical trials in ischaemic heart disease. VEGF also has therapeutic potential in a second area of cardiovascular gene therapy, the enhancement of arterioprotective endothelial functions to prevent post-angioplasty restenosis and bypass graft arteriopathy. The endothelial cell growth and survival functions of VEGF promote endothelial regeneration, whereas VEGF-induced endothelial production of NO and prostacyclin inhibits vascular smooth muscle cell proliferation. Inhibition of neointimal hyperplasia may also be achieved by gene transfer of endothelial NO synthase, prostaglandin I synthase, or cell cycle regulators (retinoblastoma, cyclin or cyclin-dependent kinase inhibitors, p53, growth arrest homeobox gene, fas ligand) or anti-sense oligonucleotides to c-*myb*, c-*myc*, proliferating cell nuclear antigen, and transcription factors such as nuclear factor kappaB and E2F. An improved understanding of aetiologically complex pathologies involving the interplay of genes and the environment, such as atherosclerosis and systemic hypertension, has led to the identification of new targets for gene therapy, with the potential to alleviate inherited genetic defects such as familial hypercholesterolaemia. The use of vasodilator gene overexpression and anti-sense knockdown of vasoconstrictors to reduce BP in animal models of systemic and pulmonary hypertension offers the prospect of gene therapy for human hypertensive disease. The renin–angiotensin system has been the target of choice for antihypertensive strategies because of its wide distribution and additional effects on fibrinolytic and oxidative stress pathways.

INTERPRETATION. Gene therapy in cardiovascular disease has an exciting future but remains at an early stage. Further developments in gene transfer vector technology and the identification of additional target genes will be required before its full therapeutic potential can be realized.

The future of hypertension therapy: sense, antisense, or non-sense?

Pachori AS, Huentelman MJ, Francis SC, *et al. Hypertension* 2001; **37**(part 2): 357–64.

BACKGROUND. Hypertension is a debilitating disease with significant socio-economic and emotional impact. Despite recent success in the development of traditional pharmacotherapy for the management of hypertension, the incidence of this disease is on the rise and has reached epidemic proportions by all estimates. This has led many to conclude that traditional pharmacotherapy has reached an intellectual plateau, and novel approaches for the treatment and control of hypertension must be explored. We have begun to investigate the possibility of treating and/or curing hypertension by using genetic means.

INTERPRETATION. This review provides evidence in favour of targeting of the renin–angiotensin system by antisense gene therapy as an effective strategy for the lifelong prevention of hypertension in the spontaneously hypertensive rat model. In addition, the properties of an ideal vector for the systemic delivery of genes and the potential experimental hurdles that must be overcome will take this innovative approach to the next level of evaluation.

Comment

Are we ready for this yet? All the existing data indicate that gene therapy based on either the overexpression of vasodilatory genes or the inhibition of vasoconstrictor genes is an exciting pharmacotherapeutic approach, which holds great potential for the treatment of hypertension in the future. It appears that this gene therapy approach is conceptually sound and may provide a means for the permanent control and possible cure of hypertension. However, we must use extreme caution and restraint. Extensive experiments must be carried out to establish the mechanisms, and new and safe viral vectors that have a high transduction efficiency must be developed. An *in vivo*-regulated system must be tested. Each of these components must be completed before we can attempt to try the gene therapy approach in human hypertension.

The review by Phillips (2001) provides some thought provoking arguments for us to consider phase I trials of gene therapy for hypertension, based on pre-clinical data available (see Table 4.4). However, the review by Khurana *et al.* (2001) advocates a more cautious approach.

Table 4.4 Preclinical data of gene therapy for hypertension vasodilator genes

Target gene	Delivery	Model	Max Δ BP, mmHg	Duration of effect
Human tissue Kallikrein	Adenovirus	Dahl salt-sensitive		4 weeks
		5/6 renal mass	−37	5 weeks
		SHR	−30	36 days
	Adenovirus, intramuscular	SHR		5 weeks
		2K1C	−26	24 days
	Adenovirus, intravenous	DOCA-salt		23 days
Adrenomedullin	Adenovirus	DOCA-salt	−41	9 days
	Intravenous	SHR		
	Intravenous	Dahl salt-sensitive		4 weeks
Atrial natriuretic peptide (ANP)	Adenovirus	Dahl salt-sensitive	−32	5 weeks
NO	Plasmid	SHR	−21	5 to 6 weeks (first injection) 10 to 12 weeks (second injection)

Source: Phillips (2001).

Endothelin rules, OK

Endothelin-1 gene variant associates with blood pressure in obese Japanese subjects: the Ohasama study.
Asai T, Ohkubo T, Katsuya T, *et al. Hypertension* 2001 Dec 1; **38**(6): 1321–4.

BACKGROUND. A recent report based on the results of two epidemiological studies, the Etude Cas-Temoin de l'Infarctus Myocarde (ECTIM) and the Glasgow Heart Scan Study, revealed that a G/T polymorphism with an amino acid substitution (Lys–Asn) at codon 198 in exon 5 of the endothelin-1 gene (ET-1) is associated with BP in overweight people. They suggested that G/T polymorphism of ET-1 strongly interacted with body mass index in the determination of BP levels. To examine interaction among G/T polymorphism of ET-1, body mass index and BP, the present study performed an association study in a general Japanese population.

INTERPRETATION. Lys198Asn polymorphism of ET-1 is involved in the determination of BP levels in obese subjects.

Renal endothelin ETA/ETB receptor imbalance differentiates salt-sensitive from salt-resistant spontaneous hypertension.
Rothermund L, Luckert S, Koβmehl P, Paul M, Kreutz R. *Hypertension* 2001; **37**: 275–80.

BACKGROUND. It is unclear why a subgroup of patients with essential hypertension develop salt-sensitive hypertension with progression of target organ damage over time. This study evaluated the role of the renal ET system in the stroke-prone spontaneously hypertensive rat (SHRSP) model of salt-sensitive spontaneous hypertension (SS-SH) compared with the spontaneously hypertensive rat (SHR) model of salt-resistant spontaneous hypertension (SR-SH).

INTERPRETATION. Activation of the renal ET system together with an increased ETA/ETB receptor ratio may contribute to the development and progression of SS-SH.

Comment
ET originally was isolated in 1988 from a supernatant of porcine aortic endothelial cell cultures and demonstrated strong vasoconstrictive peptide. ET has three isoforms (ET-1, ET-2 and ET-3) translated from three independent genes and is produced by endothelium and many tissues.

ET-1 plays a part in increasing BP, cell proliferation and modulation of vasomotor tone; it also interacts with the pathophysiology of a variety of vascular diseases, such as hypertension, arteriosclerosis and ischaemic heart disease. Because ET-1 concentration in the blood is increased by standing and decreased by volume overload, it is considered to be modulated by body fluid volume through the RAAS. Because of its vasoconstrictive actions for vessels and hypertrophic actions for heart, ET-1 has been examined as an important risk for hypertension.

Plasma level of ET-1 was higher in patients with essential hypertension than in normotensive subjects and paralleled the level of target organ damage. ETA receptor gene was overexpressed in arteries of hypertensive patients, which suggests that ET-1 contributes to the pathogenesis of hypertension by means of endothelial dysfunction or proliferation of vascular smooth muscle cell. Chronic treatment by use of an ET receptor antagonist for hypertensive patients reduced BP also provides supporting data for the correlation between ET-1 and hypertension. Even with these supporting data, the causal relationship between ET-1 and hypertension has yet to be clarified.

On the other hand, the full length of the human ET-1 gene was cloned and sequenced in 1989 and mapped on 6p24–p23. The 2026-nucleotide mRNA of ET-1, excluding the poly(A) tail, is encoded in five exons distributed over 6836 bp. Indeed, a G/T polymorphism with an amino acid substitution (Lys–Asn) at codon 198 in exon 5 of ET-1 was associated with BP in overweight European people in two epidemiological studies, the ECTIM Study and the Glasgow Heart Scan Study. Asai *et al.* report similar results in a Japanese population, which suggests that the Lys198Asn polymorphism of ET-1 is involved in the determination of BP levels in obese subjects from different populations. Rothermund *et al.* add to the data on the ET gene, suggesting that activation of the renal ET system together with an increased ETA/ETB receptor ratio may contribute to the development and progression of salt-sensitive spontaneous hypertension.

Maybe atrial natriuretic peptide as well, in hypertension

Polymorphisms in the hANP (human atrial natriuretic peptide) gene, albuminuria, and hypertension.

Nannipieri M, Manganiello M, Pezzatini A, *et al. Hypertension* 2001 Jun; **37**(6): 1416–22.

BACKGROUND. ANP jointly affects kidney function and BP homeostasis and is a candidate susceptibility gene for both essential hypertension and kidney disease. This study evaluated the relation between the *Sca*I and *Bst*XI polymorphisms of the human ANP (hANP) gene, hypertension and albuminuria in a clinical cohort of 1033 subjects, including type 1 and type 2 diabetic patients, non-diabetic subjects with essential hypertension and non-diabetic normotensive control subjects.

INTERPRETATION. The mutated genotypes of the *Sca*I polymorphism are negatively associated with overt nephropathy, whereas the mutated genotypes of *Bst*XI polymorphism are positively associated with microalbuminuria. hANP gene variants may exert a protective effect against the development and progression of kidney damage in diabetes.

Comment

Several lines of evidence indicate that familial predisposition to hypertension increases the susceptibility to diabetic nephropathy, thus implying that inherited factors distinct from hyperglycaemia play a part in the development and progression of kidney damage. Both diabetic nephropathy and hypertension probably have a significant genetic basis. However, the number and the kind of genes involved in the pathogenesis of kidney damage and hypertension are still unknown.

ANP is an endogenous vasoactive peptide, produced mainly in cardiac atria, which plays a central part in the regulation of BP by modulating sodium homeostasis and the RAAS. ANP also affects renal haemodynamics and microvascular permeability to macromolecules. The ANP gene has thus been included in the list of candidate genes for familial susceptibility to hypertension and diabetic nephropathy.

Indeed, disruption of the ANP gene leads to salt-sensitive hypertension in transgenic animals. However, the results of association studies between DNA polymorphisms at the hANP locus and hypertension or diabetic nephropathy have been conflicting.

Nannipieri *et al.* examine the simultaneous association of two (*Sca*I and *Bst*XI) polymorphisms of hANP with hypertension and proteinuria in a large cohort,

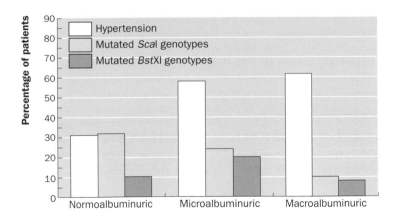

Fig. 4.2 Prevalence rates of hypertension and mutated *Sca*I $(A^2A^1 + A^2A^1)$ and *Bst*XI $(C^{TOB}/T + T^{TOB}/T)$ genotypes according to albumin excretion rate in a whole study cohort $(n = 1033)$. Source: Nannipieri *et al.* (2001).

including patients with type 2 diabetes and non-diabetic subjects with essential hypertension. They found that the mutated genotypes of the *Sca*I polymorphism are negatively associated with overt nephropathy, whereas the mutated genotypes of *Bst*XI polymorphism were positively associated with microalbuminuria. Thus hANP gene variants may exert a protective effect against the development and progression of kidney damage in diabetes.

... and many, many more genes, as well

Genetic dissection of region around the *Sa* gene on rat chromosome 1: evidence for multiple loci affecting BP.

Frantz S, Clemitson J-R, Bihoreau M-T, Gauguier D, Samani NJ. *Hypertension* 2001 Aug; **38**(2): 216–21.

BACKGROUND. A region with a major effect on BP is located on rat chromosome 1 in the vicinity of the *Sa* gene, a candidate gene for BP regulation. Previously, we observed a single linkage peak for BP in this region in second filial generation rats derived from a cross of the SHR with the Wistar-Kyoto rat (WKY), and we have reported the isolation of the region containing the BP effect in reciprocal congenic strains (WKY.SHR-Sa) and (SHR.WKY-Sa) derived from these animals.

INTERPRETATION. Two congenic substrains each were derived from WKY.SHR-Sa (WISA1 and WISA2) and SHR.WKY-Sa (SISA1 and SISA2) by backcrossing to WKY and SHR, respectively. Although there was some overlap of the introgressed regions retained in the various substrains, the segments in WISA1 and SISA1 did not overlap. Furthermore, although the Sa allele in WISA1, WISA2 and SISA2 remained donor in origin, recombination in SISA1 reverted it back to the recipient (SHR) allele. Surprisingly, all four substrains demonstrated a highly significant BP difference compared with that of their respective parental strain, which was of a magnitude similar to those seen in the original congenic strains. The findings strongly indicate that there are at least two quantitative trait loci (QTLs) affecting BP in this region of rat chromosome 1. Furthermore, the BP effect seen in SISA1 indicates that at least a proportion of the BP effect of this region of rat chromosome 1 cannot be due to the *Sa* gene. SISA1 contains an introgressed segment of <3 cM, and this will facilitate the physical mapping of the BP QTL(s) located within it and the identification of the susceptibility-conferring genes. Our observations serve to illustrate the complexity of QTL dissection and the care needed to interpret findings from congenic studies.

Comment

As evident from the wide variety of genes 'linked' to hypertension discussed in this chapter, this paper by Frantz *et al.* provides evidence for multiple loci affecting BP. This is not unsurprising, and hypertension is likely to be multifactorial.

Polymorphism in the beta(1)-adrenergic receptor gene and hypertension.

Bengtsson K, Melander O, Orho-Melander M, *et al. Circulation* 2001; **104**(2): 187–90.

BACKGROUND: **The Arg389 variant of the β₁-adrenergic receptor gene mediates a higher isoproterenol-stimulated adenylate cyclase activity than the Gly389 variant** *in vitro*. **We investigated whether the Arg389Gly or the Ser49Gly polymorphism is associated with hypertension in Scandinavians.**

INTERPRETATION. Data suggest that individuals homozygous for the Arg389 allele of the β₁-adrenergic receptor gene are at increased risk to develop hypertension.

Comment

The β₁-adrenergic receptor, a seven-transmembrane Gs-protein-coupled receptor, is expressed in cardiac myocytes. On agonist stimulation, it elicits excitatory reactions in the heart, leading to higher cardiac output through increased cardiac inotropy and chronotropy. In addition, β-blocking agents are widely used in the treatment of hypertension, and their antihypertensive effect is mediated by blocking the β₁-adrenergic receptor.

In 1987, the β₁-adrenergic receptor gene was cloned, and it is localized to chromosome 10. Two common polymorphisms, Ser49Gly and Arg389Gly, were identified in 1999. Arg389Gly is located in the intracellular cytoplasmic tail near the seventh transmembrane region of the receptor, which is a putative Gs-protein binding domain. The Arg389 variant mediates a higher isoproterenol-stimulated adenylate cyclase activity than the Gly389 variant *in vitro*. The Ser49Gly polymorphism is located in the extracellular amino-terminal region of the receptor, but no studies have been published on the potential functional consequences of this polymorphism.

Bengtsson *et al.* investigate whether the functionally important Arg389Gly polymorphism or the Ser49Gly polymorphism of the β₁-adrenergic receptor gene was associated with hypertension in a case–control study. They suggest that individuals homozygous for the Arg389 allele of the β₁-adrenergic receptor gene are at increased risk to develop hypertension.

Association between a polymorphism in the G protein beta3 subunit gene (GNB3) with arterial hypertension but not with myocardial infarction.

Hengstenberg C, Schunkert H, Mayer B, *et al. Cardiovasc Res* 2001; **49**(4): 820–7.

BACKGROUND. **A polymorphism at position C825T of the G protein β3 (GNB3) gene was found to be associated with enhanced transmembrane signalling as well as with an** increased prevalence of arterial hypertension. The aim of this study was to investigate further the association of the GNB3 C825T allele status with arterial hypertension in a large population-based sample and its association with specific end organ damage, i.e. myocardial infarction.

INTERPRETATION. In male individuals from a large population-based sample, the T allele of the GNB3 polymorphism was associated with arterial hypertension. However, the effects of the GNB3 825T allele on BP were small and did not translate to a clinically relevant increase of risk for myocardial infarction.

Comment

Heterotrimeric guanosine triphosphate-binding proteins (G proteins) are essential partners of multiple transmembrane receptors for the activation or inhibition of intracellular signalling cascades. Specifically, most vasoactive or growth stimulating factors communicate via G proteins in virtually all cardiovascular tissues. Recently, a polymorphism in GNB3 exchanging cytosine to thymidine (C825T) has been discovered in selected patients with essential hypertension and considered as a candidate mutation for both, arterial hypertension and atherosclerosis. The T allele of the GNB3 polymorphism was related to an RNA splice variant that results in the deletion of nucleotides 498–620 of exon 9 and structural changes in the β-subunit. Moreover, an enhanced signal transduction via pertussis toxin-sensitive G proteins was observed in lymphoblast lines from hypertensive individuals carrying the T allele, which suggests that this genetic variation may indeed affect signal transduction. In recent studies, the association of the T allele of the GNB3 polymorphism with arterial hypertension has been confirmed in smaller cohorts. Based on the originally reported relative risk of arterial hypertension of 1.44 for individuals carrying the TT genotype, none of the previous studies was sufficiently powered to document conclusively a positive association with arterial hypertension.

Hengstenberg *et al.* investigate the association of the GNB3 C825T allele status with arterial hypertension in a large, sufficiently powered population-based sample ($n = 2052$). They found that in male individuals from a large population-based sample, the T allele of the GNB3 polymorphism was associated with arterial hypertension. However, the effects of the GNB3 825T allele on BP were small and did not translate to a clinically relevant increase of risk for myocardial infarction.

Scientific contributions

Interaction of α1-Na,K-ATPase and Na,K,2Cl-cotransporter genes in human essential hypertension.
Glorioso N, Filigheddu N, Troffa C, *et al. Hypertension* 2001; **38**(2): 204–9.

BACKGROUND. Essential hypertension is a common disease the genetic determinants of which have been difficult to unravel because of its clinical heterogeneity and complex, multifactorial, polygenic aetiology. **Based on our observations that α1-Na, K-ATPase (ATP1A1) and renal-specific, bumetanide-sensitive Na,K,2Cl-cotransporter (NKCC2) genes interactively increase susceptibility to hypertension in the Dahl salt-sensitive hypertensive (Dahl S) rat model, we investigated whether parallel molecular genetic mechanisms might exist in human essential hypertension in a relatively genetic homogeneous cohort in northern Sardinia.**

INTERPRETATION. The data are compelling that ATP1A1 and NKCC2 genes are candidate interacting hypertension-susceptibility loci in human essential hypertension and affirm gene interaction as an important genetic mechanism underlying hypertension susceptibility. Although corroboration in other cohorts and identification of functionally significant mutations are imperative next steps, the data provide a genotype-stratification scheme, with fourfold predictive value (odds ratio 4.28; 95% confidence interval 2.29 to –8.0), which could help decipher the complex genetics of essential hypertension.

Comment

Studies on the ATP1A1 and NKCC2 genes as a putative hypertension-susceptibility interacting gene pair based on data suggesting that interaction of ATP1A1 and NKCC2 genes increases susceptibility to salt-sensitive hypertension in Dahl S rats. In this paper by Glorioso *et al.*, they suggest that the ATP1A1/D1S453 and NKCC2 loci interactively increase susceptibility to hypertension in humans in a northern Sardinian population.

Conclusion

In recent years, we have seen enormous advances in the molecular genetic aspect of hypertension research. Pharmacogenomic research based on interindividual differences, i.e. genetic polymorphisms in therapeutic responses and drug metabolisms. Individual patients can be targeted or predicted according to genetic and specific individual 'drug response markers', and thus selection of medications and optimization of dosages, and hence improve safety and efficacy, i.e. personalize prescriptions. The ACE gene has been recognised as a top candidate gene for pharmacogenomic research in hypertension.

Gene therapy takes further steps than pharmacogenomic approach. Culprit gene can be identified and specifically targeted. Gene therapy for hypertension is needed for the next generation of antihypertensive drugs. Indeed, new techniques have been developed to inhibit target gene expression. In particular, targeting of the renin–angiotensin system (RAS) by antisense gene therapy as an effective strategy for the lifelong prevention of hypertension has been the main focus. The basic principle of the antisense approach is that it blocks the formation of targeted proteins rather selectively, either at the transcriptional or translational level. Both gene targeting and transgenic studies in mice have clearly suggested a critical role of the ACE gene in BP regulation. Furthermore, the use of antisense oligonucleotides to angiotensinogen and the angiotensin II receptor type 1 (AT1) subtype in various animal models of hypertension have reported promising results. Although antisense gene therapy target those genes that encode enzymes and peptides of the RAS or other proteins related to sodium handling or vascular function, recent gene therapy strategies either insert genes to overexpress products associated with vasodilation or inhibit genes that are associated with vasoconstriction and growth promotion such as Ca2+ channels, signaling molecules-related genes, or genes relevant to matrix proteins may also be potential sites for hypertension gene therapy.

Finally, effective vector delivering systems have been crucial to the development of effective gene therapy strategies directed at the vasculature and myocardium in animal models. Fundamental research to improve the safety profile and route of gene delivery vectors must continue.

References

1. Giner V, Poch E, Bragulat E, Oriola J, González D, Coca A, de la Sierra A. Renin–angiotensin system genetic polymorphisms and salt sensitivity in essential hypertension. *Hypertension* 2000; **35**: 512–17.

2. Turner ST, Schwarz GL, Chapman AB, Boerwinkle E. C825T polymorphism of the G protein beta(3)-subunit and antihypertensive response to a thiazide diuretic. *Hypertension* 2001 Feb; **37**(2 Part 2): 739–43.

3. Turner ST, Schwartz GL, Chapman AB, Hall WD, Boerwinkle E. Antihypertensive pharmocogenetics: getting the right drug into the right patient. *J Hypertens* 2001 Jan; **19**(1): 1–11. Review.

4. Chao J, Chao L. Kallikrein gene therapy: a new strategy for hypertensive diseases. *Immunopharmacology* 1997; **36**: 229–36.

5

Target organ damage: the cellular and molecular mechanisms

Introduction

Hypertensive heart disease (HHD) is a progressive condition in which the compensatory left ventricular hypertrophy (LVH) that maintains cardiac output leads to myocardial remodelling. At some point in the evolution of this adaptation, the increase in LV mass ceases its positive compensatory function and becomes a potent marker of cardiovascular risk. Structural abnormalities in the myocardial wall accelerate the development of diastolic and systolic dysfunction, resulting in heart failure.

The cause of end-organ dysfunction in hypertensive individuals is multifactorial. Most studies suggest that end-organ damage in hypertension is diffuse and affects organs to different degrees within individual patients. The renin–angiotensin system (RAS), in particular the angiotensin II (Ang II) and the angiotensin-1 receptor have emerged as one of the essential links in the pathophysiology of hypertension and hypertensive target organ damage. Data from basis experimental studies have clearly shown that functionally complete local RAS are operative within organs/tissues in both autocrine and paracrine fashion. Ang II is a potent vasoconstrictor with growth-promoting properties. It is generally accepted that locally formed Ang II could activate the cells regulating the expression of many substances, including growth factors, cytokines, chemokines and adhesion molecules, which are involved in cell growth/apoptosis, fibrosis and inflammation. On the other hand, nitric oxide (NO) is a vasodilator with antigrowth and antithrombogenic effects that plays a part in maintaining vascular integrity and preventing end-organ damage. The pathogenesis of hypertensive end-organ injury is affected by both an NO deficit and an Ang II increase.

In addition, a growing number of reports have provided an important role for oxidative stress in the pathogenesis of hypertension. Ang II stimulates the production of reactive oxygen species by inducing the vascular NADP/NADPH oxidase system. Increased vascular reactive oxygen species production, especially superoxide anion, contributes significantly to endothelial dysfunction and hypertrophy of vascular cells in hypertension, and influence the mechanisms that trigger inflammation in the vessel wall in response to Ang II. Emerging data also suggest a potential role of nuclear factor (NF)-κB as a mediator of Ang II-induced inflammatory process.

Thus, it seems clear that Ang II is more than just a vasoactive hormone. The following articles will show the complexity of the RAS and the multiplicity role of Ang II in pathological processes, and provide some mechanistic responses of the beneficial effects of the treatment with RAS blockers in preventing and slowing down the progression of end-organ damage.

Hypertension and cardiovascular risk factors. Role of the angiotensin II–nitric oxide interaction.
Raij L. *Hypertension* 2001 Feb; **37**(2 Part 2): 767–73.

BACKGROUND. The role of the renin–angiotensin (Ang) II system, particularly of Ang II, holds high interest in the areas of cardiovascular and renal physiology and pathology. Recently, more interests are directed to the Ang II's non-haemodynamic effects rather than its better-known haemodynamic effect as a vasopeptide. The L-arginine–NO pathway, particularly NO as an endothelial-derived relaxing factor, has also been an area of keen interest. The interactions of and balance between Ang II and NO are of key importance in cardiovascular and renal injury and are the focus of this review.

INTERPRETATION. An understanding of the relations between hypertension, cardiovascular risk factors, end-organ damage and the NO–Ang II axis leads one to believe that the combination of therapeutic agents capable of reinstating the homeostatic balance of these vasoactive molecules within the vessel wall would be most effective in preventing or arresting end-organ disease.

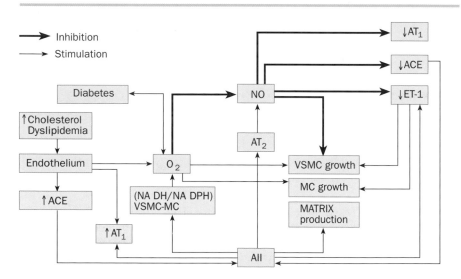

Fig. 5.1 Schematic representation of the pathophysiology of the interaction between Ang II and NO. Source: Raij (2001).

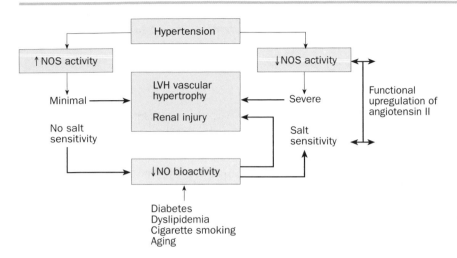

Fig. 5.2 Schematic representation of the relationship between hypertension, end-organ injury, salt sensitivity and the NO–Ang II interaction. Source: Raij (2001).

Comment

This article opened another arena of the role Ang II, in particular, its non-haemo-dynamic effects on the pathogenesis of cardiovascular diseases. This time the emphasis is on the balance between Ang II and NO. Indeed, the presence or the relative bioavailability of either one can make it either injurious or protective of target organs (Fig. 5.2). Although NO–Ang II imbalance may not explain all the vascular patho-physiology of hypertension, it certainly appears to be an important component. The interaction of Ang II and NO in the regulation of vascular tone, in cardiovascular and renal injury, in diabetes and insulin resistance and finally in salt-sensitivity were discussed.

Cardioreparation in hypertensive heart disease.
Weber KT. *Hypertension* 2001 Sep; **38**(3 Part 2): 588–91.

BACKGROUND. The normal myocardium is composed of a variety of cells. Cardiac myocytes, tethered within an extracellular matrix of fibrillar collagen, represent one-third of all cells; non-cardiomyocytes account for the remaining two-thirds. Ventricular hypertrophy involves myocyte growth. Hypertensive heart disease (HHD) includes myocyte and non-myocyte growth that leads to an adverse structural remodelling of the intramural coronary vasculature and matrix.

INTERPRETATION. In HHD, it is not the quantity of myocardium but rather its quality that accounts for increased risk of adverse cardiovascular events. Structural homogeneity of cardiac tissue is governed by a balanced equilibrium existing between stimulator and inhibitor signals that regulate cell growth, apoptosis, phenotype and matrix turnover. Today's management of hypertension should not simply focus on a reduction in blood pressure, it must also target the adverse structural remodelling that begets HHD.

Comment

There is growing evidence from both laboratory and clinical experiments to support the ideation that certain antihypertensive agents such as angiotensin-converting enzyme inhibitors (ACEIs) achieve cardioprotection or renoprotection beyond that that can be predicted from its blood pressure (BP) lowering property. This paper raised some interesting and innovative pathological concepts that may explain the former. The cardiac structural homogeneity is governed by a balanced equilibrium existing between stimulators (e.g. Ang II, aldosterone and endothelins) and inhibitors (e.g. bradykinin, NO and prostaglandins). Accordingly, to reduce the risk of cardiovascular events, its adverse structural remodelling must be targeted for pharmacological intervention that include cardioprotective agents (ACE and endopeptidase inhibitors and respective receptor antagonists) that counteract the imbalance between stimulators and inhibitors. On the other hand, cardioreparative agents reverse the growth-promoting state and regress existing abnormalities in coronary vascular and matrix structure. ACE inhibition has achieved this outcome with favourable impact on vasomotor reactivity and tissue stiffness. Indeed, the cardioreparative concept has undergone experimental and clinical validation.

Hence, it is time to revisit the current management of HHD, to focus on quality, not quantity, of myocardium in HHD. Cardioprotective and cardioreparative interventions specifically target such remodelling with the view toward, respectively,

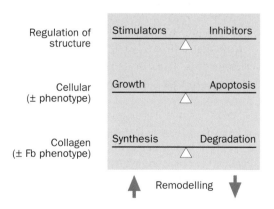

Fig. 5.3 Cardiac remodelling in HHD. Source: Weber (2001).

preventing or regressing cardiac fibrosis in HHD and in so doing favourably influencing adverse risk.

Mechanisms and cardiovascular damage in hypertension.
Luft FC. *Hypertension* 2001; **37**: 594–8.

BACKGROUND. As the growing role of 'oxidative stress' in the pathogenesis of hypertension becomes more appreciated, our impression of hypertension as a rather indolent, solely haemodynamic process is being revised. Reactive oxygen species not only influence both normal and abnormal cellular processes, they can also act as intracellular signalling molecules. Various signal-related kinases include NF-κB are potential targets for reactive oxygen species in endothelial and vascular smooth muscle cells. NF-κB activation has been associated with vascular inflammation and cell survival. Overall, Ang II plays an important part in the regulation of these processes.

INTERPRETATION. Evidence has recently accrued showing that Ang II is important in stimulating the production of reactive oxygen species and the activation of ancient inflammatory mechanisms. The transcription factor NF-κB is pivotal to these processes. NF-κB activation stimulates the expression of a gene menagerie important to chemoattraction, surface adhesion molecule expression, coagulation and inflammation. Anti-inflammatory interventions may have therapeutic utility.

Comment

Ang II has traditionally been considered as a regulatory hormone stimulating vascular smooth muscle cell constriction, aldosterone release from the adrenal gland, and sodium reabsorption in the renal tubule, hence hypertension. Recently, Ang II has been shown to form and act locally as a chemokine, inducing tyrosine phosphorylation, cell growth, hypertrophy and differentiation. The central role of Ang II in the regulation of these complex processes is gradually becoming better appreciated. This paper summarizes these latest developments. The complexity of the various molecular interactions leading to target organ damage was dissected in detail but simplified by schematic diagrams.

With such multiplicity of the role of Ang II, Luft has provided us with some insights into the cellular mechanisms that agents such as ACEIs may exert important vascular protective effects independent of BP reduction, and why 'statins' stabilize atherosclerotic plaques, diminished inflammation and confer cardiovascular event reduction. Thus, from conventional signalling pathways, our attention was directed toward signal transduction involving specific tyrosine kinases, inducing not only vasoconstriction but also proto-oncogene expression, protein synthesis, hypertrophy and growth as well as the inflammatory reactions involving NF-κB activation and related gene expression.

Local haemodynamic changes in hypertension: insights for therapeutic preservation of target organs.

Frohlich ED. *Hypertension* 2001; **38**(6): 1388–94.

BACKGROUND. As a result of antihypertensive therapy, there has been a remarkable decrease in morbidity and mortality from cardiovascular end-points, such as stroke, coronary heart disease and major hypertensive emergencies. In contrast, there has been no relenting in the increasing prevalence of cardiac failure and end-stage renal disease (ESRD) associated with hypertensive cardiovascular disease.

INTERPRETATION. Experiments in spontaneously hypertensive rats demonstrated that the natural history and pathophysiological lesions associated with hypertensive-related cardiac failure and ESRD may be vastly different from the heretofore more pressure-dependent brain and other cardiac end-points reported in earlier years. Older antihypertensive agents (e.g. diuretics, β-adrenergic receptor inhibitors) had minimal anti-ischaemic and antifibrotic effects on heart and kidney and did not exert the cardiac and nephroprotective haemodynamic effects of the newer classes of agents (i.e. ACEIs, Ang II type 1 receptor antagonists, certain calcium antagonists, and perhaps L-arginine), which may reverse these pathophysiological lesions through improving blood flow and flow reserve, their antifibrotic and other actions.

Comment

As suggested by the author, there may be important pathophysiological explanations for the disparate effects on the major target organs of hypertensive disease. Summarizing the recent reports from his laboratory that focused on naturally occurring hypertensive coronary heart disease and ESRD in hypertensive rats with specific pathophysiological alterations, their responses to various hypertensive agents, and ageing, the author managed to link closely the pathophysiological experiment observations with very recent clinical trial and meta-analysis reports in patients with

Table 5.1 Angiotensin II, oxidative stress and atherosclerosis

Pathogenic	Effect mechanism
Vascular smooth muscle growth	Intracellular ROS and p38
Generation of O^2	Increased expression of NADH oxidase and stimulation of mono-oxygenases
Activation of adhesion molecules	NF-κB induction by ROS
Monocyte/macrophage activation	Direct effect on macrophages
Oxidation of LDL	Stimulates 12 lipoxygenase in macrophages
Procoagulant	Stimulates platelet aggregation (decreased NO)
	Stimulates PAI-1

Source: Frohlich (2001).

hypertension, especially those involved with ACEIs, angiotensin receptor blockers and calcium channel blockers.

Conclusion

Target organ damage in hypertension—the focus is on Ang II. Stimulation of the angiotensin-1 receptor by Ang II leads to a cascade of signalling pathways in several cell types, which finally leads to processes such as vasoconstriction, inflammation and proliferation. These processes are of great importance in various cardiovascular diseases, including hypertension, atherosclerosis and ventricular hypertrophy. ACE inhibitors and Ang II receptor blockers block Ang II and recent large-scale, randomized, controlled clinical trials have demonstrated that these agents offer cardiovascular and renal protective benefits independent of their effects on systemic BP. The most recently published Losartan Intervention For Endpoint (LIFE) reduction in hypertension study confirmed the superiority of Ang II receptor blockers against beta-blockers in a large-scale prospective trial (see Chapter 16).

6

Surrogate markers in hypertension

Introduction

Many imaging modalities are now available to monitor the progress of structural vascular abnormalities, most commonly, atherosclerotic plaques. Refinement of these techniques and innovation in the field are progressing fast, although their applications in clinical practice are still debatable in many aspects. The use of imaging methods to quantify the progression and regression of atherosclerosis represents an evolution in our thinking about drug development. Many years ago, high blood pressure (BP), cholesterol, glucose were considered as 'surrogate markers' of cardiovascular disease (CVD), now they are classic risk factors, whereas newer markers/predictors of disease such as carotid intima-media thickness (IMT), endothelial dysfunction, arterial stiffness, pulse pressure and microalbuminuria are considered as 'surrogates', and plasma indices, such as C-reactive protein, homocysteine, fibrinogen, etc. are considered as 'predictors' of future cardiovascular events. It seems that left ventricular hypertrophy (LVH), previously considered as a 'surrogate', has been regarded as a significant risk factor in the Framingham risk equation, WHO/ISH guideline and other risk scoring algorithms.

Details have been discussed in Chapter 2 (Endothelial function in hypertension), and Chapter 3 (Pulse pressure and arterial stiffness). We shall see below the expansion of our current direction in search of a better surrogate marker that is noninvasive, reproducible, easy to perform as well as more powerful in its 'indicative value' for underlying disease or its 'predictive value' for future cardiovascular events. Many methods have been developed to 'visualize' structural disease as well as to measure its functional impairment at the same time. Alongside we begin to explore the inter-relationships between endothelial dysfunction, atherogenesis, central and peripheral arterial stiffness and hypertrophy and, finally, vascular haemodynamic—pulse pressure and systolic pressure load. Accordingly, methods for measuring arterial stiffness have now been explored to relate that of measuring endothelial function—a surrogate for another surrogate? How far are we heading to in search of a better disease 'marker' or 'predictor'?

A surrogate for another surrogate? ... Where and how far are we heading to?

Relation between brachial artery reactivity and non-invasive large and small arterial compliance in healthy volunteers.

Parvathaneni L, Harp J, Zelinger A, Silver MA. *Am J Cardiol* 2002; **89**(7): 894–5.

BACKGROUND. Brachial artery reactivity or flow-mediated vasodilation is an established non-invasive method believed to reflect endothelial function using high-resolution ultrasonography; however, this method is time-consuming, subject to measurement error, and requires technical expertise. New methods of measuring vascular compliance are non-invasive, easy to perform, and may also reflect aspects of vascular function, which may parallel or represent endothelial function.

INTERPRETATION. Non-invasive computer-based analysis of large and small artery compliance using the CardioVascular Profiling Instrument (CVPI) may provide useful single and serial determinations of vascular compliance that parallel those measured with ultrasonographic flow-mediated brachial artery dilation, and may similarly serve as a surrogate of endothelial function in a wide variety of clinical situations.

Comment

Arterial stiffness is an important, independent determinant of cardiovascular risk. New methods of measuring vascular compliance are non-invasive, easy to perform, and may provide assessment of endothelial function at the same time. The aim of this study was to evaluate the relation between computer-based measurement of arterial compliance and brachial artery reactivity to determine if it paralleled information obtained by flow-mediated brachial artery dilation, and therefore, might potentially be used as a surrogate measure of endothelial function.

The authors studied 26 healthy volunteers (16 men, aged 25–51 years) who are free of CVD or risk factors. Percentage change of flow-mediated dilatation (FMD) was obtained in a standard fashion at the brachial artery. Method for measurement of arterial compliance was based on analysis of the radial arterial pressure pulse waveforms using the CVPI following modified Windkessel model allowing determination of proximal 'capacitative' compliance (large artery elasticity compliance) and distal 'oscillatory' compliance (small artery elasticity compliance) as well as an inductance and a resistance (systemic vascular resistance) during the diastolic portion of the cardiac cycle. The results showed a significant linear regression relation between per cent change in FMD at 60 s and both large (multiple $R = 0.53$, $P = 0.006$) and small (multiple $R = 0.39$, $P = 0.05$) artery compliance.

Indeed, early identification of abnormal vascular compliance may provide better assessment of cardiovascular risk and therefore the opportunity to reduce individuals' overall risk and delay or reverse the disease process, which emphasizes the need for developing a simple method to measure it with broader applications. But, the physiology and pathophysiology of vascular compliance and endothelial function may be fundamentally different, but they may also be related due to the effect of 'subclinical' atherosclerosis, i.e. early vascular disease, which is a prime target for primary prevention.

Although structural changes in arteries are thought to be a major factor in the age-related increase in arterial stiffness, several lines of evidence suggest that the endothelium may play an important part in the local functional regulation of stiffness by releasing vasoactive substances, such as nitric oxide (NO) (see Wilkinson IB, Qasem A *et al.* below)

Of note, as already pointed out above, changes in FMD may not be solely due to altered endothelial function, but may also be due to underlying structural vascular changes and thus reduced vasodilatory capacity, or vice versa.

Clinical evaluation of a non-invasive, widely applicable method for assessing endothelial function. Pulse wave analysis.

Wilkinson IB, Hall IR, MacCallum H, *et al. Arterioscler Thromb Vasc Biol* 2002; **22**: 147–52.

BACKGROUND. Current methods for assessing vasomotor endothelial function are impractical for use in large studies. We tested the hypothesis that pulse-wave analysis (PWA) combined with provocative pharmacological testing might provide an alternative method. Radial artery waveforms were recorded and augmentation index (AIx) was calculated from derived aortic waveforms.

INTERPRETATION. This methodology provides a simple, repeatable, non-invasive means of assessing endothelial function *in vivo*.

Comment

In a further search for a better method that is simple, reproducible, non-invasive and allows broader applications in assessing endothelial function, the authors proposed that PWA combined with provocative pharmacological testing might provide such an attractive method.

Radial artery waveforms were recorded with a high-fidelity micromanometer from the wrist of the dominant arm. PWA was then used to generate a corresponding central (aortic) waveform and AIx and heart rate were determined by using the integral software. These were compared with the forearm venous occlusion plethysmography commonly used for brachial endothelial function assessment. They divided their study into four parts: test for repeatability of the technique in 13 healthy subjects, then the effects of inhibition of NO Synthase by NG-monomethyl-L-arginine (L-NMMA) infusion in another 12 healthy subjects, and in a similar fashion in 27 hypercholesterolaemic subjects (compared with 27 matched normo-cholesterolaemics), and finally 27 subjects with a range of serum cholesterol values but no other cardiovascular risk factors were tested using forearm venous occlusion plethysmography.

The results showed that albuterol (a β2 agonist) and nitroglycerin produce qualitatively and quantitatively similar and repeatable effects on AIx, that the effect of albuterol but not of nitroglycerin is inhibited by L-NMMA and reduced in hyper-cholesterolaemic subjects, and that the response to albuterol is correlated with the effect of acetylcholine (ACh) in the forearm vascular bed. These data indicate that the effect of albuterol is, in part, NO and endothelium dependent and are consistent with the presence of endothelial dysfunction in hypercholesterolaemic subjects. Moreover, they suggest that PWA and administration of albuterol and nitroglycerin provide a simple, reliable, non-invasive method for assessing endothelial function, as the authors and others have previously hypothesized.

The authors believe that PWA may provide a more suitable means of assessing endothelial function in large numbers of patients, thus answering the important question of the predictive value of endothelial function testing. PWA has already been included in the substudies of Anglo-Scandinavian Cardiac Outcomes Trial (ASCOT), Study of the Effectiveness of Additional Reductions in Cholesterol and Homocysteine (SEARCH), the Edinburgh Artery Study, and Fenofibrate Intervention and Event Lowering in Diabetes (FIELD) trial. These will address the importance of basal arterial distensibility as a predictor of risk. Hence, it is attractive to include the non-invasive assessment of both endothelial function and arterial stiffness in future large intervention studies.

Pulse wave analysis for 'global' endothelial function assessment?

Assessment of endothelial function using peripheral waveform analysis. A clinical application.
Hayward CS, Kraidly M, Webb CM, Collins P. *J Am Coll Cardiol* 2002; **40**(3): 521–8.

BACKGROUND. It is known that β2-receptor stimulation results in endothelial release of NO. Furthermore, for over a century glyceryl trinitrate (GTN) has been known to affect markedly the arterial pressure waveform, even in the absence of significant BP changes. Therefore, it was hypothesized that the change in the peripheral pressure waveform, as measured using tonometry and quantified using the AIx and in response to salbutamol, would allow assessment of global endothelial function.

INTERPRETATION. The peripheral arterial pressure waveform is sensitive to β2 stimulation. Changes are related to NO release, are reproducible and can distinguish between clinical subject groups. Arterial waveform changes following salbutamol may thus provide a non-invasive method of measuring 'global' arterial endothelial function.

Comment

To investigate whether radial artery applanation tonometry could be used as a non-invasive method of assessing global endothelial function, Hayward *et al.* divided their study into three pilot parts. In the first study (protocol validation), salbutamol (400 µg) was administered to 11 healthy subjects via inhalation after either intra-venous L-NMMA (3 mg/kg over 5 min) or control solution (normal saline) in the supine, rested, fasted condition. The BP, heart rate and waveform responses were recorded each 5 min following salbutamol for 20 min. Next, GTN was given and responses recorded 5 min later. In the second study (reproducibility assessment), both the reproducibility of salbutamol and the GTN responses were assessed in nine subjects studied twice on separate days. In the third study (clinical validation), the salbutamol and GTN responses of 12 subjects with angiographic coronary artery disease (CAD) were compared with 10 age-matched control subjects with no athero-sclerotic risk factors.

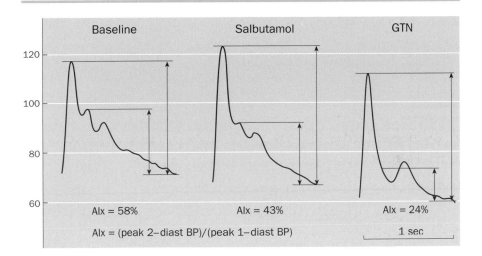

Fig. 6.1 An example of the effect of salbutamol and GTN on the radial waveform in a single individual. It can be seen that the second systolic peak, obvious at baseline, is diminished by salbutamol and almost completely abolished following GTN. The changes in the wave-shape are quantified using the AIx, calculated as the ratio of the pulse pressure at the second systolic peak to that at the first systolic peak. Source: Hayward *et al.* (2002).

After control infusion, AIx decreased following salbutamol, from $50.8 \pm 4.3\%$ to $44.8 \pm 4.2\%$, a change of $-11.8 \pm 3.7\%$, $P < 0.01$. After L-NMMA, AIx did not significantly change following salbutamol ($54.2 \pm 5.1\%$ vs $52.9 \pm 5.3\%$, $-2.0 \pm 3.1\%$). The GTN-induced decreases in AIx were similar after either infusion ($35.1 \pm 3.3\%$ vs $36.5 \pm 3.3\%$). Reproducibility of salbutamol-induced changes in AIx between studies performed on separate days was good ($r = 0.80$, $P < 0.01$). Salbutamol-induced changes in AIx in CAD patients were significantly less compared with control subjects ($-2.4 \pm 1.9\%$ vs. $-13.2 \pm 2.4\%$, respectively, $P < 0.002$). The GTN-induced changes were not significantly different (-27.6 ± 4.2 vs $-38.9 \pm 4.4\%$, $P = 0.07$).

This study shows that the peripheral arterial pressure waveform is sensitive to low-dose inhaled β2 stimulation. The changes induced are related to NO release, are reproducible over the short term, and can distinguish between clinical subject groups. As such, the analysis of salbutamol-induced changes in the peripheral arterial pressure waveform may provide a non-invasive method of assessing 'global' arterial endothelial function. The potential benefits of this technique are that it is non-invasive, readily portable and is quickly learned. It thus provides a method for assessing endothelial function that may be suitable for large-scale population studies. A further benefit of this technique is that the use of salbutamol to induce endothelial NO release will allow a global assessment of endothelial function rather than assessment of a single vascular bed (usually the brachial arterial tree). This has not previously been available; therefore, it represents a potential significant improvement on current techniques. As pointed out, further studies are needed to document effects in larger patient groups, the elderly, subjects with hypercholesterolaemia, diabetes, hypertension, smoking, etc., and to examine the effect of therapies.

Endothelial dysfunction, arterial stiffness, vascular hypertrophy, atherosclerosis and cardiovascular risk: Where are the inter-relationships? ... Nitric oxide?

Nitric oxide regulates local arterial distensibility *in vivo*.
Wilkinson IB, Qasem A, McEniery CM, Webb DJ, Avolio AP, Cockcroft JR.
Circulation 2002; **105**: 213–17.

BACKGROUND. Arterial stiffness is an important determinant of cardiovascular risk. Several lines of evidence support a role for the endothelium in regulating arterial stiffness by release of vasoactive mediators. The objective of this study was to test the hypothesis that NO acting locally regulates arterial stiffness *in vivo*, and the aim of this experiment was to test this hypothesis in an ovine hind-limb preparation.

INTERPRETATION. These results demonstrate, for the first time, that basal NO production influences large-artery distensibility. In addition, exogenous ACh and GTN both increase arterial distensibility, the former mainly through NO production. This may help explain why conditions that exhibit endothelial dysfunction are also associated with increased arterial stiffness. Therefore, reversal of endothelial dysfunction or drugs that are large artery vasorelaxants may be effective in reducing large-artery stiffness in humans, and thus cardiovascular risk.

Comment

In this study, Wilkinson *et al.* investigated the importance of basal and stimulated NO production in regulating muscular artery distensibility. They have shown that local arterial distensibility is reduced by blockade of endogenous NO synthesis with the NO synthase inhibitor L-NMMA in the ovine common iliac artery. Indeed, they have also extended previous observations by demonstrating that the increase in arterial distensibility produced by an endothelium-dependent but not endothelium-independent agonist can be substantially inhibited by L-NMMA.

They conducted their studies in anaesthetized sheep. Pulse wave velocity (PWV) was calculated by the foot-to-foot methodology from two pressure waveforms recorded simultaneously with a high-fidelity dual pressure-sensing catheter placed in the common iliac artery. According to the authors, the use of an intravascular catheter to measure PWV, a robust measure of distensibility, and eliminates inaccuracies in determining the path length and provides a high degree of resolution to detect small but significant differences in transit time. Their results showed that intra-arterial infusion of L-NMMA increased iliac PWV significantly, by 3 ± 2% ($P < 0.01$). Infusion of ACh and GTN reduced PWV significantly, by 6 ± 4% ($P = 0.03$) and 5 ± 2% ($P < 0.01$), respectively. Only the effect of ACh, however, was significantly inhibited during coinfusion of L-NMMA ($P = 0.03$). There was no change in systemic arterial pressure throughout the studies. Importantly, infusion of

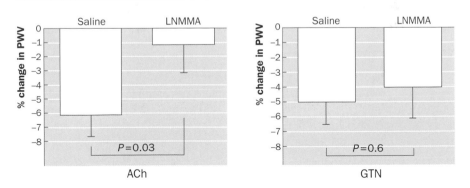

Fig. 6.2 Effect of ACh and GTN on iliac PWV during co-infusion of saline or L-NMMA. Values are mean ± SEM. Source: Wilkinson *et al.* (2002).

L-NMMA or ACh distal to the common iliac artery (via the sheath) did not affect PWV.

Admittedly, this study was conducted in the ovine iliac artery; therefore, the applicability of the results to human muscular arteries requires confirmation. However, the ovine and human systemic responses to L-NMMA are similar. They also pointed out that they are unable to identify the precise mechanism responsible for changes in distensibility brought about by modulation of the L-arginine–NO pathway in the present study.

The demonstrations that basal NO production influences muscular artery distensibility *in vivo* and that the effect of ACh on large arteries is mainly NO dependent are novel. Such findings support the concept of local functional regulation of large-artery stiffness. Accordingly, drug therapies that improve NO bioavailability or act directly to relax large-artery smooth muscle may prove to be efficient strategies for reducing arterial stiffness and cardiovascular risk in patients at high risk, such as those with diabetes mellitus and isolated systolic hypertension.

Endothelium-derived nitric oxide regulates arterial elasticity in human arteries *in vivo*.

Kinlay S, Creager MA, Fukumoto M, *et al. Hypertension* 2001; **38**: 1049–53.

B A C K G R O U N D . Arterial elasticity is determined by structural characteristics of the artery wall and by vascular smooth muscle tone. The identity of endogenous vasoactive substances that regulate elasticity has not been defined in humans. We hypothesized that NO, a vasodilator released constitutively by the endothelium, augments arterial elasticity.

I N T E R P R E T A T I O N . Loss of constitutively released NO associated with cardiovascular risk factors may adversely affect arterial elasticity in humans.

Comment

This study is comparable with the above study by Wilkinson *et al.* The idea is the same, but in a different vascular bed, this time—human brachial artery. The hypothesis tested was similar—whether endogenous endothelium-derived NO plays a significant physiological role in regulating arterial elasticity/stiffness.

Seven healthy young men were investigated in this rigorous study set-up. Indices of elasticity (pressure–area relationship, instantaneous compliance, and stress–strain, pressure–incremental elastic modulus (Einc), and pressure–PVW relationships) and artery cross-sectional area, wall thickness, and intra-arterial pressure were measured by using an intravascular ultrasound (IVUS) catheter inserted into the brachial artery and was examined over a range of distending pressures (0–100 mmHg transmural pressure) obtained by inflation of an external cuff. Thereafter, the basal production of endothelium-derived NO was inhibited by L-NMMA (4 and 8 mg/min). Finally, nitroglycerin (2.5 and 12.5 µg/min), an exogenous donor of NO, was given to relax the vascular smooth muscle. Elasticity was measured under all of these conditions.

The results showed that L-NMMA (8 mg/min) decreased brachial artery area ($P = 0.016$) and compliance ($P <0.0001$) and increased Einc ($P <0.01$) and PWV ($P <0.0001$). Nitroglycerin (12.5 µg/min) increased brachial artery area ($P <0.001$) and compliance ($P <0.001$) and decreased PWV ($P = 0.02$). NO, an endothelium-derived vasodilator, augments arterial elasticity in the human brachial artery.

Indeed, the novel finding of this study is that the constitutive release of NO contributes to arterial elasticity in healthy humans. The findings have important implications. As pointed out, risk factor modification may take years to alter arterial structure favourably, but loss of constitutive NO can be corrected more rapidly, and therefore, by inference, restore functional impairment to 'normality'. Importantly, future studies need to define the contribution of NO to elasticity in other arterial 'beds', including the aorta, and in patients at high cardiovascular risk. That these are more 'pathophysiologically' relevant, would put the concerns to 'bed' |**1**|.

Vasodilatory capacity and vascular structure in long-standing hypertension: a LIFE substudy.
Olsen MH, Wachtell K, Aalkjaer C, Dige-Petersen H, Rokkedal J, Ibsen H.
Am J Hypertens 2002; **15**(5): 398–404.

BACKGROUND. FMD, which is considered a measure of endothelial function, has been found impaired in hypertension. However, it is unclear whether this impairment is explained solely by endothelial dysfunction, or whether it is associated with structural vascular changes and reduced vasodilatory capacity.

INTERPRETATION. Low FMD as well as low nitroglycerin-induced dilatation (NID) were related in parallel to high systolic BP (SBP) and to the severity of vascular changes in different vascular beds, suggesting that elevated BP load in hypertension induces parallel abnormalities in conduit artery structure and overall vasodilatory capacity. Therefore, the decrease in FMD observed in severe hypertension may be caused by endothelial dysfunction as well as by structural vascular changes, suggesting difficulties in interpreting FMD solely as a measure of endothelial dysfunction in hypertensive patients with LVH.

Comment

It is believed that impaired FMD is due to endothelial dysfunction, as it has been shown to be dependent on endothelial release of NO in healthy subjects. Indeed, endothelial dysfunction has been related to high carotid IMT and to LVH in never-treated hypertensive patients, and has been suggested to promote vascular hypertrophy. The authors hypothesized that reduced FMD in hypertension may also be due to vascular hypertrophy with reduced vasodilatory capacity as well as endothelial dysfunction.

They studied 42 unmedicated patients (34 men, aged 56–76 years) recruited from the Insulin Carotids US Scandinavia (ICARUS) substudy of the Losartan Intervention

For Endpoint-Reduction in Hypertension (LIFE) trial, all with essential hypertension and ECG LVH. All participants had 24-hour ambulatory BP, minimal forearm vascular resistance (MFVR) by plethysmography, intima-media cross-sectional area of the common carotid arteries (IMA), FMD and NID in the brachial artery by ultrasound. They found that FMD was correlated positively with NID ($r = 0.38$, $P < 0.05$). However, FMD as well as NID correlated negatively to 24-hour SBP ($r = -0.41$, $P = 0.01$ and $R = -0.52$, $P = 0.001$), IMA/height ($r = -0.41$, $P < 0.01$ and $R = -0.53$, $P < 0.001$) and $MFVR_{men}$ ($r = -0.44$, $P < 0.05$ and $R = -0.42$, $P < 0.05$).

As would be expected, a high BP load promotes atherosclerosis and vascular hypertrophy. The former may be represented by impaired endothelial function (reduced % FMD), and the latter by increased IMA of the carotid artery. Accordingly, as in this study, hypertensive patients with higher SBP had higher carotid artery IMT and IMA/height, that is, elevated BP load in long-standing hypertension induces vascular hypertrophy. Interestingly, these patients had not only reduced dilatation of the brachial artery in response to increased blood flow but also in response to nitroglycerin infusion. The latter observation was in fact previously reported by Strauer *et al.* |2,3| that reduced endothelium-independent vasodilatation in forearm resistance arteries was related to high BP in previously treated hypertension.

As pointed by the authors, FMD is dependent upon the magnitude of the vasodilatory stimuli as well as the vasodilatory capacity through the NO-cyclic guanosine monophosphate (cGMP) pathway of the brachial artery. Therefore, as the relationships of low FMD to vascular hypertrophy as well as to high SBP were not independent of the flow velocity integral reserve or NID, the study can conclude only that hypertensive patients with high SBP or vascular hypertrophy have reduced FMD, but not to what extent this is due to endothelial dysfunction in the brachial artery.

In this study, low FMD and low NID were related to high SBP as well as to the degree of vascular hypertrophy in different vascular beds. Elevated BP load in long-standing hypertension induces abnormalities in vascular structure and reduces the overall vasodilatory capacity through the NO-cGMP pathway as well as endothelial dysfunction. The data suggest difficulties in interpreting FMD solely as a measure of endothelial dysfunction in patients with long-standing hypertension and ECG LVH.

The study by Lopez-Farre *et al.* (2002, see below) highlights the possibility that processes underlying impaired vasodilation in hypertension extend beyond the endothelium and that altered vascular smooth muscle behaviour may be of importance. While the exact mechanisms remain elusive, the suggestion that α_1-adrenergic receptors might play a part is significant, especially as alpha-1-receptor blockers are effective antihypertensive agents.

Reduction of the soluble cyclic GMP vasorelaxing system in the vascular wall of the stroke-prone spontaneously hypertensive rats. Effects of the alpha-receptor blocker doxazosin.

Lopez-Farre A, Rodriguez-Feo JA, Garcia-Colis E, *et al. J Hypertens* 2002; **20**: 463–70.

BACKGROUND. The aim of this study was to analyse the NO/cGMP relaxing system in spontaneously hypertensive rats of the stroke-prone substrain (SHRSP)

INTERPRETATION. Independently of the endothelial NO-generating system, impaired vasorelaxation could also result from vascular smooth muscle cell layer dysfunction. Doxazosin treatment improved the endothelial-independent relaxation and preserved the cGMP generating system in the vascular wall of SHRSP rats.

Comment

Impaired vascular relaxation, a characteristic feature in CVD, including hypertension in rats and humans, is associated with impaired endothelium-dependent vasodilation (endothelial dysfunction) due, in large part, to reduced NO signalling, through the NO/cGMP pathway. This has been attributed mainly to increased oxygen free radical activity and a reduced activity of endothelial nitric oxide synthase (eNOS) due to an insufficient presence of cofactors of eNOS (i.e. tetrahydrobiopterin). However, recent studies in experimental animals have challenged this concept. Growing evidence indicates that endothelium-independent, NO/cGMP-mediated processes also play a part in the modulation of vascular tone and that abnormalities in these events contribute to aberrations in vasorelaxation in hypertension.

To test this hypothesis and the possible underlying mediator, they divided their experiment into two parts: (i) to analyse in spontaneously hypertensive SHRSP rats the endothelium-dependent (to ACh) and independent vasorelaxing (sodium nitroprusside-induced) responses, analysing the level of expression of both soluble guanylate cyclase (sGC) and eNOS in the vascular wall, and (ii) as these rats have increased plasma catecholamine levels and increased sympathetic tone, the authors questioned the putative regulatory role of α_1-adrenergic receptors on the NO/cGMP relaxing system using the α_1-receptor blocker doxazosin.

The first part of the experiment basically confirmed the existence of an impaired endothelium-dependent and endothelium-independent vasodilatory response in SHRSP rats that endothelium-dependent relaxation, as well as sodium nitroprusside-induced dilation, were blunted in SHRSP. This was accompanied by reduced expression of soluble guanylate cyclase (β1 subunit) in the aortic wall and decreased generation of vascular cGMP. These data suggest that, independent of the endothelial NO-generating system, reduced vasorelaxation in hypertension could also result from abnormal vascular smooth muscle function.

The novel results came from the second experiment, which demonstrated that doxazosin, preserved endothelium-independent vasorelaxation. This suggests that α_1-adrenergic receptors play an important part in processes underlying endo-thelium-independent NO/cGMP-mediated relaxation in SHRSP aorta. However, the precise mechanisms remain unknown. This phenomenon certainly warrants further consideration.

Thus, it appears from these experiments that endothelial dysfunction may result from an impaired vascular smooth muscle cell functionality that is independent of the NO-generating system. Doxazosin treatment improved endothelium-independent relaxation and preserved the cGMP generating system in the vascular wall of SHRSP rats, suggesting α1-receptor may play a part in mediating this effect.

Despite these data from experimental hypertensive animals implicating endo-thelium-independent processes in impaired vasodilation, there is little convincing data to support these findings in human hypertension. In fact, clinical studies demonstrate, for the most part, that vasodilatory responses to ACh, but not to sodium nitroprusside, are attenuated in human hypertension. However, it is difficult to reconcile that human hypertension is invariably characterized by impaired endothelial-mediated vasorelaxation. Indeed, it may be possible that factors other than the endothelium, such as vascular smooth muscle, could be important in altered vascular tone, as suggested in the present study.

Carotid plaques, but not common carotid intima-media thickness, are independently associated with aortic stiffness.

Zureik M, Temmar M, Adamopoulos C, et al. J Hypertens 2002; **20**: 85–93.

BACKGROUND. It has been suggested that non-invasive aortic stiffness measurements can be used as an indicator of atherosclerosis. The relationships of arterial stiffness with arterial wall hypertrophy and atherosclerosis, however, have rarely been investigated in large-scale studies. This study reports the associations of carotid arterial structure assessed by B-mode ultrasound with carotid-femoral PWV in hypertensive and non-hypertensive subjects.

INTERPRETATION. This study shows that there is a differential association of PWV with CCA-IMT and carotid plaques (CCA stands for common carotid arteries). The nature of the independent positive association between atherosclerosis and arterial stiffness should be thoroughly investigated.

Comment

Vascular structure and function are closely linked, and functional impairment usually precedes visible structural abnormalities. Endothelial dysfunction is an early marker of atherosclerosis formation. Endothelial dysfunction can be detected in patients with cardiovascular risk factors such as smoking, hypercholesterolaemia, diabetes, etc. Endothelial dysfunction is related to atherosclerotic processes at the endothelial intima, whereas arterial stiffness appears to be more related to medial degeneration and/or vascular hypertrophy associated with ageing, a process of which may be accelerated by hypertension or diabetes and in patients with end-stage renal disease. Indeed, arterial stiffness is emerging as the most important determinant of increased systolic and pulse pressure in our ageing community, and both systolic and pulse pressure have been shown to be independent predictors of mortality.

Indeed, prospective studies have demonstrated that coronary and forearm circulation endothelial dysfunction are independent predictors of future cardiovascular events, highlighting the prognostic importance of identifying abnormalities in vascular function in individual patients. Similarly, Boutouyrie et al. |3a| has reported the first direct evidence in a longitudinal study that aortic stiffness measured through PWV is an independent predictor of primary coronary events in patients with essential hypertension. Thus, it appears that both arterial stiffness and endothelial dysfunction are not only predictors for future CHD events but also markers of significant underlying vascular disease. Although endothelial dysfunction and arterial stiffness may be different in terms of pathophysiology, they may be closely related to one another by a yet unknown mechanism. Hence, few investigators have investigated the relationship between endothelial dysfunction and peripheral arterial stiffness, and postulated possible links. It is not clear whether their possible inter-relationships are entirely due to their associations with common factors, particularly age and hypertension, or whether atherosclerosis process may be involved in arterial stiffening or vice versa.

In this cross-sectional study, Zureik et al. examined the relationship between carotid structure (IMT, lumen diameter and plaques) assessed by B-mode ultrasound and aortic stiffness assessed by carotid–femoral PWV (Complior) in 564 subjects (age 58 ± 11 years, 32% of women, 53% of all were hypertensive) attended free health examinations. They found that the mean sex-adjusted values of PWV were significantly higher in subjects with carotid plaques than those without carotid plaques (12.7 ± 0.2 vs 11.1 ± 0.1 m/s, $P <0.001$). The difference remains significant after adjustment for age, mean BP and pulse pressure, and other conventional cardiovascular risk factors ($P <0.009$). These associations were observed in many subgroups according to gender, hypertensive status and antihypertensive treatment status, although the relationship of carotid plaque with arterial stiffness was more pronounced in men than in women. Interestingly, increased carotid lumen diameter also independently associated with PWV. On the other hand, the associations between aortic arterial stiffness and CCA-IMT were wholly explained by age and elevated BP and pulse pressure. Thus, there was a differential association of PWV with CCA-IMT and carotid atherosclerotic plaques.

Their findings corroborate the recent results of the Rotterdam Study |4|, showing that arterial stiffness was strongly related to abdominal aortic and carotid atherosclerotic plaques. In subjects with end-stage renal disease, carotid and aortic stiffness were also related to the presence and the extent of arterial calcified plaques in three arterial sites (carotid, aorta, femoral) in another study |5|. The authors explained that atherosclerotic changes in the arterial wall could include smooth muscle cell proliferation, deposition of lipid and accumulation of collagen, elastin and proteoglycans, and changes in the ratio of collagen to elastin have been known to structurally affect the elastic behaviour of the arterial wall. Thus, in addition to the primary role of ageing and hypertension, some atherogenic stimuli may be involved in arterial stiffening. However, the mechanisms and precise role of arterial stiffness in the promotion of atherosclerosis are largely unknown. Admittedly, their results were obtained from an observational population-based study. The inter-relationships between the arterial structure and function should be complementarily investigated by the use of other research techniques and methods, which are currently beyond reach of epidemiological investigations.

The list of independent predictors of cardiovascular events is increasing. Future prospective studies are needed to determine which of the following is the best predictor of cardiovascular events: SBP, pulse pressure (brachial or central), carotid-femoral PWV (aortic stiffness), endothelial dysfunction, CCA-IMT, carotid plaques, and so on. What complicates the analysis further is the fact that these surrogate markers appear to be highly correlated to each other.

Non-invasive surrogate markers of atherosclerosis.
Feinstein SB, Voci P, Pizzuto F. *Am J Cardiol* 2002; **89**(5A): 31–43C.

BACKGROUND. Non-invasive imaging techniques offer a unique opportunity to study the relation of surrogate markers to the development of atherosclerosis. These non-invasive imaging modalities include: (i) carotid artery, coronary, and aorta imaging; (ii) LV echocardiography imaging; (iii) electron-beam computed tomography; (iv) magnetic resonance imaging (MRI); and (v) ankle–brachial index. Because the incidence of CAD is a function of the development and progression of atherosclerosis, the use of non-invasive surrogate markers of atherosclerosis can aid in the diagnosis of CVD through the identification of subclinical disease.

INTERPRETATION. In enabling the measurement of subclinical disease, non-invasive surrogate markers of atherosclerosis provide an approach for identifying high-risk individuals who may benefit from active intervention to prevent clinical disease. Non-invasive imaging techniques hold promise for expanding the diagnostic armaments available to bring new insight into the pathophysiology and treatment of CAD.

Comment

Drug prevention of cardiovascular events is effective but costly, leading to a debate about who should receive this treatment. Patient selection is often based on surrogate markers, such as prior cardiovascular events, number of risk factors and lipid levels, but quantification of atherosclerosis severity is desirable. Aggressive risk factor reduction, formerly used exclusively in secondary prevention, may be pivotal to optimal patient management in high-risk primary prevention. A number of non-invasive imaging modalities have the potential to measure and to monitor atherosclerosis in asymptomatic individuals and include exercise ECG testing, electron beam computed tomography, high-resolution magnetic resonance coronary angiography, positron emission tomography, ankle–brachial index, and B-mode ultrasound for measuring carotid IMT. In addition, transthoracic coronary Doppler echocardiography as already discussed has also showed promising results. The use of these non-invasive methods to measure subclinical atherosclerosis and its progression or regression offers a unique opportunity to improve preventive strategies as well as to study and to bring new insight into the pathophysiology and development of new treatment for CAD. This article summarizes the clinical applications of all the above.

A discussion of modalities for assessing regression and progression in vascular disease.

Black DM. *Am J Cardiol* 2002; **89**(4A): 40–1B.

B A C K G R O U N D . Many groups are currently seeking to validate new techniques on invasive and non-invasive measurement of structural vascular disease. Several of these new methods continue to improve yearly and alter our perception of the atherosclerotic process. The question is, do these methods quantify the same or different aspects of the atherosclerotic process? And if they characterize different aspects, which are most promising for the study of vascular disease progression and regression, and are most likely to correlate with clinical events and thus to be developed to enhance earlier diagnosis and treatment?

I N T E R P R E T A T I O N . Large trials are needed that can link changes in vascular disease as measured by EBCT (electron beam computerised tomography), IVUS, MRI, endothelial function, transoesophageal echocardiography, and so on, to clinical end-points, or at least to accepted vascular measurements, such as quantitative coronary angiography (QCA) and IMT. Several ongoing studies sponsored by the US government and the pharmaceutical industry should help us understand these effects in the future.

Comment

In search of many other better 'markers/predictors' of CVD, besides measuring various plasma markers, we are heading towards visualizing structural damage and measuring functional impairment of both macrovasculatures and microvasculatures. Unlike plasma markers, assessing the vessel directly brings us closer to the insult. Indeed, as advocated by the author, these new 'toys' are also a very powerful tool for drug development.

New methods of quantifying vascular structure, including quantification of atherosclerosis by IVUS of the coronary arteries, MRI of the coronary and carotid arteries, and quantification of coronary calcification, provide different estimates of vascular structure. Computed tomography has gained wide popularity for quantifying coronary calcium, but it has not yet been accepted as a measurement technique for

quantifying progression and regression of atherosclerosis. The assessment of endothelial function is non-invasive and reproducible. Positron emission tomography
may provide a non-invasive technique that is more robust than brachial plethysmography. Measuring vascular function is an easy and, in the right hands, a very
sensitive (perhaps too sensitive) and specific modality. Newer computerized devices
and software are being develop to facilitate assessment and may even allow more
widespread application in population studies, and alongside with the development of
these new techniques is our evolving understanding of the pathogenesis of vascular
disease.

The static measures of vascular structure (QCA, IVUS, MRI quantification of
atherosclerosis, coronary calcification and B-mode ultrasound) all have strengths
related to their robust association with a history of risk factor exposure but weak-
nesses in that they reflect long-term exposure and do not capture change over
months or years before the non-invasive evaluation. These changes might modify
risk of events but not acutely change the volume of atherosclerosis. On the other
hand, measures of vascular function (vascular reactivity) are highly sensitive indices
of current risk but may be so non-specific as to preclude quantification of future risk.
Small changes in the environment may make large changes in vascular function.

Most importantly, large trials are needed that can link changes in vascular disease
as measured by EBCT, IVUS, MRI, endothelial function, transoesophageal echocardiography, and so on, to clinical end-points, or at least to accepted vascular
measurements, such as QCA and IMT. Let's illustrate some of these points with one
of most recent trial below, European Lacidipine Study on Atherosclerosis (ELSA).

Intima-media thickness. A tool for atherosclerosis imaging and event prediction.
O'Leary DH, Polak JF. *Am J Cardiol* 2002; **90**(10C): 18–21L.

B ACKGROUND . Multiple studies have shown that the carotid artery IMT, as measured
non-invasively by ultrasonography, is directly associated with an increased risk of CVD.
Because it has been shown to be an independent predictor of CVD after adjustment for
traditional risk factors, it is the only non-invasive imaging test currently recommended
by the American Heart Association (AHA) for inclusion in the evaluation of risk.
However, it remains unclear how much additional information beyond that afforded by
traditional risk factors is gained by inclusion of IMT in risk profiles. Change in IMT is
increasingly being used as the end-point in interventional trials.

I NTERPRETATION . Meaningful differences in progression rates have been shown in
progression rates in trials of either lipid-lowering drugs or calcium channel blockers
involving several hundred subjects over a period of several years. Acceptance of a
standardized protocol for measuring IMT change would facilitate comparison of results
from the many trials using this technique. However, uncertainty about which measure of
IMT offers the best end-point has inhibited methodological standardization.

Comment

Carotid IMT, as a marker of vascular disease progression (or regression), as a predictor for future cardiovascular events, and as an outcome measure in clinical trials is well recognized. However, controversy regarding its use as a clinical tool for risk assessment continues in spite of recommendation from the AHA. This article reviews current controversies and clinical evidence in support of its values as a disease marker as well as an event predictor. It provides excellent up to date background information for anyone who wishes to embark on using the technique.

Intima-media thickness: a new tool for diagnosis and treatment of cardiovascular risk.
Simon A, Gariepy J, Chironi G, Megnien JL, Levenson J. *J Hypertens* 2002; **20**(2): 159–69.

BACKGROUND. Increased IMT is a non-invasive marker of early arterial wall alteration, which is easily assessed in the carotid artery by B-mode ultrasound, and more and more widely used in clinical research.

INTERPRETATION. Methodological standardization of IMT measurement still needs to be implemented before routine measurement of IMT can be proposed in clinical practice as a diagnostic tool for stratifying cardiovascular risk in primary prevention and for aggressive treatment decisions. It can be anticipated, however, that the presence of increased carotid IMT in one individual with intermediate cardiovascular risk would lead to his classification into the high-risk category and thus influence the aggressiveness of risk factor modifications.

Comment

This review provides both practical guides to the technique and normal reference values, and summarizes epidemiological evidence of IMT as risk marker and predictor, as well as regression trials with different classes of antihypertensive and lipid lowering agents.

Table 6.1 Methodological criteria taken into account for measuring carotid IMT

Image acquisition	Segment: CCA, bulb, ICA, right/left
	Wall: far, near
Type of measure	Mean of several maximum measures (from 2 to 12)
	Mean of randomly selected measures (from 3 to 5)
	Mean of measures over 1 cm (≥ 100)
Methods of analysis	Manual cursor placement
	Automated computerized edge-detection

CCA, common carotid artery; ICA, internal carotid artery.
Source: Simon *et al.* (2002).

Basically, IMT measurement can be categorized by two approaches: (i) measurement at multiple extracranial carotid sites in near and far walls, and (ii) computerized measurement restricted to the far wall of the distal common carotid artery.

Because IMT reflects global cardiovascular risk, its normal value might be better defined in terms of increased risk rather than in terms of statistical distribution within a healthy population. The available epidemiological data indicate that increased IMT (at or above 1 mm) represents a risk of myocardial infarction and/or cerebrovascular disease.

Close relationships have been shown between: (i) most traditional cardiovascular risk factors; (ii) certain emerging risk factors, such as lipoproteins, psychosocial status, plasma viscosity, or hyperhomocysteinaemia; and (iii) various cardiovascular

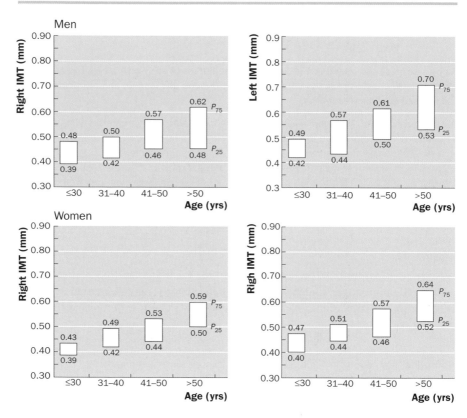

Fig. 6.3 Distribution of 'normal' values of common carotid artery far wall IMT (both scales) in a population of healthy men and women by age range; AXA Study (Gariepy et al., 1998) |6|. Upper and lower limits of bars are 75th upper (P_{75}) and 25th lower percentiles (P_{25}) of IMT distribution within the age range indicated in the x-axis. Abnormal increased IMT are values above the 75th upper percentile in each category of age. Source: Simon et al. (2002).

Table 6.2 Relation of carotid intima-media thickness (IMT) with cardiovascular events in asymptomatic subjects

Increase in IMT	Site of measure	Study (country)	Subject (sex, age)	Follow-up duration (years)	Outcome	Risk ratio (95% confidence interval)
At or above 1 mm	CCA	KIHD |8| (Finland)	M, 40–60	3	AMI	2.2 (0.07–6.7)
At or above 1 mm	Mean maximum 6 sites	ARIC |9,10| (USA)	M, 45–64	4–7	CHD	1.9 (1.3–2.7)*
			W, 45–64	4–7	CHD	5.1 (3.1–8.4)*
			M, 45–64	6–9	Stroke	3.6 (1.5–9.2)*
			W, 45–64	6–9	Stroke	5.5 (3.5–20.7)*
At or above 1.18 mm	CCA	CHS |11| (USA)	M-W, ≥64	6	AMI and stroke	2.0 (2–4)†
Per 0.16 mm	CCA	Rotterdam |12| (Holland)	M-W, ≥55	3	AMI	1.4 (1.2–1.8)†
			M-W, ≥55	3	Stroke	1.4 (1.3–1.8)†

KIHD, Kuopio Ischaemic Heart Disease; ARIC, Atherosclerosis Risk in Communities; CHS, Cardiovascular Health Study; CCA, common carotid artery; AMI, acute myocardial infarction; CHD, coronary heart disease. *Adjusted for age and race; †adjusted for age and sex.
Source: Simon et al. (2002).

Table 6.3 Effect of calcium antagonism and angiotensin-converting enzyme inhibition on carotid intima-media thickness (IMT) in randomized double-blind trials

Treatment	Study	Outcome	Patients	Follow-up years	IMT progression rate (mm/year)		
					Drug	Control	P
Isradipine versus hydrochlorothiazide	MIDAS |13|	Mean maximum 12 sites	Hypertensive	3	0.04 ± 0.002	0.05 ± 0.002	NS
Verapamil versus chlortalidone	VHAS |14|	Mean maximum 6 sites	Hypertensive	4	0.015 ± 0.005	0.016 ± 0.005	NS
Lacidipine versus atenolol	ELSA |7|	Mean maximum 4 sites	Hypertensive	4	–	–	
Nitedipine versus hydrochlorothiazide/amiloride	INSIGHT |17| IMT	Mean CCA	Hypertensive	4	−0.007 ± 0.002	0.0077 ± 0.002	0.002
Amlodipine versus placebo	PREVENT |15|	Mean maximum 12 sites	Coronary	3	−0.012 ± 0.012	0.033 ± 0.012	0.007
Ramipril versus placebo	SECURE |16|	Mean maximum 12 sites	High risk	4.5	0.014 ± 0.002	0.022 ± 0.003	0.03

Source: Simon et al. (2002).

or organ damage, such as white matter lesions of the brain, LVH, microalbuminuria or decreased ankle to brachial systolic pressure index.

Prospective primary and secondary prevention studies have also shown that increased IMT is a powerful predictor of coronary and cerebrovascular complications (risk ratio from 2 to 6) with a higher predictive value when IMT is measured at multiple extracranial carotid sites than solely in the distal common carotid artery.

Therapeutic double-blind trials have shown that lipid-lowering drugs, such as resin and overall statins, and to a lesser extent antihypertensive drugs, such as calcium antagonists, may have a beneficial effect on IMT progression in asymptomatic or in coronary patients.

Calcium antagonist lacidipine slows down progression of asymptomatic carotid atherosclerosis. Principal results of the European Lacidipine Study on Atherosclerosis (ELSA), a randomized, double-blind, long-term trial.

Zanchetti A, Bond MG, Hennig M, *et al.* European Lacidipine Study on Atherosclerosis Investigators. *Circulation* 2002; **106**(19): 2422–7.

BACKGROUND. Most cardiovascular events associated with hypertension are complications of atherosclerosis. Some antihypertensive agents influence experimental models of atherosclerosis through mechanisms independent of BP lowering.

INTERPRETATION. The greater efficacy of lacidipine on carotid IMT progression and number of plaques per patient, despite a smaller ambulatory BP reduction, indicates an antiatherosclerotic action of lacidipine independent of its antihypertensive action.

Comment

ELSA was the largest prospective randomized, double-blind trial to use carotid artery wall IMT as the primary end-point. The study compared 2334 patients with mild-to-moderate hypertension, who were randomized to the β-blocker atenolol or lacidipine on the changes of carotid atherosclerosis (mean of the maximum IMT in far walls of common carotids and bifurcations [CBMmax]) over 4 years. CBMmax has been shown by epidemiological studies to be predictive of cardiovascular events. It was measured by ultrasound scan at baseline, and then at 1, 2, 3 and 4 years.

Among the 1519 patients who completed the 4-year treatment period, lacidipine had a significant treatment effect (P <0.0001), with a treatment difference in 4-year CBMmax progression of –0.0227 mm (intention-to-treat population) and –0.0281 mm (completers). The yearly IMT progression rate was reduced by 40% with lacidipine compared with atenolol. Carotid IMT progression was 0.0145 mm/year with atenolol vs 0.0087 mm/year with lacidipine (P = 0.0073). Patients with plaque progression were significantly less common, and patients with plaque regression were significantly more common in the lacidipine group.

Table 6.4 Changes from baseline in lacidipine- and atenolol-treated patients

Measurement	Lacidipine	Atenolol	P
Yearly IMT progression rate (mm/year)	0.0087	0.0145	0.0073
Patients with plaque progression	25.3%	31.3%	*
Patients with plaque regression	20.4%	14.8%	*
In-clinic change in SBP/DBP (mmHg)	−21.8/−15.5	−21.6/−15.6	NS
Ambulatory change in SBP/DBP (mmHg)	−6.8/−4.9	−10.3/−8.7	<0.0001

*ψ^2 tests $P = 0.0036$. DBP, diastolic BP. All values refer to ELSA patients who completed the 4-year study.
Source: Zanchetti *et al.* (2002).

Interestingly, clinic BP reductions were identical with both treatments, but 24-hour ambulatory SBP/diastolic BP changes were greater with atenolol (−10/−9 mmHg) than with lacidipine (−7/−5 mmHg). No significant difference between treatments was found in any cardiovascular events, although the relative risk for stroke, major cardiovascular events, and mortality showed a trend favouring lacidipine.

Based on these findings, the investigators concluded that lacidipine has anti-atherosclerotic effects in addition to its antihypertensive effect.

To strengthen their argument on the suitability of IMT as a surrogate marker of atherosclerosis, the investigators measured not only at the common carotid but also at four different sites, including the carotid bifurcation 'where most plaques occur', as well as counting the number of plaques at these sites. In view of strong epidemiological evidence of a relationship between carotid wall thickness and cardiovascular events, the slowdown of carotid atherosclerosis progression should translate into better cardiovascular outcomes. However, they saw no significant differences in terms of the number of cardiovascular events or deaths per 1000 person-years between patients in the two arms of the study. Although ELSA was not powered to test these long-term end-points, they did see a trend towards improved outcomes (a lower incidence of strokes and cardiovascular death) in the lacidipine patients. The argument for 'antiatherosclerotic' effects independent of BP lowering may be further strengthened by the fact that ambulatory BP measurements indicated significantly greater BP lowering in atenolol-treated patients than in the lacidipine group, despite BP measurements taken in-clinic were identical for the two treatment groups.

These arguments may further be supported by other studies that have shown similar findings with other calcium blockers—the Verapamil in Hypertension and Atherosclerosis Study (VHAS) with verapamil and the Prospective Randomized Evaluation of the Vascular Effects of Norvasc Trial (PREVENT) trial with amlodipine. The latter showed that amlodipine had a significant effect on a secondary measure—carotid atherosclerosis measured by ultrasound—although it was conducted in patients with angiographic evidence of CAD rather than a hypertensive population.

While lacidipine may have an effect on atherogenesis, the debate will remain whether this translates into an improved clinical outcome.

Role of echocardiography and carotid ultrasonography in stratifying risk in patients with essential hypertension: the Assessment of Prognostic Risk Observational Survey.

Cuspidi C, Ambrosioni E, Mancia G, et al. J Hypertens 2002; **20**(7): 1307–14.

B A C K G R O U N D. Echocardiography and carotid ultrasonography, by providing a more accurate assessment of cardiac and vascular damage related to hypertension, may lead to a more precise stratification of the global cardiovascular risk. However, current guidelines do not recommend systematic use of ultrasound examination of heart and large arteries in evaluating the cardiovascular risk in patients with hypertension.

I N T E R P R E T A T I O N. Ultrasound assessment of the heart and carotid wall helps to obtain a more valid assessment of global cardiovascular risk in hypertensive patients without evidence of target organ damage after routine examination.

Comment

Non-invasive imaging techniques can be used to directly identify and monitor pre-clinical atherosclerosis in human arteries. The additional information, when added to the basic risk information already available, has the potential to substantially improve our ability to identify individuals at risk for the development of CVD. Non-invasive imaging can also be used to monitor changes in rates of atherosclerosis progression in response to treatment.

Indeed, initiation of drug treatment should not be based on BP alone, but on a global/absolute risk of the individual. The WHO/ISH guidelines on global cardio-vascular risk stratification into four classes: low, medium, high and very high. Treatment is indicated when patient's BP is particularly high (grade 3) and when a more moderate increase in BP is accompanied by (i) three or more additional risk factors, organ damage or diabetes (high risk), or (ii) clinical cardiovascular complications (very high risk), thus presenting a global cardiovascular risk profile predicting an incidence of at least 20% for major cardiovascular events over 10 years. In patients at low or medium risk (<20% in 10 years), WHO/ISH guidelines recommend wait and see policy.

The objective of this study was to assess the impact of echocardiography and carotid ultrasonography on global risk stratification in hypertensive patients classified as being at low or medium risk according to routine clinical work-up as suggested by current hypertension guidelines. A total of 8502 consecutive patients screened at 44 out-patient hypertension hospital clinics in different parts of Italy, 1074 untreated individuals with low-to-medium risk essential hypertension (i.e. without diabetes or target organ damage) were selected according to the 1999 WHO/ISH guidelines criteria. The extent of risk for the 1074 individuals was reassessed by adding the results of ultrasound examinations of heart and carotid arteries: LVH (defined as LV mass index >120 g/m^2 in men and >100 g/m^2 in women), carotid-IMT (defined as diffuse thickening if ≥0.8 mm), and presence of plaque (defined as focal thickening >1.3 mm).

The results showed that the percentage of subjects classified as 'low risk' decreased from 19 to 11% and those classified as 'medium' risk decreased from 81 to 36%. On the other hand, 53% of patients previously classified as 'low' or 'medium' risk were reclassified as 'high' absolute risk. When the reclassification was based on either cardiac or carotid ultrasound alone, the number reclassified as high risk was reduced by approximately one-third with echocardiography alone and by approximately one-half with carotid ultrasound alone. According to a multivariate analysis, age, grade of hypertension, male sex and serum cholesterol concentration were the variables with the greatest impact on risk class change.

This study provides good evidence that echocardiography and carotid ultrasound refine our risk stratification substantially as a larger group of hypertensive patients with target organ damage, i.e. into the high-risk stratum, could be selected for intervention, be it life-style changes and/or drug therapy. Accordingly, these patients who were initially stratified as low or medium risk on the WHO/ISH criteria will have the greatest potential gain from a more accurate stratification of their absolute risk status.

There have been multiple prospective epidemiological studies that have shown that increases in carotid artery IMT are associated with increased risk of myocardial infarction and stroke in adults without a history of CVD. Indeed, carotid IMT measurement obtained with B-mode ultrasound is currently recommended by the AHA for inclusion in the evaluation of risk. Despite its recommendation, the routine use of this technique is still controversial and in fact many still regard it as merely a surrogate marker rather than a risk factor of CVD. On the other hand, echocardiographic LVH has been regarded as a powerful risk factor, predictor and marker of CVD. Up until recently, LVH regression has not been linked with reduction in hard end-point such as stroke or cardiovascular death. By contrast, there is so far no evidence that carotid IMT regression leads to reduction of cardiovascular events. Furthermore, carotid IMT has been regarded as a 'less' powerful predictor than LVH for cardiovascular event. These factors plus the lack of agreement in the standardization of carotid IMT measurement protocol may explain the lack of acceptance of IMT as a cardiovascular risk factor as compared with echocardiographic LVH.

It is important to note that patients in this were drawn from a population referred to specialized hospital-based hypertension clinics, and thus may not be representative of the wider population of hypertensive patients managed at the primary care level. Furthermore, to recommend routine use of these examinations for these patients is costly including training for staffs, treatment and follow-up, etc. Accordingly, further studies are needed in a primary care or general practice situation at community level. Next, is the need for careful and detailed cost–benefit analysis, weighing up the costs of the investigations and of the additional drug treatment entailed against the savings generated from reductions in morbidity and mortality. It should be noted that the presence of hypertensive retinopathy and proteinuria are also evidence of target organ damage, and thus indicate a 'high-risk' category. It would seem cheaper and simpler to perform fundoscopy and 24-hour urine collection routinely for this matter.

Conclusion

Measurements of endothelial function, arterial stiffness, vascular and myocardial hypertrophy are surrogate markers of cardiovascular risk. We have witnessed an increasing number of therapeutic strategies aimed at improving these markers in a variety of CVD states. The next decade will witness an exponential interest in developing reliable, non-invasive and easy to use methods of measuring these as a potential predictor of CVD in a wider scale in population studies. Several large non-invasive studies would be underway to determine the predictive value of these markers and they are likely to find their way into risk assessment algorithms. As measures of these markers become clinically applicable, this may translate into improved methods of risk assessment and equip physicians with yet another tool to predict, prevent and treat CVD.

References

1. Wilkinson IB, Webb DJ, Cockcroft JR. Nitric oxide and the regulation of arterial elasticity: right idea, wrong vascular bed? *Hypertension* 2002; **39**: e26–7.
2. Kelm M, Preik M, Hafner DJ, Strauer BE. Evidence for a multifactorial process involved in the impaired flow response to nitric oxide in hypertensive patients with endothelial dysfunction. *Hypertension* 1996; **27**: 346–53.
3. Preik M, Kelm M, Feelisch M, Strauer BE. Impaired effectiveness of nitric oxide-donors in resistance arteries of patients with arterial hypertension. *J Hypertens* 1996; **14**: 903–8.
3a. Boutouyrie P, Tropeano AI, Asmar R, Gautier I, Benetos A, Lacolley P, Laurent S. Aortic stiffness is an independent predictor of coronary events in hypertensive patients: a longitudinal study. Hypertension. 2002 Jan; **39**(1): 10–15.
4. van Popele NMN, Grobbee DE, Bots ML, Asmar R, Topouchian J, Rencman RS *et al.* Association between arterial stiffness and atherosclerosis: The Rotterdam study. *Stroke* 2001; **32**: 454–60.
5. Guerin AP, London GM, Marchais SJ, Metivier F. Arterial stiffening and vascular calcifications in end-stage renal disease. *Nephrol Dial Transplant* 2000; **15**: 1014–21.
6. Gariepy J, Salomon J, Denarie N, Laskri F, Megnien JL, Levenson J, Simon A. Sex and topographic differences in associations between large-artery wall thickness and coronary risk profile in a French working cohort: the AXA Study. *Arterioscler Thromb Vasc Biol* 1998; **4**: 584–90.

7. Zanchetti A, Bond MG, Henning M, Neiss A, Mancia G, Dal Palu C *et al*. Risk factors associated with alterations in carotid intima-media thickness in hypertension: baseline data from the European Lacidipine Study on Atherosclerosis. *J Hypertens* 1998; **16**: 949–61.

8. Salonen JT, Salonen R. Ultrasonographically assessed carotid morphology and the risk of coronary heart disease. *Arterioscler Thromb* 1991; **11**: 1245–9.

9. Chambless LE, Heiss G, Folsom AR, Rosamond W, Szklo M, Sharrett AR, Clegg LX. Association of coronary heart disease incidence with carotid arterial wall thickness and major risk factors: the Atherosclerosis Risk in Communities (ARIC) Study, 1987–1993. *Am J Epidemiol* 1997; **146**: 483–94.

10. Chambless LE, Folsom AR, Clegg LX, Sharrett AR, Shahar E, Nieto FJ *et al*. Carotid wall thickness is predictive of incident clinical stroke: the Atherosclerosis Risk in Communities (ARIC) study. *Am J Epidemiol* 2000; **151**: 478–87.

11. O'Leary DH, Polak JF, Kronmal RA, Manolio TA, Burke GL, Wolfson SK. Carotid-artery intima and media thickness as a risk factor for myocardial infarction and stroke in older adults. Cardiovascular Health Study Collaborative Research Group. *N Engl J Med* 1999; **340**: 14–22.

12. Bots ML, Hoes AW, Koudstaal PJ, Hofman A, Grobbee DE. Common carotid intima-media thickness and risk of stroke and myocardial infarction: the Rotterdam Study. *Circulation* 1997; **96**: 1432–7.

13. Borhani NO, Mercuri M, Borhani PA, Buckalew VM, Canossa-Terris M, Carr AA *et al*. Final outcome results of the Multicenter Isradipine Diuretic Atherosclerosis Study (MIDAS). A randomized controlled trial. *JAMA* 1996; **276**: 785–91.

14. Zanchetti A, Rosei EA, Dal Palu C, Leonetti G, Magnani B, Pessina A. The Verapamil in Hypertension and Atherosclerosis Study (VHAS): results of long-term randomized treatment with either verapamil or chlorthalidone on carotid intima-media thickness. *J Hypertens* 1998; **16**: 1667–76.

15. Pitt B, Byington RP, Furberg CD, Hunninghake DB, Mancini GB, Miller ME, Riley W (for The PREVENT Investigators). Effect of amlodipine on the progression of atherosclerosis and the occurrence of clinical events. *Circulation* 2000; **102**: 1503–10.

16. Lonn EM, Yusuf S, Dzvik V, Doris CI, Yi Q, Smith S. *et al.*, for the SECURE investigators. Effects of Ramipril and vitamin E on Atherosclerosis. The study to evaluate ultrasound changes in patients treated with Ramipril and vitamin E (SECURE). Circulation 2001; 103: 919–25.

17. Simon A, Gariepy J, Moyse D, Levenson J. Differential effects of nifedipine and co-amilozide on the progression of early carotid atherosclerosis. A four-year randomized, controlled clinical study of intima-media thickness measured by ultrasound. *Circulation* 2001; **103**: 2949–54.

Part II

Clinical management

7

Blood pressure measurement: traditional versus contemporary

Introduction

Blood pressure (BP) measurement based on conventional mercury sphygmomanometer and Korotkoff sounds at the brachial artery has been regarded as the gold standard for over a century. Epidemiological studies have established the prognostic value of BP measured by conventional methods. Moreover, therapeutic trials using the conventional method for measuring BP have shown that a reduction in BP is associated with a reduction in cardiovascular morbidity and mortality. However, the methods used for measuring BP are evolving rapidly with the advent of automatic electronic devices and the 'gold standard' based on the former has recently been questioned. Manual BP measurement has the disadvantage of being prone to observer bias, error, terminal digit preference, and inadequate or erroneous techniques. Furthermore, with the increasing popularity of the newer electronic devices for BP measuring and the pressure from environmentalists to ban mercury as a toxic substance, mercury sphygmomanometers are gradually phasing out of clinical practice, both from the hospital and doctor's surgery.

Nevertheless, BP measurement based on occluding the brachial artery with an inflatable cuff introduced over a century ago by Riva-Rocci in 1896, is still the fundamental principle of BP measuring regardless of whether the device is mercury-based or oscillometrically aneroid sphygmomanometers, determined by the change of Korotkoff sounds, or automatic sphygmomanometer with electronic digital readings displayed. Furthermore, the accuracy of BP measurement by newer devices has still to be validated by comparing with the traditional mercury-based auscultatory method, although the degree of reproducibility of the former might be higher than the traditional method due mainly to observer bias. Indeed, the first generation of automated devices have had a poor record for accuracy, with many failing to satisfy the stringent criteria (see below) of the validation protocols of the British Hypertension Society (BHS) and the Association for the Advancement of Medical Instrumentation (AAMI).

Previous reports indicate that self-measured BPs are better predictors for prognosis of hypertension than office BP and provide a more accurate evaluation of the effect of treatment. Indeed, with increasing awareness of high BP as a major cardiovascular risk factor and the increasingly affordable wide range of portable automated

BP measuring instruments, self-measurement of BP at home is becoming increasingly popular, not only to subjects with hypertension, but also those who are apparently healthy. The increased popularity of home self-BP measuring is indeed reflected by the growing sale figures from the manufacturers of these devices, especially wrist cuff devices. As the matter of fact, more than one-third of the automated BP measuring devices recently sold in the world are wrist-cuff devices. Although many of the arm-cuff automated devices are now beginning to meet the validation protocols of the BHS and/or AAMI |1–3|, none of the wrist devices are recommended regardless of their accuracy because they do not measure BP at heart level as specified by both protocols. It is of note that the international consensus conference that recommended self-measurement of BP only referred to studies that were made with upper arm-cuff devices. However, BP measurement by wrist-cuff device equipped with a position sensor (see below) to guide the users to adopt the correct position of the forearm and wrist at the heart level may be comparable with self-measurements with upper arm-cuff devices (see below). Finger-cuff devices are also available but their accuracy and reproducibility are poor. Inaccurate self-measured BP inevitably leads to an incorrect diagnosis in practice, hence inappropriate treatment and an erroneous conclusion in hypertension research. It is therefore of paramount importance that users of these devices are aware of their limitations and the risks that may be associated with the inaccurate self-measurement of BP. Certainly, independent validation studies are needed to approve formally the BP instrument for clinical use; in particular, when the device is used to manage patients with BP problems in out-patient settings. In addition, regular calibration of the device against a mercury manometer is important; most manufacturers of aneroid and electronic instruments recommend calibration every 6 months |4|.

The advent of ambulatory BP monitoring (ABPM) devices has allowed BP to be measured away from the clinic/medical environment, and thus the identification of the phenomenon of 'white-coat or isolated office hypertension'. In addition, the correlation between the BP level and target organ damage, cardiovascular risk and long-term prognosis has been shown to be closer for ABPM than for BP measured at the clinic. However, controversy remains on whether 'white coat or isolated office hypertension' is a benign clinical condition or is linked with an increased risk of target organ damage (about 10% of these subjects show echocardiographic evidence of increased left ventricular hypertrophy) and a worse prognosis. It is also unknown whether self-measurement of BP at home can reveal the 'white coat' phenomenon equivalent to that demonstrated by the 24-hour BP profiles. Nevertheless, the issue of equipment accuracy is very much better for ABPM devices than for other automated devices, with a large number of devices fulfilling the criteria of the BHS and AAMI protocols. Indeed, ABPM seems particularly useful for defining the efficacy of anti-hypertensive medication in clinical trials.

No matter which device is used to measure BP, it must be recognized that BP is a variable haemodynamic phenomenon, which is influenced by many factors, not least being the circumstances of measurement itself. Body posture and arm positions are two obvious subject's factors affecting the accuracy and reliability of BP measurement, as we will discuss below. It is important to realize that BP readings in different positions are not interchangeable and that BP readings taken in different positions may yield different prognostic and therapeutic implications. For example, the tendency for a higher pressure measured in the right arm may contribute to the difference between office BP, which is generally measured on the right arm, and the self-measured or ambulatory values, which are generally measured on the left arm, and hence overestimation of the prevalence of 'white-coat hypertension'.

Blood pressure measuring devices: recommendations of the European Society of Hypertension.

O'Brien E, Waeber B, Parati G, Staessen J, Myers MG, on behalf of the European Society of Hypertension Working Group on Blood Pressure Monitoring. *Br Med J* 2001; **322**(7285): 531–6.

BACKGROUND. There is a large market for BP measuring devices not only in clinical medicine but also among the public where the demand for self-measurement of BP is growing rapidly. For consumers, whether medical or lay, accuracy should be of prime importance when selecting a device to measure BP. However, most devices have not been evaluated for accuracy independently using the two most widely used protocols: the BHS protocol and the standard set by the US AAMI.

INTERPRETATION. The European Union and international organizations of specialists in hypertension have unanimously recommended that all devices for measuring BP should be independently validated. The European Society of Hypertension Working Party on Blood Pressure Monitoring agreed proposals to simplify the BHS protocol without compromising the integrity of the procedures. This will help manufacturers to market devices world-wide, expedite validation procedures, reduce the expense of performing studies, and permit more centres to undertake validation procedures; all of which would enable manufacturers to have all devices validated independently before they are marketed.

Comment

Problems with the many different BP measuring devices available on the market have long been raised and debated by not only the medical professionals but also by other scientific communities as well as by those who manufactured them and the public. As the number of devices available in the market especially those for self-measurement has increased dramatically but comparatively few have been validated, serious concerns with the accuracy of these devices are apparent.

This is the first thorough expert review by the Working Group on Blood Pressure Monitoring of the European Society of Hypertension (which was first set up in 1998) on the validation of these devices. Only BP measuring devices that have published evidence of independent validation using the BHS protocol and the standard set by the US AAMI, and only literature published up to December 1999 were identified and reviewed in this study. The authors noted that devices that have been validated recently for which results have not yet been fully published were not included in the present survey. However, this shortcoming will be addressed in a future study. It is important to note that the number of devices that have undergone independent validation is only a fraction of the devices available on the market world-wide.

In order to fulfil the criteria of the BHS protocol, devices must achieve at least grade B (where A denotes greatest agreement with mercury standard and D denotes least agreement) for systolic (SBP) and for diastolic (DBP) pressures (Table 7.1). To fulfil the criteria of the AAMI protocol, the test device must not differ from the

Table 7.1 Grading criteria used by the British Society of Hypertension. Grades represent the cumulative percentage of readings falling within 5 mmHg, 10 mmHg, and 15 mmHg of the mercury standard. All three percentages must be greater than or equal to the values shown for a specific grade to be awarded. Values are mmHg

		Absolute difference between standard and test device (%)		
	Grade	≤5	≤10	≤15
	A	60	85	95
	B	50	75	90
	C	40	65	85
	D		Worse than C	

Source: O'Brien et al. (2001).

Table 7.2 Manual blood pressure measuring devices validated using the protocols of the Association for the Advancement of Medical Instrumentation and the British Hypertension Society

Device	Protocol		Use	Recommendation
	AAMI*	BHS (systolic/ diastolic)†		
PyMah mercury	Passed	A/A	At rest	Recommended
Hawksley RZS (US model)	Failed	B/D	At rest	Not recommended
Hawksley RZS (UK model)	Failed	C/D	At rest	Not recommended
Aneroid device	NA	Failed	At rest; only abstract available	Questionable recommendation

AAMI, Association for the Advancement of Medical Instrumentation; BHS, British Hypertension Society; RZS, random zero sphygmomanometer; NA, not applied. *To meet AAMI criteria the mean difference between the device and the mercury standard must be ≤5 mmHg or the standard deviation must be ≤8 mmHg. †To meet BHS criteria devices must achieve a grade of at least B for both systolic and diastolic measurements. Grade A denotes greatest agreement with mercury standard and D denotes least agreement.
Source: O'Brien et al. (2001).

Table 7.3 Automated blood pressure measuring devices for clinical use in hospitals validated using the protocols of the Association for the Advancement of Medical Instrumentation and the British Hypertension Society. Devices were validated in oscillometric mode unless otherwise indicated

Device	Protocol		Use	Recommendation
	AAMI*	BHS (systolic/ diastolic)†		
Datascope Accutorr Plus	Passed	A/A	At rest	Recommended
CAS Model 9010	Passed	NA	At rest in adults	Recommended
			In neonates	Recommended
Tensionic Mod EPS 112	Passed	B/A	At rest; only abstract available	Questionable recommendation
Colin Pilot 9200 (tonometric mode)	Passed	NA	At rest; intra-arterial	Questionable recommendation
Dinamap 8100	Failed	B/D	At rest	Not recommended

AAMI, Association for the Advancement of Medical Instrumentation; BHS, British Hypertension Society; NA, not applied. *To meet AAMI criteria the mean difference between the device and the mercury standard must be ≤5 mmHg or the standard deviation must be ≤8 mmHg. †To meet BHS criteria devices must achieve a grade of at least B for both systolic and diastolic measurements. Grade A denotes greatest agreement with mercury standard and D denotes least agreement.
Source: O'Brien et al. (2001).

Table 7.4 Automated blood pressure measuring devices for self measurement at the wrist validated using the protocols of the Association for the Advancement of Medical Instrumentation and the British Hypertension Society

Device	Protocol		Use	Recommendation
	AAMI*	BHS (systolic/ diastolic)†		
Omron R3	NA	NA	Intra-arterial comparison	Questionable recommendation
Omron R3	Failed	D/D	At rest	Not recommended
Boso-Mediwatch	NA	C/C	At rest; protocol violation	Not recommended
Omron Rx	Failed	B/B	At rest; only abstract available	Questionable recommendation

AAMI, Association for the Advancement of Medical Instrumentation; BHS, British Hypertension Society; NA, not applied. *To meet AAMI criteria the mean difference between the device and the mercury standard must be ≤5 mmHg or the standard deviation must be ≤8 mmHg. †To meet BHS criteria devices must achieve a grade of at least B for both systolic and diastolic measurements. Grade A denotes greatest agreement with mercury standard and D denotes least agreement.
Source: O'Brien et al. (2001).

Table 7.5 Ambulatory blood pressure measuring devices validated using the protocols of the Association for the Advancement of Medical Instrumentation and the British Hypertension Society

Device	Mode	Protocol		Use	Recommendation
		AAMI*	BHS (systolic/ diastolic)†		
Accutracker II (30/23)	Auscultatory	Passed	A/C	At rest	Not recommended
CH-DRUCK	Auscultatory	Passed	A/A	At rest	Recommended
Daypress 500	Oscillometric	Passed	A/B	At rest	Recommended
DIASYS 200	Auscultatory	Passed	C/C	At rest	Not recommended
DIASYS Integra	Auscultatory	Passed	B/A	At rest	Recommended
	Oscillometric	Passed	B/B	At rest	Recommended
ES-H531	Auscultatory	Passed	A/A	At rest	Recommended
	Oscillometric	Passed	B/B	At rest	Recommended
Medilog ABP	Auscultatory	Passed	NA	At rest	Questionable recommendation
Meditech ABPM-04	Oscillometric	Passed	B/B	At rest	Recommended
Nissei DS-240	Oscillometric	Passed	B/A	Only abstract available; details missing	Questionable recommendation
OSCILL-IT	Oscillometric	Passed	C/B	At rest	Not recommended
Pressurometer IV	Auscultatory	Failed	C/D	At rest	Not recommended
Profilomat	Auscultatory	Passed	B/A	At rest	Recommended
Profilomat	Auscultatory	Passed	B/C	In pregnancy	Not recommended
Profilomat II	Oscillometric	Failed	C/B	At rest	Not recommended
QuietTrak	Auscultatory	Passed	B/B	At rest	Recommended
QuietTrak	Auscultatory	Passed	B/B	At rest; only abstract	Questionable recommendation
QuietTrak	Auscultatory	Failed	D/D	In pre-eclampsia	Not recommended
QuietTrak	Auscultatory	Failed	B/B	In pregnancy	Not recommended
QuietTrak51	Auscultatory	Passed	A/A	At rest	Recommended
			A/A	During exercise	Recommended
			A/A	Different postures	Recommended
			A/A	In elderly people	Recommended
			A/A	In children	Recommended
			A/A	In pregnancy	Recommended
Save 33, Model 2	Oscillometric	Passed	B/B	At rest	Recommended
Schiller BR-102	Auscultatory	Passed	B/B	At rest	Recommended
	Oscillometric	Failed	D/B	At rest	Not recommended
SpaceLabs 90202	Oscillometric	Passed	B/B	At rest	Recommended
SpaceLabs 90207	Oscillometric	Passed	B/B	At rest	Recommended
SpaceLabs 90207	Oscillometric	Passed	A/C	In pregnancy	Not recommended
SpaceLabs 90207	Oscillometric	Passed	B/B	In pregnancy	Recommended
SpaceLabs 90207	Oscillometric	Passed	B/C	In pregnancy	Not recommended
SpaceLabs 90207	Oscillometric	Failed	D/D	In pre-eclampsia	Not recommended
SpaceLabs 90207	Oscillometric	Passed	C/C	In pre-eclampsia	Not recommended
SpaceLabs 90207	Oscillometric	SBP Pass	C	In children	Not recommended
SpaceLabs 90207		DBP Fail	D	In children	Not recommended

Table 7.5 *(continued)*

Device	Mode	Protocol		Use	Recommendation
		AAMI*	BHS (systolic/diastolic)†		
SpaceLabs 90207	Oscillometric	Passed	B/A	Elderly people standing and sitting (SBP ≤160 mmHg)	Recommended
SpaceLabs 90207	Oscillometric	Passed	D/A	Elderly people supine; tested at all pressures	Not recommended
SpaceLabs 90207	Oscillometric	Passed	C/B	During haemodialysis	Not recommended
SpaceLabs 90217	Oscillometric	Passed	A/A	At rest	Recommended
TM-2420/TM-2020	Oscillometric	Failed	D/D	At rest	Not recommended
TM-2420 Model 6	Oscillometric	Passed	B/B	At rest	Recommended
TM-2420 Model 7	Oscillometric	Passed	B/B	At rest	Recommended
TM-2421	Oscillometric	Passed	B/A	At rest	Recommended
TM-242167	Oscillometric	NA	A/B	In children aged 7–8 years sitting	Questionable recommendation
			A/B	In children of all ages sitting	Questionable recommendation
TM-2421	Auscultatory	NA	C/C	In children in different postures	Not recommended
Takeda 2430	Oscillometric	Passed	A/A	At rest	Recommended

AAMI, Association for the Advancement of Medical Instrumentation; BHS, British Hypertension Society; NA, not applied. *To meet AAMI criteria the mean difference between the device and the mercury standard must be ≤5 mmHg or the standard deviation must be ≤8 mmHg. †To meet BHS criteria devices must achieve a grade of at least B for both systolic and diastolic measurements. Grade A denotes greatest agreement with mercury standard and D denotes least agreement. Source: O'Brien *et al.* (2001).

mercury standard by a mean difference >5 mmHg or a SD >8 mmHg. A device is not recommended if it fails the AAMI criteria for either SBP or DBP and achieves a grade of C or D for either SBP or DBP pressure under the BHS protocol. Devices are given a questionable recommendation if there is an element of doubt in interpreting the results of a validation study.

Two broad categories of BP measuring devices were identified: manual sphygmo-manometers (including mercury and anaeroid devices), and automated sphygmo-manometers (including devices for clinical use in hospitals, for self-measurement of BP, for ABPM, and for measuring BP in community settings).

Two manual sphygmomanometers have been validated, one is recommended. The standard anaeroid sphygmomanometers are susceptible to becoming inaccurate with time as the calibration procedure of the BHS protocol is not made apparent to the user.

Automated sphygmomanometers may be divided into three groups:

1. Devices for clinical use in hospitals: five devices for clinical use in hospitals have been validated, two are recommended.

2. Devices for self-measurement of BP: 23 devices for self-measurement of BP have been validated, five are recommended. Virtually all automated devices for self-measurement of BP employed the oscillometric technique. Wrist devices are not recommended regardless of their accuracy because they do not measure BP at heart level. Digital finger devices are considered inaccurate and thus are not reviewed in this study.

3. Devices for ambulatory measurement of BP: 24 devices for ambulatory measurement of BP have been validated, 16 are recommended. Most are dependent on intermittent measurements. Validation studies with ambulatory devices have many methodological difficulties, and the inaccuracies found during static conditions may be amplified during ambulatory conditions. Devices for continuous (beat to beat monitoring) non-invasive BP monitoring of a finger such as the Portapres (TNO, Amsterdam, the Netherlands), which can give 24-hour waveform measurements similar to intra-arterial recordings is still awaiting formal validation.

The authors repeatedly emphasize the importance of accuracy in BP measurement. Accuracy of a particular measurement clearly relies on the reliability of the device and the user. Both carry equal weights.

Accuracy and reliability of wrist-cuff devices for self-measurement of blood pressure.

Kikuya M, Chonan K, Imai Y, Goto E, Ishii M on behalf of the Research Group.
J Hypertens 2002; **20**(4): 629–38.

BACKGROUND. Self-measurement of BP might offer some advantages in diagnosis and therapeutic evaluation and in patient management of hypertension. Recently, wrist-cuff devices for self-measurement of BP have gained more than one-third of the world market share.

INTERPRETATION. Wrist-cuff devices in the present form are inadequate for self-measurement of BP and, thus, are inadequate for general use or clinical and practical use. However, there is much possibility in wrist-cuff device and the accuracy and reliability of wrist-cuff device are warranted by an improvement of technology.

Comment

The demand for self-measurement of BP using automated electronic devices is growing rapidly |5|. Indeed, the increased popularity for wrist devices is more pronounced and is reflected by their current high rate of sale. It is estimated that wrist devices for self-measurement have gained 50% of the market share of the 1.2 million BP measuring devices sold annually in Germany |6|, and 30% of the 2 million BP measuring devices sold annually in Japan. In fact, wrist devices have gained as much as 30% of the market share for all automated BP measuring devices world-wide. Not surprisingly, more than 90% of patients performing self-BPM seem to prefer wrist rather than arm devices. This is probably due to the fact that wrist devices are more convenient to use and cause less discomfort to the subjects. It also may be more suitable for those who are obese and with extremely large or with cone-shape upper arms. Surprisingly, however, the majority of these automated devices distributed have not yet been properly validated.

In the present validation study by Kikuya *et al.*, two wrist-cuff and two arm-cuff devices for self-BP measuring were compared with those obtained through traditional auscultatory readings in 13 institutes in Japan. They used a cross-over method, where the comparison was done between auscultation, by two observers by means of a double stethoscope on one arm and the device on the opposite arm or wrist. Simultaneous same arm validation is not possible with wrist devices. The factors affecting the accuracy and reliability of wrist measuring devices were also assessed. The results demonstrated that the SD of the mean difference between auscultation and the wrist-cuff device was extremely large when compared with that between auscultation and arm-cuff device. The BP values provided by wrist devices differ from auscultation by more than 10 mmHg in SBP and/or more than 5 mmHg in DBP in approximately 30 and 50% of the measurements, respectively. In other words, if subjects defined their BP level on the basis of a wrist-cuff device, a large proportion of subjects were judged to be as hypertensive and normotensive, although they are actually normotensive and hypertensive, respectively. Such inaccuracy in BP measurements, as emphasized by the authors, could have serious consequences for clinical practice, clinical science and public health.

Although the study was carried out under stringently controlled validation conditions and has the merit of including a fairly large number of subjects, an important limitation was that none of the requirements of established validation protocols (BHS or AAMI) has been fulfilled |7–9|. If AAMI validation criterion were followed and applied as a *post-hoc* procedure (according to which the mean difference between tested and reference method should be >5 mmHg with a SD >8 mmHg) to the total of the data provided by each device, both wrist devices and one of the arm devices would be rejected as inaccurate. Furthermore, the large between-centre differences in the results observed for the same device cannot be explained simply on the basis of device inaccuracy but could most likely be attributed to observer variability in some centres. Indeed, training of observers to a very high standard is of critical importance in validation studies. The importance of this methodological aspect is greatly emphasized in the BHS protocol. Other methodological factors such as the inclusion of subjects with a rather narrow range of pressures (fewer than 10% of participants with DBP >100 mmHg and SBP >180 mmHg) and improper positioning of the wrist to heart level could possibly bias the results. However, the novel demonstrations of the significant influence of the 'wrist–forearm angle' (besides the wrist–heart hydrostatic height difference) on wrist BP measurements are methodologically important and should be investigated further in future validation studies. As pointed out by the authors it is doubtful that users can strictly control the measurement conditions during measurements by wrist-cuff devices, such as the position of the wrist, angle of the hand joint and fitness of the cuff. Thus the divergence between BP estimated by auscultation and BP provided using a wrist-cuff device would become larger in daily use than that in the validation study.

Based on the available evidence from several validation studies in the last few years and that of the current paper, the general use of wrist-cuff devices in clinical practice (both in the doctor's office and at the patients' home) should not at present be recommended. However, the fact that the use of wrist BP devices is widespread, additional validation studies to be carefully carried out according to established protocols are urgently needed, certainly taking into account the methodological issues raised by Kikuya *et al.* Furthermore, manufacturers are responsible for this validation process and should publish it for consumers as well as practitioners.

Evaluation of the performance of a wrist blood pressure measuring device with a position sensor compared with ambulatory 24-hour blood pressure measurements.

Uen S, Weisser B, Wieneke P, Vetter H, Mengden T. *Am J Hypertens* 2002; **15**(9): 787–92.

BACKGROUND. This randomized, single-centre, open, within-subject study evaluated the performance of the Braun PrecisionSensor 2000 BP measurement wrist device (BP 2000, Braun GmbH, Germany) with and without the position sensor, and compared the results with data obtained from 24-hour ambulatory BP measurement (ABPM, A&D TM 2430).

INTERPRETATION. Self-BP measurements with BP 2000, by untrained subjects, produced results consistent with those found recently with self-BP measurements with upper arm devices, when both data sets are compared with ABPM. The rates of false classification of normotension/hypertension with the wrist device were small and at least as reliable as office measurements.

Comment

As pointed out in the earlier paper (Kikuya *et al.*), correction of hydrostatic pressure is one of the most important issues when subjects use a wrist-cuff device for BP measurement. It is known that a 10 cm difference between heart and cuff is equivalent to 7 mmHg difference. An inappropriate correction of difference in hydrostatic pressure between heart and cuff can seriously affect BP value. It is hoped that a wrist-cuff device equipped with a position sensor would be able to guide the user to adopt the correct position of the forearm and wrist, and thus more accurate and reproducible measurement. However, owing to the fact that only a minority of patients who purchase self-measurement BP devices receive specific training in the use of the devices (especially wrist-cuff devices), the accuracy and reliability of these devices should be evaluated under routine clinical practices (in addition to evaluating accuracy under controlled laboratory conditions with a AAMI or BHS protocol) using subjects with no prior training in self-BP measurement.

Indeed, the objectives of the present study were to validate the performance of the Braun PrecisionSensor wrist device (BP 2000, Braun GmbH, Germany) with the position sensor in comparison without the position sensor in subjects with no training in self-BP measurement, and to compare the results of these BP measurements with and without the position sensor with data obtained from one profile (24 h) ABPM. Importantly, the BP 2000 wrist device has been validated using the AAMI protocol SP10 and has satisfied the criteria for accuracy both for SBP and DBP. A cross-over design was used in this study in which 43 subjects performed BP measurements with the BP 2000 during two 7-day periods, one with the position sensor and the other without the position sensor. The correlation coefficients between self-measurement at the wrist and ambulatory 24-hour BP measurements were 0.73 for SBP and 0.65 for DBP (with position sensor) compared with 0.70 and 0.60 for readings without position sensor, respectively. The categorization of subjects as normotensive or hypertensive, using the BP 2000 without specific training in the use of the device, achieved a correct classification of 84% (with position sensor) and 81% (without position sensor) in comparison with ABPM. When the measurements were performed in the clinic by an experienced observer, the correct classification was 79% in comparison with ABPM. The cross-over study design did not reveal any significant variation between the two devices with regard to reproducibility of readings at the wrist. The measurement of BP with the Braun PrecisionSensor wrist device by untrained subjects was considered to be equally as good as that by an experienced observer. However, the use of a position sensor only slightly increased (not statistically significant) the accuracy of the device. This may be due to the fact that a selection bias of mainly subjects with high compliance were included and thus influenced the quality of readings with both BP 2000 with and without position sensor devices.

Mercury sphygmomanometers should not be abandoned: an advisory statement from the Council for High Blood Pressure Research, American Heart Association.

Jones DW, Frohlich ED, Grim CM, Grim CE, Taubert KA for the Professional Education Committee, Council for High Blood Pressure Research.
Hypertension 2001; **37**(2): 185–6.

BACKGROUND. In health-care institutions around the world, mercury sphygmomanometers are being removed. In many situations, the decision to replace the instruments is being made without significant input from involved clinicians or consideration of the health risks that will follow if they are replaced by less accurate devices.

INTERPRETATION. There is a constant need for caution in the selection of BP measuring devices. We recommend that clinicians: (i) educate themselves on the instruments available for use in their clinics and hospitals; (ii) engage in the process of selection of instruments through dialogue with administrators and through hospital committees; (iii) encourage the general use of mercury manometers as the instrument of choice until other instruments are better validated; (iv) where aneroid or electronic instruments are used, ensure that instruments are validated through the AAMI or a similar organization; and (v) ensure a programme of regular maintenance and calibration of all instruments.

Comment

While there is enthusiasm for the change from mercury sphygmomanometers to electronic devices, some caution is needed |10,11|. Care is required when choosing machines, as evident from papers discussed above. Secondly, disposal of old mercury devices requires care to avoid environmental contamination.

  We should not lose sight that the detection, appropriate measurement, treatment and achievement of control and treatment targets are crucial in our management of hypertension. It is not a question of 'do we treat' hypertension, but 'how and who to treat'.

Practice audits: reliability of sphygmomanometers and blood pressure recording bias.
S Ali, A Rouse. *J Hum Hypertens* 2002; **16**(5): 359–61.

BACKGROUND. It is well established that numerous errors, biases and omissions in recording BP exist.

INTERPRETATION. Sphygmomanometers used in general practice are very likely to be inaccurate and some may well be so deteriorated that they should be withdrawn from service. The results of the BP audit showed digit bias in SBP and DBP readings to the nearest 10 mmHg. The implications for clinical care—both overdiagnosis and underdiagnosis—although not assessed are likely to be appreciable. PCG Clinical Governance teams in conjunction with Practice Clinical Leads must address these basic issues.

Comment

The BHS recommends that the accuracy of BP readings should be 'within 2 mm of mercury'. It goes without saying that unreliable, poorly maintained machines will not do this.

Body position and blood pressure measurement in patients with diabetes mellitus.

Netea RT, Elving LD, Lutterman JA, Thien Th. *J Intern Med* 2002; **251**: 393–9.

BACKGROUND. **World Health Organization (WHO) guidelines recommend that the BP should be routinely measured in sitting or supine followed by standing position, providing that the arm of the patient is placed at the level of the right atrium in each position.**

INTERPRETATION. The data from this study indicate that the WHO recommendation with regard to the equivalence of sitting and supine BP readings is incorrect at least in diabetic patients, as the sitting BP is lower than the supine BP when the arm was positioned at the right atrial level. In addition, incorrect positioning of the arm in a standing position results in an underestimation of prevalence of orthostatic hypotension. Therefore, during BP measurement the arm should be placed at the right atrial level regardless of the body position.

Comment

This is yet another study looking at how the ways we measured BP may significantly influence BP readings and thus may result in overdiagnosis and underdiagnosis of hypertension with its associated lack of appropriate treatment.

The aim of the present study was to test the effects of different body and arm positions on BP readings in diabetic patients. The following five positions that are often used in daily clinical practice were investigated in 142 diabetic patients: (i) sitting with the arms supported at the right atrial level; (ii) sitting with the arm supported on the arm support of the chair; (iii) lying on a bed; (iv) standing with the arm supported at the right atrial level; and (v) standing with the arm pending, parallel to the body. The average of the three readings for the BP and heart rate in both sitting and supine positions was considered as the representative value for the respective position. The right atrial level was estimated at the level of the mid-sternum. All measurements were performed by one trained observer, simultaneously at both arms, during each position using two specimens of the same semiautomated oscillometric devices. The study demonstrated that both SBP and DBP were significantly lower in the sitting position with the arm at the right atrial level than in the supine position (by 7.4 and 6.6 mmHg, respectively, $P < 0.01$). In sitting and standing positions, SBP and DBP were higher when the arm was placed either on the arm support of the chair or vertical, parallel to the body, than when the arm was supported at the level of the right atrium (by 6–10 mmHg, $P < 0.001$). It has been suggested that BP measurement after at least 2 min of standing would estimate more accurately the evidence of orthostatic hypotension. However, in this study the influence of the arm level in the standing position was more important than the duration of standing for the estimation of the BP response to orthostasis.

It seems that the lower the arm level with respect to the reference right atrial level, the higher the BP and vice versa. This suggests that hydrostatic rather than autonomic factors are responsible for these differences in BP measured with the arm at different levels. However, due to the study design, it is not known how much of the BP difference between the two arms at different levels is contributed by the actual inter-arm BP difference as demonstrated in the study by Lane *et al.* (2002).

None the less, as BP measurement is one of the most frequently performed clinical procedures, this and the study by Lane *et al.* support the urgent need to standardize BP measurement guidelines especially when conducting clinical trials on which most therapeutic decisions are based. Medical students, student nurses and other medical personnel should be taught to follow the standardized guidelines at an early stage of their medical education: BP should be measured with the arm placed at the right atrial level, regardless of the body position.

Comparison of acceptability of and preferences for different methods of measuring blood pressure in primary care.

Little P, Barnett J, Barnsley L, Marjoram J, Fitzgerald-Barron A, Mant D.
Br Med J 2002a; **325**(7358): 258–9.

BACKGROUND. **BP is probably the most common measurement used in clinical practice and the most common reason for the initiation of long-term treatment. Recent guidelines for the use of ABPM recommend its use in both initial diagnosis (before starting treatment) and assessing control. No study has yet explored the main issues for patients about the acceptability of the different methods of measuring BP or compared the acceptability of all the available methods.**

INTERPRETATION. Patients rated most methods as causing few problems and being worth the trouble to get accurate readings. Few patients regarded measurement by a doctor as the most acceptable method. Ambulatory monitoring performed less well than other methods, largely owing to discomfort and disturbance of life and sleep; there may be a trade-off between the accuracy of ambulatory monitoring and its acceptability. Overall, home measurements may be the most promising option, as they are the most acceptable method to patients and were preferred to either readings in the surgery or ambulatory monitoring.

Comparison of agreement between different measures of blood pressure in primary care and daytime ambulatory blood pressure.

Little P, Barnett J, Barnsley L, Marjoram J, Fitzgerald-Barron A, Mant D.
Br Med J 2002b; **325**(7358): 254–7.

BACKGROUND. **Six prospective studies have shown that ABPM may be a much better predictor of target organ damage and subsequent adverse events than measurements** made in a clinic. As these results were found in research studies and mostly not in typical primary care settings, however, patients may have had a higher 'alerting response' than in everyday settings with their family doctor or nurse. Further evidence is needed from typical primary care settings to explore the implications of using ambulatory pressures and other alternatives, both in the initiation of treatment and in monitoring controls.

INTERPRETATION. The 'white coat' effect is important in diagnosing and assessing the control of hypertension in primary care and is not a research artefact. If ambulatory or home measurements are not available, repeated measurements by the nurse or patient should result in considerably less unnecessary monitoring, initiation or changing of treatment. It is time to stop using high BP readings documented by general practitioners (GPs) to make treatment decisions.

Comment

This paper has clearly highlighted several uncertainties currently surrounding the issue of BP measurements by different methods, and its implications in daily clinical practice. In this study, 200 patients (54% women, 33% >65 years of age) with either newly diagnosed or borderline essential hypertension (96 patients) or established hypertension being treated but with poor control (104 patients) were recruited from three general practices in England. BPs were measured in all patients by repeated measurements by a nurse, by the patient at home, ambulatory monitoring, and measurement by a doctor. Interestingly, the final 70 patients also had their BP taken by themselves in a room at the GP practice. Overall agreement with the 24-hour ambulatory pressure, prediction of high ambulatory pressure (>135/85 mmHg) and treatment thresholds were assessed as outcome measures. The data showed that doctors' and recent BP readings in the clinic ranked worst in all three outcome measures when compared with repeated readings by nurse and repeated self-measurements by patients at the practice as well as at home. The authors concluded that BP measurements by the nurse or patients can be an alternative to ambulatory monitoring and that treatment decisions should not rely on high BP readings by the GPs.

There are several important points for discussion we can raise from this study:

1. It is important to realize that the assessment of cardiovascular risk attributable to high BP and the efficacy of antihypertensive therapies are based on BP measurements in the clinic, obtained by doctors and/or nurses in clinical trials or epidemiological studies.

2. Current advice regarding the treatment targets and thresholds of high blood pressure, published by the BHS, Joint National Committee (JNC-VI) and the WHO/ISH, are based on clinical studies using clinic readings |12–14|.

3. A number of studies have shown that ABPM is superior to clinic BP in the diagnostic and prognostic evaluation of hypertensive patients. In other words, the correlation between the BP level and target organ damage, cardiovascular risk and long-term prognosis is closer for ABPM than for clinical measurements |15|.

4. However, ABPM over a 24-hour span cannot be assumed as the gold standard in the assessment of a subject's BP and of the risk associated with high BP level |16|.

5. Multiple/repeated clinic BP measures may be as good as if not superior to ABPM in predicting risk |17,18|.

6. Morbidity or mortality outcome data to support ambulatory readings is still lacking in subgroup patients, such as those with diabetes mellitus or chronic renal failure.

7. The risk levels of an average BP done by the patient, nurse or ambulatory monitoring; at home or in clinic are different. Accordingly, our threshold for intervention and target levels have also been set differently for each method |12,19,20|.

8. There is no published evidence suggesting that ABPM has a greater predictive value for outcome than BP measured by the nurse or by the patient at home or in the clinic.

9. At present, it remains difficult to know which kind of measurement is closest to the measurements taken in clinical trials.

10. In terms of reproducibility, ABPM may be better than clinic BP. However, home BP seems to have superior reproducibility compared with both clinic BP and ABPM but at present the prognostic value of home BP remains largely unproved |21|. The reproducibility of BP measured by the nurse or by the patient in the clinic also remains unclear (see Stergiou *et al.* 2002, below).

11. 'White coat' hypertension can only be revealed by BP measured at home either by ambulatory machine or other validated devices when compared with a higher clinic BP. It should be noted that, however, 'white coat' hypertension may not necessarily be related to the true pressor response to BP measurements by a doctor, which was accurately quantified by having the patients on beat-to-beat prolonged BP monitoring |22|. Thus it should be more appropriately termed as 'isolated office hypertension', as indicated in the WHO/ISH Guidelines.

12. There is evidence indicated that 'white coat' hypertension or 'isolated office hypertension' is not a benign phenomenon and its risk seems to lie in between true hypertension and normotension |22–25|. More questions follow: At what level should we intervene? With what therapy, drug or psychotherapy? Would such treatment(s) alter the risk, etc.

13. Recent study indicates that home BP measurement may be able to predict 'white-coat' hypertension more precisely than does ABPM |26|.

As we are moving into the electronic era, more BP measuring electronic devices will be available to the public domain in addition to clinical use. Though many of these devices have not been subjected to scientific validation study, they are increasingly popular as reflected by their sale statistics. Indeed, more and more patients are bringing in their own BP readings chart to the clinic and would expect their physicians to know what these readings actually mean |5|.

There are many questions still unanswered regarding the values of self-measurement of BP at home or in the clinic and how it will be incorporated into patient management |5|. None the less, it is just a matter of time that these uncertainties would become clearer as more clinical studies are being carried out. Therefore we should welcome newer BP measurement methods as we welcomed ABPM when it was first introduced. Indeed, the values of ABPM in hypertension management are increasingly appreciated. As a matter of fact, many more BP measuring gadgets are here to stay; researchers and clinicians should continue to explore their roles in the management of hypertension, not to deny their existence. Interestingly, an earlier paper by Little *et al.* (2002a) demonstrated that self-measurement at home appears to be the most acceptable method to patients when compared with doctors' readings or ABPM.

However, we must caution against the conclusion by Little *et al.* (2002b) that 'It is time to stop using high BP readings documented by GPs to make treatment decisions' as from no part of their data can they infer such a dogmatic interpretation. Indeed, it is wrong to encourage clinicians to discard their sphygmomanometer or other BP measuring devices to nurses or patients. But, the best rational approach would perhaps be to 'calibrate' each patient's clinic readings taken on multiple occasions against their 24-hour ABPM readings or self-measurements at diagnosis, and set their treatment target accordingly.

Reproducibility of home, ambulatory, and clinic blood pressure: implications for the design of trials for the assessment of antihypertensive drug efficacy.

Stergiou GS, Baibas NM, Gantzarou AP, *et al. Am J Hypertens* 2002; **15**(2 Pt 1): 101–4.

BACKGROUND. Although clinic BP remains the reference method of measurement, it has several major drawbacks, including observer bias, white coat effect, and placebo effect, and therefore has limited reproducibility. Home BP monitoring is increasingly being used, and the accumulating evidence suggests it provides highly reproducible measurements free of the white coat and placebo effects.

INTERPRETATION. The study shows that home BP seems to have superior reproducibility compared with both clinic BP and ambulatory BP. In addition, home BP can improve the accuracy of antihypertensive drug trials, thereby reducing the sample size required.

Comment

The aims of this study were to compare the reproducibility of BP measured in the clinic, at home, and by ambulatory monitoring, and to assess its implications on the accuracy of antihypertensive drug trials. The study also has highlighted some of the points we have discussed in the previous paper. Indeed, high reproducibility of a particular measurement is important in assessing the efficacy of therapies over time in clinical trials |27,28|. Indeed, as has been pointed out by the authors in this regard, home BP has superior reproducibility over both clinic BP and ambulatory BP, and thus not only the efficacy of antihypertensive therapy would be more reliably assessed over time, the number of subjects needed for this to be reliably assessed is also comparatively smaller for home BP than clinic BP and ambulatory BP. Indeed, the results showed that home BP provided the lowest standard of deviation of differences values (6.9/4.7 mmHg, SBP/DBP, compared with 8.3/5.6 for ambulatory BP and 11.0/6.6 for clinic BP). For a parallel trial aiming to detect a difference in the effect of two drugs of 10 mmHg SBP, 51 subjects would be required when using clinic BP compared with 29 using ambulatory BP and 20 using home BP (73, 53 and 37 subjects, respectively, for the detection of a 5 mmHg difference in DBP). For a cross-over design, no more than 10 patients would be required |29|.

However, one possible bias for home BP is that a patient may voluntarily discard low or high home BP readings and therefore underestimate actual risk. This problem can easily be resolved by using validated memory-equipped devices that automatically store measurements. Another limitation with home BP is that its readings (measure with standardized posture, i.e. sitting for at least 5 min rest) may not actually relate to BP response to usual daily activities, which may be better assessed with ABPM that cannot only provide measurements during daily life stresses, at home, but also during sleep. Clinicians and researchers should bear these limitations in mind |30,31|.

An interesting finding of this study is the need for home BP monitoring on ≥2 days as the minimum schedule of measurements in order to provide a reliable estimate of the level of home BP. The readings recorded during the first day may be regarded as training.

Evaluation of the extent and duration of the 'ABPM effect' in hypertensive patients.

Hermida RC, Calvo C, Ayala DE, Fernandez JR, Ruilope LM, Lopez JE. *J Am Coll Cardiol* 2002; **40**(4): 710–17.

B ACKGROUND . The use of ABPM has provided a method of BP assessment that compensates for some of the limitations of office values. While a 'white-coat' pressor effect on conventional measurements has been defined and frequently used for the improved evaluation of hypertensive patients, there has been no clear indication that the ambulatory technique could also influence BP.

I NTERPRETATION . Ambulatory monitoring for 48 consecutive hours reveals a statistically significant pressor response that could reflect a novelty effect in the use of the monitoring device for the first time. This effect has marked implications in both research and clinical daily practice for a proper diagnosis of hypertension and evaluation of treatment efficacy by the use of ambulatory monitoring.

Comment

The 'white-coat' pressor effect associated with conventional clinic BP measured by doctors has been well defined |**32,33**|. It was recognized when the BPs measured in the clinic or office by the doctors are significantly higher than those measured by ABPM or patients at home, i.e. away from the stressful environment of the clinic setting. It is indeed interesting of this study to be able to demonstrate a statistically significant pressor effect associated with first time use of ABPM device at home. Importantly, subjects with 'white-coat' hypertension, according to the definitions provided by the JNC-VI and the WHO/ISH were not included in this study. Indeed, this 'ABPM pressor effect' could have marked implications in both research and clinical daily practice in view of the fact that definitions of 'normal' ABPM, ABPM criteria for diagnosis of hypertension and assessment of antihypertensive therapy have been established from data gathered with ABPM over 24 h |**34,35**|.

A large number of subjects, 538 (233 men and 305 women; age 54.2 ± 14.2 years, range, 22–88 years), with diagnoses of mild-to-moderate essential hypertension were recruited in this study. BP and heart rate were measured at 20-min intervals during the day and at 30-min intervals at night for 48 consecutive hours. The mean physical activity for the 5 min before each ABPM reading measured was also recorded simultaneously by a wrist actigraph. The data suggested a significant 'ABPM pressor effect'—for the first 4 h of measurement, both SBP and DBP were significantly increased by an average of 7 mmHg and 4 mmHg, respectively. Interestingly, such 'pressor or alerting reaction effect, possibly elicited by the monitoring device', was documented in about 73% of all hypertensive patients evaluated by 48-hour ABPM in this study, and remained as statistically significant for up to 9 h after patients start wearing the device. Intriguingly, the differences between consecutive days of ABPM were no longer significant when about 30% of the hypertensive patients were evaluated for the second or successive times, 3 months apart. Furthermore, this 'pressor response' to ABPM seems to be independent of any change in the physical activity pattern or any apparent modification in heart rate, as well as independent of possible confounding factors such as gender, days of the week of monitoring or number of antihypertensive drugs used by the treated patients.

In addition, it is also important to note that the nocturnal mean of BP was similar between both days of sampling, although the diurnal mean of SBP and DBP were significantly different. This is particularly relevant in the classification of patients into dippers and non-dippers with ABPM, in relation to target-organ damage |**36**|. Accordingly, the total number of non-dippers would be considerably higher when the classification is obtained on the basis of data sampled during the second day of ABPM as compared with the first in a 48-hour ABPM. The 'ABPM effect' could, thus, provide an underestimation of the real percentage of non-dippers among patients with mild-to-moderate hypertension when a 24-hour ABPM was used.

However, it is of note that a study by Parati *et al.* |**37**| have shown that, except for a short-lasting initial period, automatic ABPM do not trigger any alerting reaction and pressor response. In view of the increased use of 24-hour ABPM in the management of hypertensive patients, and the implications of the possible 'ABPM pressor effect', further study is needed in another population group in order to confirm or refute the phenomenon. Change in the guidelines for the use of 24-hour or 48-hour ABPM may then be recommended accordingly.

To stretch the hypothesis further, one may wonder: Are subjects with 'white-coat or in-office' hypertension or the 'ABPM effect' more anxious people? It has been shown that subjects with an anxiety trait are more at risk of cardiovascular disease. If so, subjects with white-coat hypertension (isolated office hypertension) or 'ABPM effect' may be at an intermediate cardiovascular risk as they are inherently more anxious relatively to those who are truly normotensives. Furthermore, the observation in those subjects with the so-called 'reverse white coat hypertension' (i.e. mean daytime 24-hour ABPM readings are higher than clinic or office BP) may well be due to the fact that we are seeing the 'pressor effect' in these individuals elicited only when they are wearing the ABPM device for the first time.

Inter-arm differences in blood pressure: when are they clinically significant?

Lane D, Beevers M, Barnes N, *et al. J Hypertens* 2002; **20**(6): 1089–95.

BACKGROUND. As hypertension is a modifiable risk factor, the accurate assessment of BP is vital for correct diagnostic and therapeutic decisions. The most recent guidelines for the management of hypertension by the BHS, the JNC-VI, and the WHO, make no mention of which arm to measure BP in or of inter-arm BP differences. However, earlier guidelines recommended that BP should be measured in both arms at the initial assessment of the patient and that if there is a difference, the arm with the higher pressure should be used for all future measurements.

INTERPRETATION. Significant differences in mean inter-arm SBP, and mean absolute inter-arm SBP and DBP are present. This emphasizes the importance of measuring BP in both arms initially to prevent this misdiagnosis of hypertension, due to normal differences in BP between the arms.

Comment

BP is routinely measured in daily clinical practice. Most clinicians have been taught since medical school that BP should be measured in both arms as a BP different of ≥20 mmHg could be a sign of an important anatomical abnormality such as coarctation, subclavian stenosis, dissection, etc., which requires further investigations. But these conditions are uncommon and only very few clinicians bother to measure BP from both arms routinely unless there is clinical suspicion. However, 'normal' inter-arm BP exists |**38**|.

The authors are to be praised for carrying out such rigorous clinical study to answer a simple yet important question of 'normal' inter-arm BP differences. Though the results were not a big surprise to many of us that BP readings are indeed

Table 7.6 Inter-arm differences in blood pressure

	0–5 mmHg	6–10 mmHg	11–15 mmHg	16–20 mmHg	>20 mmHg
Systolic	231	89	50	16	14
	57.8%	22.3%	12.5%	4.0%	3.5%
Diastolic	284	71	16	14	15
	71.0%	17.8%	4.0%	3.5%	3.8%

Reference: Eoin O'Brien, Gareth Beevers, and Gregory YH Lip. ABC of hypertension: Blood pressure measurement. *BMJ* 2001.
Source: Lane *et al.* (2002).

significantly different between the two arms, such findings emphasize the importance of measuring BP in both arms (especially during initial assessment) and further support continuation or resumption of the older practice of measuring BP from both arms. Such recommendation should be encouraged in clinical guidelines as we base our diagnosis, therapeutic target, conclusions of clinical trials and even health economics on BP values, we should get the basics right and be consistent.

The methodology of this study is indeed rigorous. In order to be able to identify a small but statistically significant inter-arm BP difference and to have a reliable estimate of the phenomenon and to seek factors that might be linked to it, the authors recruited a sufficiently large sample size (200 men and 200 women, aged 18–92 years) and a mixed population (of whom 20% had a history of hypertension and 15% were diabetic). Two sets of bilateral simultaneous BP measurements were obtained using two validated automatic brand new Omron HEM-705CP devices and thus observer biases were minimized. Swapping of the devices between series also avoided machine bias and reduced any variability inherent in the equipment. The relative and absolute differences in values of BP measured from the right and left arms were analysed.

The results showed significant mean inter-arm SBP differences, with higher SBPs (1.81 ± 8.6 mmHg, $P < 0.0001$) but not DBPs in the right arm compared with the left. This variation in mean inter-arm BP was unrelated to age, sex, ethnicity, arm circumference, handedness, being hypertensive, diabetic or previous history of cardiovascular disease. However, this study only included 10% of left-handed individuals and could not assess whether lateral dominance was the main factor for the difference between right and left arms. The authors did find that BP was higher in the right arm in the 361 right-handed subjects with no significance difference between the two arms in the 39 left-handed subjects. Of greater significance is the absolute difference in value between the two arms, in both SBP (6.32 ± 6.12 mmHg, $P < 0.0001$) and DBP (5.06 ± 6.57 mmHg, $P < 0.0001$). Clinically significant inter-arm differences in SBP of >10 and >20 mmHg were found in 20 and 3.5%, respectively; diastolic differences of >10 and >20 mmHg were present in 11 and 3.5%, respectively. Age was the only significant predictor of clinically significant variations in inter-arm BPs and mean absolute BP differences. Certainly it is possible that the 3% of patients with a difference of more than 20 mmHg between arms had unrecognized arterial disease that should prompt clinicians to investigate further. As in other studies that have investigated inter-arm BP differences, no diagnostic tools such as angiography or radiological imaging was used in this study to exclude anatomical anomalies or congenital causes of disparity in BP as possible explanations for inter-arm differences in BP.

Conclusion

BP is a dynamic, multidimensional, cardiovascular indicator of a person's state, but the well-established cardiovascular risk associated with BP has been derived from many epidemiological studies that only included one or two BP measurements obtained in the clinic. The advent of 24-hour ABPM has enabled us to fine-tune individual BP profiles and thus associated risk. However, the interpretations of ABPM data require physician attention and thus limit its accessibility to a wider general population. ABPM further allows stratification of BP profiles, such as 'white-coat hypertension' and 'non-dipping nocturnal BP' states, which have yet to establish their associated cardiovascular risk.

Automatic devices are increasingly used in the hospital and clinic as well as at home. It appears that these devices are gradually replacing the traditional mercury-based sphygmomanometer. Most clinical studies now use automatic devices and many have been clinically validated according to strict criteria. However, many of these devices are now increasingly affordable and used at home as health consciousness improves. Devices that measure arterial pressure at the wrist or even finger are increasingly popular due to their portability and comfort, although many of these devices have not been properly validated and most failed to meet the validation criteria. Despite these facts, home BP measurements may soon be integrated into hypertension management in the clinic.

References

1. O'Brien E, Petrie J, Littler WA, de Swiet M, Padfield PL, Altman D, *et al.* The British Hypertension Society protocol for the evaluation of blood pressure measuring devices. *J Hypertens* 1993; **11**(Suppl. 2): S43–63.

2. Association for the Advancement of Medical Instrumentation. American national standard. Electronic or automated sphygmomanometers. ANSI/AAMI SP 10-1992. Arlington, VA. AAMI 1993: 40.

3. O'Brien E, Atkins N. A comparison of the BHS and AAMI protocols for validating blood pressure measuring devices: can the two be reconciled? *J Hypertens* 1994; **12**: 1089–94.

4. Canzanello VJ, Jensen PL, Schwartz GL. Are aneroid sphygmomanometers accurate in hospital and clinic settings? *Arch Intern Med* 2001; **161**: 729–31.

5. Asmar R, Zanchetti A. Guideline for the use of self-blood pressure monitoring: a summary report of the first international conference. *J Hypertens* 2000; **18**: 493–508.

6. Eckert S, Gleichmann U, Zagorski O, Klapp A. A validation of the Omron R3 blood pressure self-measuring device through simultaneous comparative invasive measurements according to protocol 58130 of the German Institute for validation. *Blood Press Monit* 1997; **2**: 189–92.

7. O'Brien E, Petric J, Littler WA, deSwiet M, Padfied PL, O'Malley K *et al.* The British Hypertension Society Protocol for the evaluation of automated and semi-automated blood pressure measuring devices with special reference to ambulatory systems. *J Hypertens* 1990; **8**: 607–19.

8. AAMI. American national standard. Electronic or automated sphygmomanometers. ANSI/AAMI SP 10-1992. Arlington, VA: AAMI, 1993: 40.

9. O'Brien E, Mee F, Atkins N, *et al.* Evaluation of three devices for self-measurement of blood pressure: according to the revised British Hypertension Society protocol: the Omron HEM-705CP, Phillips HP5332, and Nissei DS-175. *Blood Press Monit* 1996; **1**: 55–61.

10. Markandu ND, Whitcher F, Arnold A, Carney C. The mercury sphygmomanometer should be abandoned before it is proscribed. *J Hum Hypertens* 2000; **14**: 31–6.

11. O'Brien E. Replacing the mercury sphygmomanometer. *Br Med J* 2000; **320**: 815–16.

12. Ramsay L, Williams B, Johnston G, MacGregor G, Poston L, Potter J *et al.* Guidelines for management of hypertension: report of the third working party of the British Hypertension Society. *J of Hum Hypertens* 1999; **13**: 569–92.

13. Joint National Committee on Prevention, Detection, Evaluation, and Treatment of High Blood Pressure, The sixth report of the Joint National Committee on Prevention, Detection, Evaluation, and Treatment of High Blood Pressure. *Arch Intern Med* 1997; **157**: 2413–46.

14. Guidelines Subcommittee, 1999 World Health Organization–International Society of Hypertension guidelines for the management of hypertension. *J Hypertens* 1999; **17**: 151–83.

15. Verdecchia P. Prognostic value of ambulatory blood pressure current evidence and clinical implications. *Hypertension* 2000; **35**: 844–51.

16. O'Brien E, Coats A, Owens P, Petrie J, Padfield PL, Littler WA *et al.* Use and interpretation of ambulatory blood pressure monitoring: recommendations of the British Hypertension Society. *Br Med J* 2000; **320**: 1128–34.

17. Fagard R, Staessen J, Thijs L. Prediction of cardiac structure and function by repeated clinic and ambulatory blood pressure. *Hypertension* 1997; **29**: 22–9.

18. Jula A, Puukka P, Karanko H. Multiple clinic and home blood pressure measurements versus ambulatory blood pressure monitoring. *Hypertension* 1999; **34**: 261–6.

19. Staessen JA, Thijs L. Development of diagnostic thresholds for automated self-measurement of blood pressure in adults. First International Consensus Conference on Blood pressure Self-Measurement. *Blood Press Monit* 2000; **5**(2): 101–9.

20. Pickering TG. What is the 'normal' 24 h, awake, and asleep blood pressure? *Blood Press Monit* 1999; **4**(Suppl. 2): S3–7.

21. Ohkubo T, Imai Y, Tsuji I, Nagai K, Kato J, Kikuchi N *et al*. Home blood pressure measurement has a stronger predictive power for mortality than does screening blood pressure measurement: a population-based observation in Ohasama, Japan. *J Hypertens* 1998; **16**: 971–5.

22. Parati G, Ulian L, Santucciu C, Omboni S, Mancia G. Difference between clinic and daytime blood pressure is not a measure of the white coat effect. *Hypertension* 1998; **31**: 1185–9.

23. Grandi AM, Broggi R, Colombo S, Santillo R, Imperiale D, Bertolini A, Guasti L, Venco A. Left ventricular changes in isolated office hypertension: a blood pressure-matched comparison with normotension and sustained hypertension. *Arch Intern Med* 2001 Dec 10–24; **161**(22): 2677–81.

24. Sega R, Trocino G, Lanzarotti A, Carugo S, Cesana G, Schiavina R, Valagussa F, Bombelli M, Giannattasio C, Zanchetti A, Mancia G. Alterations of cardiac structure in patients with isolated office, ambulatory, or home hypertension: data from the general population (Pressione Arteriose Monitorate E Loro Associazioni [PAMELA] Study). *Circulation* 2001 Sep 8; **104**(12): 1385–92.

25. Muscholl M, Hense H, Brockel U, Doring A, Riegger GHS. Changes in left ventricular structure and function in patients with white coat hypertension: cross sectional survey. *Br Med J* 1998; **317**: 565–70.

26. Palatini P. Too much of a good thing? A critique of overemphasis on the use of ambulatory blood pressure monitoring in clinical practice. *J Hypertens* 2002 Oct; **20**(10); 1917–23.

27. Coats AJ. Benefits of ambulatory blood pressure monitoring in the design of antihypertensive drug trials. *Blood Press Monit* 1996; **1**: 157–60.

28. Trazzi S, Mutti E, Frattola A, Imholz B, Parati G, Mancia G. Reproducibility of noninvasive and intra-arterial blood pressure monitoring. Implications for studies on antihypertensive treatment. *J Hypertens* 1991; **9**: 115–19.

29. Mengden T, Bättig B, Vetter W. Self-measurement of blood pressure improves the accuracy and reduces the number of subjects in clinical trials. *J Hypertens* 1991; **9**(Suppl. 6): S336–7.

30. Mengden T, Schwartzkopff B, Strauer BE. What is the value of home (self) blood pressure monitoring in patients with hypertensive heart disease? *Am J Hypertens* 1998; **11**: 813–19.

31. Mengden T, Medina RMH, Alvarez E, Kraft K, Vetter H. Reliability of reporting self-measured blood pressure values by hypertensive patients. *Am J Hypertens* 1998; **11**: 1413–17.

32. Pickering TG. White coat hypertension. In: Laragh JH, Brenner BM, eds. *Hypertension: Pathophysiology, Diagnosis and Management*. New York: Raven Press, 1995; 1913–27.

33. O'Brien E. White coat hypertension: how should it be diagnosed? *J Hum Hypertens* 1999; **13**: 801–2.

34. O'Brien E, Staessen J. Normotension and hypertension as defined by 24-hour ambulatory blood pressure monitoring. *Blood Press* 1995; **4**: 266–82.

35. Staessen JA, Thijs L. Development of diagnostic thresholds for automated self-measurement of blood pressure in adults. First International Consensus Conference on Blood pressure Self-Measurement. *Blood Press Monit* 2000; **5**(2): 101–9.

36. Mochizuki Y, Okutani M, Donfeng Y *et al*. Limited reproducibility of circadian variation in blood pressure dippers and nondippers. *Am J Hypertens* 1998; **11**: 403–9.

37. Parati G, Pomidossi G, Casadei R, Mancia G. Absence of alarm reactions with use of non-invasive blood pressure monitoring devices. *Clin Exp Hypertens* 1983; **1** (Suppl. 2): 299–301.

38. O'Brien E, Beevers G, Lip YH. ABC of hypertension: Blood pressure measurement. Part III – automated sphygmomanometry: ambulatory blood pressure measurement. *Br Med J* 2001 May 5; **322**(7294): 1110–14.

8

High-normal blood pressure, to treat or not to treat? . . . and the J-curve

Introduction

What should the target blood pressure (BP) be when treating hypertensives? What about patients with high-normal BP, as defined in guidelines, such as the Joint National Committee (JNC)-VI? Certainly, many studies have shown beyond doubt that a reduction of BP in hypertensive populations significantly reduces the incidence of cardiovascular mortality and morbidity. In high-risk populations, such as those with diabetes mellitus or evidence of hypertensive target organ damage, recommended target BP levels should be well below 130/80mmHg. There is some controversy as to what the target BP should be, although recent large clinical trials have tried to address this point.

Some people advocate aggressive BP control with the BP lowered to the lowest tolerated level in order to achieve maximal cardiovascular protection. Others are more conservative in their approach and are concerned that too vigorous lowering of the BP may be associated with increased cardiovascular mortality and morbidity, the so-called J-curve.

We would expect that a stage must be reached beyond which further lowering of the BP will not reduce morbidity and mortality. Instead, hypotension may even harm the patient by compromising the perfusion of vital organs. The question is, therefore, not 'to lower or not to lower' but rather 'how low should we go' with regard to BP. Certainly, this goes well with the concept that hypertension can be defined as that level of BP above which treatment does more good than harm.

One million adults' blood pressures ... the lower the better?

 Age-specific relevance of usual blood pressure to vascular mortality: a meta-analysis of individual data for one million adults in 61 prospective studies.
Prospective Studies Collaboration. *Lancet* 2002; **360**: 1903–13.

BACKGROUND. The age-specific relevance of BP to cause-specific mortality is best assessed by collaborative meta-analysis of individual participant data from the separate prospective studies.

INTERPRETATION. Throughout middle and old age, 'usual BP' is strongly and directly related to vascular (and overall) mortality, without any evidence of a threshold down to at least 115/75 mmHg.

Comment

This collaborative meta-analysis combined data from 61 prospective observational studies of BP and mortality, which involved data from as many as 1 million individuals aged 40–89 years without known vascular disease at baseline, 70% from Europe, 20% from North America and Australasia, and 10% from China and Japan. During 12.7 million person-years at risk, there were about 120 000 deaths occurred: 56 000 vascular deaths (12 000 stroke, 34 000 ischaemic heart disease [IHD], 10 000 other vascular) and 66 000 other deaths. The primary risk factors for this meta-analysis are age, and the systolic BP (SBP) and diastolic BP (DBP). The data showed that BP was strongly related to the age-specific risk of death from cardiovascular causes throughout the so-called 'normal range' (i.e. down to a pressure of 115 mmHg systolic and 75 mmHg diastolic); with the mortality rates from IHD almost as strong as the mortality rates from stroke. For example, at ages 40–69 years, each BP difference of 20 mmHg systolic or 10 mmHg diastolic was associated with more than a twofold difference in the stroke death rate and with twofold differences in the death rates from IHD and from other vascular causes. Importantly, all of these proportional differences in vascular mortality are about half as extreme at ages 80–89 years as at ages 40–49 years, but the annual absolute differences in risk are greater in old age.

The present collaborative meta-analysis differs from previous meta-analyses in several ways that increase its reliability and informativeness:

1. It is large, involving 120 000 deaths among 1 million participants in 61 prospective observational studies of BP and mortality and including parallel analyses of the Multiple Risk Factor Intervention Trial (MRFIT) observational study that involves a further 17 000 vascular deaths.

2. Individual records are available for each of the participants in each study, allowing detailed analyses.

3. Individuals with recorded history of stroke or heart disease were excluded, 'limiting any effects of disease on BP' (i.e. avoiding 'reverse causality').

4. Cause-specific mortality data, together with age at death, are generally available.

5. Information on 286 000 repeat measurements made during prolonged follow-up allows an appropriate time-dependent correction for 'regression dilution'. Measurement error, short-term biological variability (including both transient fluctuations and any diurnal or seasonal variation), or longer-term within-person fluctuations or trends in risk factor values (which may occur for several reasons, including physical activity, diet, treatment, disease or age) may contribute to the 'time-dependent regression dilution effect'.

The age-specific and sex-specific relevance of the 'usual BP' to the subsequent rates of death from stroke, IHD, other vascular causes, and the aggregate of all non-vascular causes were presented. The main analyses are age-specific, and are of cause-specific death rates during five decades of age at risk (40–49, 50–59, . . ., 80–89 years) (see Tables 8.1 and 8.2).

In general, a 20 mmHg difference in usual SBP is approximately equivalent in its hazards to a 10 mmHg difference in usual DBP. The relationship with vascular mortality risk throughout the so-called 'normal range' of usual BP is continuous, with no

Table 8.1 Hazard ratios for stroke mortality for 20 mmHg lower usual SBP

Age at risk	Hazard ratios
40–49	0.36
50–59	0.38
60–69	0.43
70–79	0.50
80–89	0.67

Source: Prospective Studies Collaboration (2002).

Table 8.2 Hazard ratios for IHD mortality for 20 mmHg lower usual SBP

Age at risk	Hazard ratios
40–49	0.49
50–59	0.50
60–69	0.54
70–79	0.60
80–89	0.67

Source: Prospective Studies Collaboration (2002).

evidence of a threshold down to at least 115 mmHg/75 mmHg (below which there is little evidence). Indeed, the data showed that the vascular mortality rates are only about half as great at 120 as at 140 mmHg usual SBP, with no apparent net adverse effect on non-vascular mortality (i.e. the absence of the so-called 'J-curve' relationship between BP and mortality at the lower end of usual BP). SBP has the most predictive value for vascular death irrespective of age, if only one single measurement of BP is to be used to predict risk.

The proportional differences in vascular death associated with a given difference in BP is greater in middle age than in old age, but the absolute annual differences in vascular mortality are greater at older ages than in middle age because of their higher absolute risk of developing a cardiovascular event. There was no difference between the sexes for age-specific proportional differences in vascular mortality.

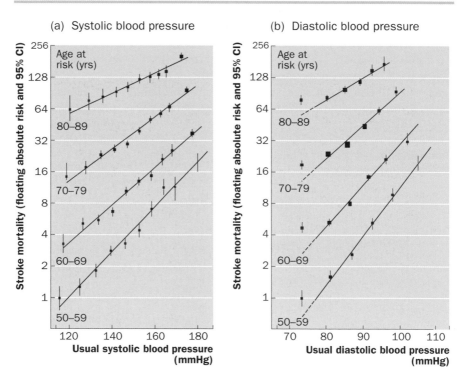

Fig. 8.1 Stroke mortality rate in each decade of age vs usual BP at the start of that decade. Rates are plotted on a floating absolute scale, and each square has area inversely proportional to the effective variance of the log mortality rate. For DBP, each age-specific regression line ignores the left-hand point (i.e. at slightly less than 75 mmHg), for which the risk lies significantly above the fitted regression line (as indicated by the broken line below 75 mmHg). Source: Prospective Studies Collaboration (2002).

Given the continuous relationship observed between BP and risk of death from vascular disease among individuals without known vascular disease at baseline, the absolute benefits of a lower BP level are likely to be greatest for those at greatest absolute risk of vascular disease, i.e. patients aged 70 years or more, and in those with pre-existing cardiovascular diseases (CVD). Hence, the authors advocated that BP-lowering treatment should be considered for a wide range of patients with evidence of vascular disease, regardless of their BP category. As have been demonstrated in previous meta-analyses of randomized trials of just a few years of BP lowering, a 10 mmHg lower usual SBP or 5 mmHg lower usual DBP would, in the long term, be associated with about 40% lower risk of stroke death and about 30% lower risk of death from IHD or other vascular causes throughout middle age with only slightly smaller proportional differences at older ages.

In relatively healthy populations included in the present analysis, the relationship between BP and events seems to be linear: lower BP is better. However, the extrapolation from the present data (of individuals without known vascular disease at baseline) to patients with CVD, especially to those ≥80 years of age requires caution

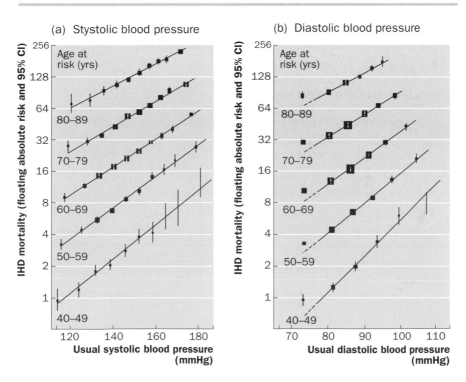

Fig. 8.2 IHD mortality rate in each decade of age vs usual BP at the start of that decade. Conventions as in fig. 8.1. Source: Prospective Studies Collaboration (2002).

as there is evidence to support that the relationship between BP and adverse events is not linear at the lower end of the curve. In older populations and in those with a prevalence of CVD, there is evidence that reducing DBP below a level of 80–85 mmHg is associated with increased risk of cardiovascular end-points and all-cause mortality, i.e. J-shaped relationship.

Nevertheless, in the present meta-analysis a 2 mmHg lower than usual SBP would involve about 10% lower stroke mortality and about 7% lower mortality from IHD or other vascular causes in middle age. These findings have important public health implications especially in places that have relatively high stroke rates (such as northern China) or high IHD rates (such as eastern Europe). Indeed, because of the large number of individuals within the stages currently classified as 'normotensive stages' according to the JNC-VI and WHO/ISH guidelines, 'high-normal' BP and 'stage 1 hypertension' have the highest population-attributable risk for future CVD. Indeed, as highlighted in the next article, recent analysis of the Framingham data have reinforced the clear gradations of risk within the 'normotensive' range, with definite stepwise increases in the risk of CVD as the BP increases from 'optimal' to 'normal' to 'high-normal' using the WHO/ISH and JNC-VI definitions.

High-normal blood pressure and cardiovascular risk

Impact of high-normal blood pressure on the risk of cardiovascular disease.
Vasan RS, Larson MG, Leip EP, *et al. N Engl J Med* 2001; **345**(18): 1291–7.

BACKGROUND. Information is limited regarding the risk of CVD in persons with high-normal BP (SBP of 130–139 mmHg, DBP of 85–89 mmHg, or both).

INTERPRETATION. High-normal BP is associated with an increased risk of CVD. The findings emphasize the need to determine whether lowering high-normal BP can reduce the risk of CVD.

Comment

This study investigated the association between BP category at baseline and the incidence of CVD on an average follow-up of 11.1 years among 6859 participants in the Framingham Heart Study who were initially free of hypertension and CVD.

When compared with optimal BP, high-normal BP was associated with an adjusted hazard ratio for CVD of 2.5 in women and 1.6 in men. The association between high-normal BP and increased risk of CVD was particularly strong in elderly patients aged over 65. A stepwise increase in cardiovascular event rates was noted across the three non-hypertensive BP categories: optimal, normal and high-normal. Hence, the

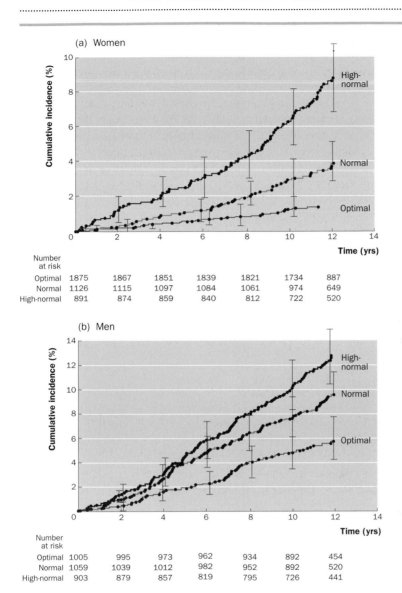

Fig. 8.3 Cumulative incidence of cardiovascular events in women (panel a) and men (panel b) without hypertension, according to BP category at the baseline examination. Vertical bars indicate 95% confidence intervals (CI). Optimal BP is a systolic pressure of less than 120 mmHg and a diastolic pressure of less than 80 mmHg. Normal BP is a systolic pressure of 120–129 mmHg or a diastolic pressure of 80–84 mmHg. High-normal BP is a systolic pressure of 130–139 mmHg or a diastolic pressure of 85–89 mmHg. If the SBP and DBP readings for a subject were in different categories, the higher of the two categories was used. Source: Vasan *et al.* (2001).

number of people at risk of hypertensive cardiovascular events is much higher than previously thought.

Such findings were really not unexpected as high-normal BP has been associated with altered cardiac morphological features, an increased thickness of the carotid intima and media and diastolic ventricular dysfunction or left ventricular hypertrophy |1–4|, all of which may be precursors of cardiovascular events. Indeed, the accompanied editorial has postulated impaired endothelial function as another possible mechanism. However, further large clinical trials are needed to determine whether lowering BP (non-pharmacological measures or drugs) in this category will actually reduce the risk of CVD and whether such treatment would be cost-effective in patients with no pre-existing CVD.

Should we treat high-normal blood pressure?
Yeo KR, Yeo WW. *J Hypertens* 2002; **20**(10): 2057–62.

BACKGROUND. To examine the risk of CVD associated with high-normal BP in English adults and estimate the proportion of these individuals who are at high cardiovascular risk.

INTERPRETATION. The findings of this study support the view that individuals with high-normal BP are at high risk for CVD should be targeted for BP-lowering treatment.

Comment

A number of risk factors for coronary atherosclerosis have been identified and interventions have been established that reduce the risk of subsequent coronary heart disease (CHD) events. Treatment of many CHD risk factors is feasible and effective, but these treatments are associated with side-effects, adverse events, and significant cost to both the individual patient and society in general. In this regard, cost–benefit and risk–benefit ratios are dependent on estimates of the absolute risk of CHD events. For example, the National Cholesterol Education Program has issued guidelines for the treatment of hyperlipidaemia that define three strata of CHD risk and use these strata to guide the intensity of therapy.

Whereas the impact of individual CHD risk factors is well documented, accurate estimation of multivariable absolute risk is more difficult. Several prediction models have been developed to generate coronary score sheets and other tools for the estimation of CHD risk in healthy subjects with measurable risk factors. Estimates of absolute CHD risk are most commonly based on risk prediction models derived from prospective, observational databases such as the Framingham Heart Study. The Framingham investigators have developed prediction algorithms that use risk factor categories. These algorithms are derived from a study sample of 2489 males and 2856 females aged 30–74 years at the time of their initial examination (1971–74). They have been adapted to create simplified score sheets that allow physicians to estimate multivariable absolute CHD risk in middle-aged subjects. The Framingham model uses age, sex, low-density lipoprotein cholesterol or total cholesterol, high-density lipoprotein cholesterol, SBP and DBP, the presence or absence of diabetes mellitus, and smoking status to predict the 10-year risk of CHD events. The European Society of Cardiology (ESC) has also issued separate recommendations in the form of a risk chart based on the Framingham model, with the β coefficients derived from this observational database. The European coronary risk chart uses total cholesterol for the estimation of risk, and assumes a high-density lipoprotein cholesterol of 1.0 mmol/L (39 mg/dL).

The meta-analysis from the Prospective Studies Collaboration (2002, see above) has not only confirmed that there is a continuous relationship with risk throughout the normal range of usual BP (down at least as far as 115/75 mmHg), they have also demonstrated that within this range the usual BP is even more strongly related to vascular mortality than had previously been supposed. Vasan *et al.* (2001, see above) have showed us data from the Framingham Heart Study that individuals with high-normal BP have significantly greater cardiovascular event rates as well as about five to 12 times more likely to progress to hypertension (SBP ≥140 mmHg or DBP ≥90 mmHg) over 4 years of monitoring, than were those with optimal BP (Vasan *et al.* 2001, see above).

The present study is timely, designed for the risk of CVD in adults with high-normal BP and explored whether these individuals should be offered BP-lowering treatment. The data were extracted from the 1998 cross-sectional Health Survey for England and analysis was restricted to a nationally representative sample of 12 341 individuals (with valid BP measurements) aged 18–80 years living in private households in England. The Framingham equation was used to estimate 10-year cardiovascular risk in the categories of mild hypertension, high-normal pressure and normal pressure. The main outcome measure was the percentage of individuals with high-normal BP who have CVD, diabetes mellitus or a 10-year cardiovascular event risk of at least 20%. Of the 12 341 participants, 2413 (19.6%) had high-normal BP. About 5.3% of these individuals with high-normal BP had CVD or diabetes, and a further 7.6% were at a predicted cardiovascular event risk of at least 20% over 10 years. The mean predicted risk was 8.7% for men and 6.3% for women in the high-normal BP category. Among men aged 61–80 years in the present study, the mean cardiovascular risk associated with high-normal BP was 28.5% and the majority of men were at a predicted cardiovascular event risk ≥20% over 10 years. For women aged 61–80 years with high-normal BP, the mean cardiovascular risk approached this threshold. This would suggest that patients in this age range would benefit from BP lowering to reduce cardiovascular risk, irrespective of their BP category.

When BP 140/90 mmHg is used as a screening threshold for primary prevention, about 29% of men and 21% of women at high cardiovascular risk (Table 8.3) would be missed from antihypertensive treatment. Furthermore, when extending the current British Hypertension Society recommendation on antihypertensive treatment to these individuals with high-normal BP who are at high cardiovascular risk, it was estimated that an additional 2.5% (on top of the 22.5%) of the English population aged 18–80 years would require treatment.

Table 8.3 Sensitivity, specificity and positive and negative predictive values (95% confidence intervals) for using blood pressure to predict risk of cardiovascular disease of 20% over 10 years in men and women aged 35–80 years

	Men ($n = 1402$)	Women ($n = 1149$)
Sensitivity	71 (66 to 75)	79 (73 to 85)
Specificity	54 (51 to 57)	57 (54 to 60)
Positive predictive value	46 (43 to 50)	25 (22 to 29)
Negative predictive value	77 (74 to 80)	94 (92 to 96)

Source: Yeo and Yeo (2002).

It is interesting that the authors used cholesterol-lowering treatment as an analogy to the current controversy as to whether patients with high-normal BP should receive treatment. Indeed, instead of targeting lipid-lowering statins to those with vascular disease and total cholesterol level ≥5 mmol/L, the Heart Protection Study has demonstrated that all high-risk patients aged 40–80 years with total cholesterol as low as 3.5 mmol/L (normal cholesterol range) could benefit from statin treatment to reduce their overall cardiovascular risk. In parallel to the recommendation of change of treatment guidelines for cholesterol lowering in high-risk patients, BP lowering treatment should be recommended to patients with vascular disease and high-normal BP, or may be even normal BP (i.e. irrespective of their initial BP category). Perhaps, two studies involving the use of antihypertensive drugs, namely the Heart Outcomes Prevention Evaluation (HOPE) study and the Perindopril Protection Against Recurrent Stroke Study (PROGRESS), have demonstrated a significant benefit in terms of cardiovascular event reduction by targeting high risk rather than high BP *per se*.

It should be noted that, however, although the baseline BP in the HOPE study was normal—139/79 mmHg—in the overall population, a history of hypertension was present in almost 50% of the study population, i.e. their background cardiovascular risk was probably much higher than those with only high-normal BP but never been categorized as frank hypertension before. Furthermore, the HOPE study was not designed to be a hypertension trial and the frequency with which BP readings were obtained makes it difficult to interpret the observed BP differences. Similarly, in PROGRESS, although both hypertensive and 'non-hypertensive' patients had similar reductions in their risk of stroke with active treatment of both perindopril and indapamide (BP was reduced by 12/5 mmHg), single-drug therapy with perindopril alone (BP reduced by 5/3 mmHg), did not lead to a reduction in the risk of stroke. This observation has generated some controversy, as a 5 mmHg reduction in SBP should translate into an approximate 20% reduction in stroke risk. Admittedly, some interesting questions have been raised as to whether the benefits in both of these studies were linked entirely to BP lowering or to some other property of the active drugs.

Therefore, there is so far no strong evidence that lowering BP will reduce the risk of CVD in this high-normal BP category. However, given the high population attributable risk for future cardiovascular events and the substantial difference in the risk of cardiovascular events between persons with high-normal BP and those with optimal BP, outcome studies designed to answer this question are feasible. Indeed, a radical change to a risk-based approach will be justified only when there are outcome trials showing it is a better way of targeting treatment than using BP thresholds alone.

Although there is a continuum of cardiovascular risk across levels of BP (a continuous variable), the classification of adults according to BP categories (into discrete variable) provides a framework for differentiating levels of risk associated with various BP categories and for defining treatment thresholds and therapeutic goals, especially in high-risk individuals for CVD, such as elderly persons or those with diabetes mellitus or multiple risk factors but has not yet had an event. Thus, the concept of total risk assessment advocated in the New Zealand guidelines, the Joint European Societies' guidelines and the 1999 WHO/ISH guidelines for the management of hypertension and CHD prevention.

The linearity of risk associated with BP may be affected by the presence of other cardiovascular risk factors or even antihypertensive drugs. Hence, individuals can move from one category to the other with time. For most patients, high BP (and certainly high-normal BP) is not a disease but, rather, one of many risk factors for the development of disease. Physicians should consider the absolute risk of a cardiovascular event (and therefore the potential benefit from therapy) on an individual basis.

The J- or U-shaped tails ... the debates continue

 ### J-shaped relationship between blood pressure and mortality in hypertensive patients: new insights from a meta-analysis of individual-patient data.
Boutitie F, Gueyffier F, Pocock S, Fagard R, Boissel JP; INDANA Project Steering Committee. INdividual Data ANalysis of Antihypertensive intervention. *Ann Intern Med* 2002; **136**(6): 438–48.

BACKGROUND. Population-based longitudinal studies of hypertension have usually shown a continuous and positive relationship between BP and mortality. However, several studies in hypertensive patients receiving treatment have described this relationship as J-shaped, with an increased risk for events in patients with low BP.

INTERPRETATION. The increased risk for events observed in patients with low BP was not related to antihypertensive treatment and was not specific to BP-related events. Poor health conditions leading to low BP and an increased risk for death probably explain the J-shaped curve.

Comment

It may be naive to believe that 'the lower the BP the better the outcome' for most hypertensive individuals. The J-curve phenomenon (i.e. that a BP threshold exists below which there is an increase in the rate of cardiovascular events) in the relationship between BP and cardiovascular morbidity and mortality has long been debated over 20 years. The linearity of the BP and mortality curve may be influenced by the presence of risk factors (cardiovascular or non-cardiovascular) or antihypertensive treatments, especially at the lower end of the log-linear curve. Indeed, many have suspected that the existence of a J-shaped relationship between BP and risk is related to antihypertensive treatment, in which overtreated patients with low BP are at increased risk for cardiovascular and total death, particularly in the very elderly individuals and in patients with previous stroke or myocardial infarction or in the presence of comorbid conditions. Low BP may cause vital organ underperfusion, especially during the diastolic phase, and may lead to cerebral or cardiac ischaemia. Elderly individuals are more prone to postural hypotension, and may lead to non-cardiovascular death. One might also argue that the rate of BP lowering by anti-hypertensive drugs could have a significant influence on the continuous log-linear relationship.

The INDANA (INdividual Data ANalysis of Antihypertensive intervention trials) project is a meta-analysis of individual patient data collected from seven randomized clinical trials of antihypertensive medication vs placebo or no intervention, with follow-up for cardiovascular events and deaths. As the study allows assessment of the evolution of risk according to achieved BP separately of both treated and untreated (controls) hypertensive patients who were subjected to the same randomization process, INDANA indeed is in a better position than has previously been possible to explore the J-curve phenomenon, especially on the issue of whether antihypertensive treatment alters the relationship at the lower BP stratum.

Data from five randomized clinical trials in 40 233 elderly (treated or control) hypertensive patients were included in the present meta-analysis. To make the results more robust, the study only focused on fatal events (both cardiovascular and non-cardiovascular death) in yearly periods of follow-up (mean follow-up, 3.9 years); 1655 participants died during the follow-up period (56% cardiovascular).

On average, patients in the treated group had a lower DBP than that of the control group. A J-shaped relationship between DBP and risk for death was observed for total and cardiovascular mortality in both treated patients (nadir, 84 and 80 mmHg, respectively) and untreated patients (nadir, 90 and 85 mmHg, respectively), and thus appears to be independent of treatment. However, there was no significant increased risk for cardiovascular death with low SBP in treated patients. For non-cardio-vascular deaths, the relationship was J-shaped in the treated group (nadir, 84 mmHg) and negative in the control group. Similar results were observed for SBP. Results remained unchanged when patients with non-fatal CHD during follow-up or those with a history of myocardial infarction were excluded. Interestingly, the magnitude of decrease in DBP from baseline did not influence the overall finding that the risk for death was increased in patients with a lower achieved DBP. The presence of patients with wide pulse pressure also did not explain these findings, thus the observed increased events are unlikely to be related to increased stiffness of arteries and atherosclerosis.

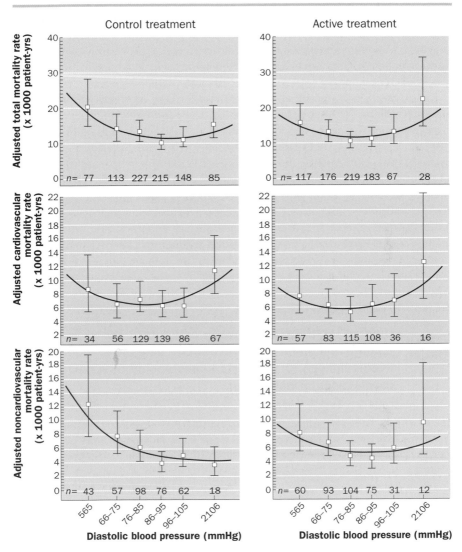

Fig. 8.4 Age- and sex-adjusted rates of events in six categories of achieved DBP and predicted continuous relationship in active treatment and control groups. Event rates (squares) and 95% CIs (bars) are shown for the following categories of achieved DBP: 65, 66–75, 76–85, 86–95, 96–105 and 106 mmHg. The number of events is shown below each bar. Source: Boutitie *et al.* (2002).

These results indicate that the lowest SBPs and DBPs are associated with increased mortality, largely regardless of antihypertensive-treatment status. The findings suggest that general health conditions associated with low BP likely are responsible for the higher death risk. It is plausible that low BP may represent an artefact of greater comorbidity. Thus, comorbidity, rather than BP *per se*, may explain observed increases in events associated with low BP. Indeed, the authors relate the observed increased mortality with a lower achieved DBP to poor health conditions and suggested the possibility of reverse causality (ill health causing low BP). Unfortunately, markers for poor health, such as body mass index and haemoglobin, were not included in the INDANA database.

Rather surprisingly, the BP at which the risk for total mortality was lowest was surprisingly high—169/94 mmHg in the control group and 156/84 mmHg in the active treatment group. Given the fact that cardiovascular risk is more related to SBP than DBP, most physicians would regard BP at these levels as unsatisfactorily controlled, especially those with vascular disease. The 1999 WHO/ISH hypertension guidelines recommended that the goal of antihypertensive treatment should be to achieve 'optimal' or 'normal' BP in young, middle-aged or diabetic subjects (below 130/85 mmHg), and at least 'high-normal' BP in elderly patients (below 140/90 mmHg). The authors made no attempt to give explanation of such an important observation in their analysis. Such observations have widespread and serious implications. Given the sharp increase of risk at the low levels of DBP demonstrated in their study, most physicians would fear to lower BP to the levels recommended by current treatment guidelines.

U-curve relationship between orthostatic blood pressure change and silent cerebrovascular disease in elderly hypertensives. Orthostatic hypertension as a new cardiovascular risk factor.

Kario K, Eguchi K, Hoshide S, *et al. J Am Coll Cardiol* 2002; **40**: 133–41.

B A C K G R O U N D . **Although orthostatic hypotension (OHYPO), often found in elderly hypertensive patients, has been recognized as a risk factor for syncope and CVD, both the clinical significance and the mechanism of orthostatic hypertension (OHT) remain unclear.**

I N T E R P R E T A T I O N . Silent cerebrovascular disease is advanced in elderly hypertensives having OHT. Elderly hypertensives with OHT or OHYPO may have an elevated risk of developing hypertensive cerebrovascular disease.

Comment

As mentioned, one possibility of higher mortality rate in patients at a lower BP range in elderly hypertensives on treatment may be related to greater comorbidity, which also may be linked to orthostatic BP dysregulation.

The objective of the present study was to investigate the clinical significance and mechanism of orthostatic BP dysregulation in elderly hypertensive patients in relation to the frequency of silent cerebrovascular disease; 241 elderly subjects (≥age 60 years) with asymptomatic hypertension (without previous or currently active CVD) identified by ambulatory BP monitoring were included. Patients with white-coat hypertension were excluded. Head-up tilting test was used to classify patients into an OHT group with orthostatic increase of SBP of ≥20 mmHg ($n = 26$), an OHYPO group with an orthostatic SBP decrease of ≥20 mmHg ($n = 23$), and a normal group with neither of these two patterns ($n = 192$). No patient had received any antihypertensive medication for at least 14 days before the study. Brain magnetic resonance imaging was used to detect silent cerebrovascular disease. They found that OHT, as well as OHYPO, is fairly frequent in elderly Japanese patients with sustained hypertension. A high prevalence (54%) of silent cerebral infarcts (SCI) was also detected in the studied group.

The data demonstrated a U-curve relationship between orthostatic BP change and hypertensive cerebrovascular disease (Fig. 8.5) after controlling for other confound-

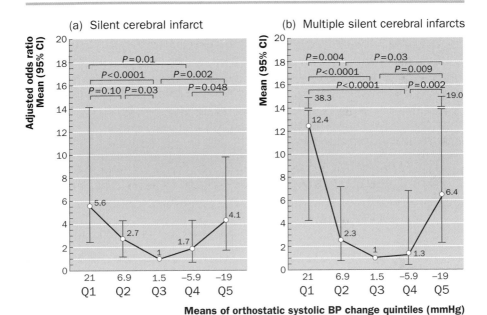

Fig. 8.5 U-curve relationship between orthostatic BP change and silent cerebral infarcts in elderly subjects with sustained hypertension. The odds ratios (mean and 95% CI) for silent cerebral infarcts: (A: 0 = subjects with no infarct; 1 = subjects with one or more infarcts) or for silent multiple cerebral infarcts (B: 0 = subjects with fewer than three infarcts; 1 = subjects with three or more infarcts) were adjusted for age (years), gender (0 = female, 1 = male), body mass index (kg/m^2), smoking status (0 = non-smoker, 1 = current smoker), presence/absence of hyperlipidaemia (0 = none, 1 = present), and 24-hour SBP (mmHg) using multiple logistic regression analysis (Q3 = the reference group). Source: Kario et al. (2002).

ing factors, including ambulatory BP levels. This association was especially marked for multiple SCIs. SCIs were more common in the OHT (3.4/person, $P < 0.0001$) and OHYPO groups (2.7/person, $P = 0.04$) than in the normal group (1.4/person). However, multiple SCIs were more common in the OHYPO than in the ONT group. The OHT (21 mmHg, $P < 0.0001$) and OHYPO (20 mmHg, $P = 0.01$) groups had higher BP variability (standard deviation of awake SBP) than the normal group (17 mmHg). Interestingly, the orthostatic BP increase was selectively abolished by α-adrenergic blocking, indicating that α-adrenergic activity is the predominant pathophysiological mechanism of OHT.

As pointed out by the authors, two large population-based prospective studies, the Atherosclerosis Risk In Communities study and the Honolulu Heart Program have reported that OHYPO is a risk factor for stroke, CAD or total death. Given the fact that SCI is a potent predictor for subsequent overt stroke, with a relative risk (RR) of about 5, in elderly hypertensives and with an RR of about 10 in all adults, OHT also may be a risk factor for future clinical stroke in elderly hypertensives.

Perhaps, we may assume that OHYPO would be more profound when these elderly hypertensives are on antihypertensive medications; theoretically, this may lead to more frequent SCIs or even overt cardiovascular events when they are on their usual antihypertensive drugs. To extend the hypothesis further, one may postulate that the J-curve's 'risk tail' may be related to OHYPO. It is of note that silent OHYPO in elderly hypertensives (9.5%) is unexpectedly less common among Japanese than in Western populations, where OHYPO is reported to occur in up to 20–30% of elderly hypertensives. Assuming that this hypothesis related to OHYPO is true, one would expect to observe a more pronounced J-curve relationship of BP and cardiovascular risk in the Western populations than in the Japanese population. It would be interesting to see whether such an observation of racial differences in the J-curve phenomenon has been reported. The paper by the Prospective Studies Collaboration (2002, as discussed above), which included 10% of the 1 million individuals' data from China and Japan, did not address this issue.

A U-shaped association between home systolic blood pressure and four-year mortality in community-dwelling older men.

Okumiya K, Matsubayashi K, Wada T, *et al. J Am Geriatr Soc* 1999; **47**(12): 1415–21.

BACKGROUND. Several studies in older people have found a U-shaped or J-shaped association of BP with mortality. The increased mortality associated with the lowest levels of BP in older people have been explained by concurrent illnesses and frailty, but previous studies used BP measured on a single occasion. Such a casual value is different from the long-term average of BP.

INTERPRETATION. This study showed a U-shaped association between the average level of SBP measured at home and mortality in older men while adjusting for potential confounding factors, including morbidity and frailty. Not only high home SBP, but also low home SBP, is an independent risk factor for mortality in older men. The mechanisms underlying the association between BP and mortality differ by levels of SBP. Cardiovascular deaths tended to be higher in the highest SBP group, and only non-cardiovascular deaths were increased in the lowest SBP group. The latter finding suggests that low SBP may be not only an independent risk of mortality but also an indicator of a subclinical non-cardiovascular comorbid condition.

Comment

This is a longitudinal study in a group of rural Japanese residents ($n = 1186$) aged 65 and older who were followed-up for 4 years. All participants had their BP measured in their home 20 times (four times per day for 5 consecutive days). The mean value of the 20 measurements was used to examine the association between home BP and subsequent 4-year mortality. The analysis was adjusted for potential confounders such as activities of daily living impairment, medical history, antihypertensive medication, smoking, use of alcohol and depression. Using repeated home BP measurements also improve the ability of their study to examine the relationship between BP and mortality.

The study demonstrated that older adults with SBP <125 mmHg had a nearly twofold higher risk of all-cause mortality compared with subjects with SBP of 125–134 mmHg while adjusting for potential confounding factors, including baseline morbidity and frailty. There was no significant evidence that frailty is more prevalent in the lowest or highest SBP group than in intermediate groups.

They also showed a U-shaped curve of the association of SBP with all-cause and non-cardiovascular mortality in the whole population and a linear association of SBP with cardiovascular mortality. Of note, the survival curve figure for men indicates that the low SBP group has the greatest mortality in the later 2 years of follow-up, whereas the highest SBP group has the most mortality in the first 2 years of follow-up. Interestingly, the cardiovascular deaths tended to be higher in the highest SBP group, and only non-cardiovascular deaths were increased in the lowest SBP group. The latter finding suggests that low SBP may not only be an independent risk of mortality but also an indicator of a subclinical, non-cardiovascular, comorbid condition.

The demonstration of a J-shaped association between home SBP and decline in cognitive function in this cohort is interesting |5|. They showed that older subjects with the highest and the lowest BP levels showed significant deterioration in Ministudy Mental State Examination scores during the 3 years of the study, whereas the group with intermediate levels of BP showed no change.

Relationship of race/ethnicity and blood pressure to change in cognitive function.

Bohannon AD, Fillenbaum GG, Pieper CF, Hanlon JT, Blazer DG. *J Am Geriatr Soc* 2002; **50**(3): 424–9.

BACKGROUND. **To determine whether there are racial/ethnic differences regarding the relationship of level of BP to change in cognitive function in older people.**

INTERPRETATION. Decline in cognitive function was associated with extremes of SBP in older white people. Although a similar but muted non-significant association was found in older African Americans, the curves for the two groups were not significantly different. Further studies in older African Americans are needed.

Comment

This longitudinal study (1986–89) found a statistically significant U-shaped relationship between SBP (but DBP) levels and changes in Short Portable Mental Status Questionnaire (SPMSQ, a screen of cognitive functioning) score over a 3-year period for older white men and women. However, these relationships were not found in older African Americans. The reason for this discrepancy between older African Americans and white people is unclear. The findings remained after adjustment for initial SPMSQ score, demographic characteristics and use of antihypertensive medication.

The analysis included a large representative, older, community-residing African Americans (*n* = 2260) and white people (*n* = 1876) in the Duke Established Populations for Epidemiologic Studies of the Elderly, aged 65–105 at baseline. BP levels were assessed and SPMSQ scoring was performed at baseline and 3 years later.

The data suggest that SBP below 110 mmHg or above 165 mmHg is a risk factor for cognitive decline in the white population, with the lower value possibly indicating poor health, but not imminent demise, because all sample members survived an additional 3 years or more. Interestingly, the use of antihypertensive medication, either as a general class or by specific type, did not contribute significantly to explaining decline in performance on the SPMSQ. The authors support the use of non-pharmacological measures before using drugs in the treatment of high BP to maintain SBP <140 and DBP <90 in this age group.

Taking this and the paper by Kario *et al.* (2002), one can hypothesize that the decline in cognitive function seen in white people at the lower SBP range may be related to the number of SCIs in these patients. Although a similar but muted non-significant association was found in older African Americans, the curves for the two groups were not significantly different.

Reverse J-curve relation between diastolic blood pressure and severity of coronary artery lesion in hypertensive patients with angina pectoris.

Hasebe N, Kido S, Ido A, Kenjiro K, Angiographical Study in Angina with Hypertension Induced Insults (ASAHI) Investigators. *Hypertens Res* 2002; **25**(3): 381–7.

BACKGROUND. The existence of the J-curve in hypertension treatment remains controversial. The major question is whether the increase in mortality from coronary disease is induced by the lowering of BP or by the severity of underlying coronary artery disease.

INTERPRETATION. There was no J-curve for DBP in hypertensive patients with angina pectoris; rather, the lower the DBP, the better was the prognosis. Interestingly, the severity of coronary lesions is in a reversed J-curve relation with DBP, suggesting that high BP plays a crucial part in serious events in hypertensive patients with moderate coronary artery lesions.

Comment

This study recruited patients with a history of hypertension (SBP >160 mmHg and/or DBP >90 mmHg) and a diagnosis of angina pectoris with angiographically confirmed coronary artery lesions. The relationship among the treated levels of SBP and DBP, the severity of coronary artery lesion, and the clinical consequences were investigated. Among the 234 enrolled patients, 115 experienced further events, 19 of which were serious. There were no significant differences in the average BP of patients with and those without events, but the coronary severity indices were significantly greater in patients with events. As a function of DBP from ≤74 to ≥105 mmHg, there was a positive association with the incidence of serious events, and a reversed J-curve in coronary severity indices with a nadir at 95–104 mmHg. A similar relationship was observed in SBP, but a potentially unfavourable outcome was suggested in the lowest SBP range of ≤124 mmHg. Contrary to some viewpoints, there was no evidence for a J-curve for DBP in hypertensive patients with angina pectoris; in fact, the lower the DBP, the better was the prognosis, in keeping with some of the more recent clinical trial data.

Conclusion

The dividing line between normal and abnormally elevated BP is arbitrary and, to a certain extent, artificial. Such limits for adults have evolved over time to the most recent recommendations of JNC-VI and WHO/ISH. BP cut-points are by and large based on data derived from long-term observations of populations, the documented relationship between elevated BP and defined target organ damage, and from clinical trials that demonstrate protection from hypertension-related risk by reducing BP. However, decisions for therapeutic intervention should be based on individual absolute global risk rather than based only on an arbitrary defined BP levels. Indeed, current guidelines recommend pharmacological therapy in diabetic or patients who have target organ damage even when SBP is less than 140 mmHg. Nevertheless, having a higher level of BP is itself a powerful risk factor for developing fixed hypertension over time. As pointed above, JNC-VI 'high-normal' BP is by no means benign in that it is associated with a much greater cardiovascular event risk over time compared with 'optimal' BP. Indeed, careful follow-up over time is the recommended approach.

On the other hand, the fear of J-curve or even U-curve relationships between BP levels and mortality risk is still one of the many factors that limit aggressive BP lowering especially in elderly patients, regardless whether such relationship is attributable to poor health or frailty that decreases SBP and increases relative risk, among the elderly. The debate continues . . . .

References

1. Black HR, Elliott WJ, Weber MA, Frishman WH, Strom JA, Liebson, PR, Hwang CT, Ruff DA, Montoro R, DeQuattro V, Zhang D, Schleman MM, Klibaner MI. One-year study of felodipine or placebo for stage 1 isolated systolic hypertension. *Hypertension* 2001; **38**: 1118–23.

2. Lonati L, Cuspidi C, Sampieri L, Boselli L, Bocciolone M, Leonetti G, Zanchetti A. Ultrasonographic evaluation of cardiac and vascular changes in young borderline hypertensives. *Cardiology* 1993; **83**: 298–303.

3. Escudero E, De Lena S, Graff-Iversen S, Almiron M, Cingolani HE. Left ventricular diastolic function in young men with high normal BP. *Can J Cardiol* 1996; **12**: 959–64.

4. Kimura Y, Tomiyama H, Nishikawa E, Watanabe G, Shiojima K, Nakayama T, Yoshida H, Kuwata S, Kinouchi T, Doba N. Characteristics of cardiovascular morphology and function in the high-normal subset of hypertension defined by JNC-VI recommendations. *Hypertens Res* 1999; **22**: 291–5.

5. Okumiya K, Matsubayashi K, Wada T, Osaki Y, Doi Y, Ozawa T. J-curve relation between blood pressure and decline in cognitive function in older people living in community, Japan. *J Am Geriatr Soc.* 1997 Aug; **45**(8): 1032–3.

Part III

Special groups and target organ damage

9

Diabetes mellitus and the metabolic syndrome

Introduction

The prevalence of diabetes mellitus (DM) is currently undergoing an unprecedented growth. It is projected to increase from the current prevalence of 150 million to 220 million affected persons world-wide by 2010 and 300 million by the year 2025. This dramatic effect is largely driven by the linked epidemic of obesity. Obesity is frequently part of a complex metabolic syndrome with coexisting dyslipidaemia, insulin-resistant, and type 2 DM. The recently released Third Report of the National Cholesterol Education Program Expert Panel on Detection, Evaluation, and Treatment of High Blood Cholesterol in Adults (NCEP ATP III) has drawn attention to the importance of the metabolic syndrome and provided a working definition of this syndrome for the first time, and highlights the importance of treating patients with the metabolic syndrome to prevent cardiovascular disease (CVD).

DM is closely aligned with the occurrence of cardiovascular, cerebrovascular and peripheral artery disease, as well as other vascular events from population studies. For example, the Framingham study showed an increased coronary heart disease (CHD) risk of 66% in men and a staggering 20% in women with DM after controlling for the other cardiovascular risk factors, while the Multiple Risk Factor Intervention Trial (MRFIT) demonstrated the amplified risk attributable to DM. Certainly, patients with DM but without CHD suffer an equivalent rate of coronary events as non-diabetics with a prior history of myocardial infarction. Whether this is simply due to a coalition of conventional factors or more specifically due to the complex metabolic effects of diabetes is not absolutely clear. What is clear is that the need for specific proactive management of cardiac and vascular risk in diabetes whether or not they have overt coronary disease or indeed any cardiac involvement.

Prevalence of the metabolic syndrome among US adults. Findings from the Third National Health and Nutrition Examination Survey.
Ford ES, Giles WH, Dietz WH. *JAMA* 2002; **287**: 356–9.

BACKGROUND. The NCEP ATP III highlights the importance of treating patients with the metabolic syndrome to prevent CVD. Limited information is available about the prevalence of the metabolic syndrome in the USA, however.

INTERPRETATION. These results from a representative sample of US adults show that the metabolic syndrome is highly prevalent. The large numbers of US residents with the metabolic syndrome may have important implications for the health care sector.

Comment

The recently released NCEP ATP III report has drawn attention to the importance of the metabolic syndrome and provided a working definition of this syndrome for the first time. The metabolic syndrome as defined by ATP III is (three of the following abnormalities): waist circumference >102 cm in men and >88 cm in women; serum triglycerides level of ≥150 mg/dl (1.69 mmol/l); high-density lipoprotein (HDL)-cholesterol level of <40 mg/dl (1.04 mmol/l) in men and <50 mg/dl (1.29 mmol/l) in women; blood pressure (BP) of ≥130/85 mmHg; or serum glucose level of ≥110 mg/dl (6.1 mmol/l). The data were derived from 8814 men and women aged 20 years or older from the Third National Health and Nutrition Examination Survey (NHANES III) 1988–94, a cross-sectional health survey of a nationally representative sample of the non-institutionalized civilian US population. The results showed that ~22% of US adults (24% after age adjustment) have the metabolic syndrome. The unrelenting increase in the prevalence of obesity in the USA suggests that the current prevalence of the metabolic syndrome is now very likely higher than that estimated from the 1988–94 NHANES III data. However, limited information is available about the prevalence of the metabolic syndrome on the other side of the Atlantic, in Europe. Because the implications of the metabolic syndrome for health care are substantial, we should seek to establish the prevalence of this condition.

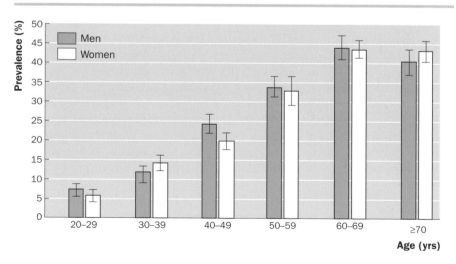

Fig. 9.1 Age-specific prevalence of the metabolic syndrome among 8814 US adults aged at least 20 years, by sex and 1988–94 NHANES III. Data are presented as a percentage (SE). Source: Ford *et al.* (2002).

Metabolic syndrome and development of diabetes mellitus: application and validation of recently suggested definitions of the metabolic syndrome in a prospective cohort study.

Laaksonen DE, Lakka HM, Niskanen LK, Kaplan GA, Salonen JT, Lakka TA.
Am J Epidemiol 2002; **156**(11): 1070–7.

BACKGROUND. The World Health Organization (WHO) and the National Cholesterol Education Program (NCEP) recently proposed definitions for the metabolic syndrome. Little is known of their validity, however.

INTERPRETATION. The WHO definition seems valid as judged by its relatively high sensitivity and specificity in predicting diabetes. The NCEP definition, including waist >102 cm also identifies persons at high risk for diabetes, but it is relatively insensitive in predicting diabetes.

Comment

Type 2 diabetes, hypertension, abdominal adiposity, dyslipidaemia and CVD are components of the insulin resistance syndrome (also known as metabolic syndrome). The syndrome is associated with an increased risk of mortality from CHD, CVD, and from all causes in these men. Its pathogenesis is multifactorial, but obesity and sedentary life-style, along with diet and still largely unknown genetic factors, interact to produce the syndrome. The threat to public health posed by the metabolic syndrome will continue to grow as the metabolic syndrome becomes epidemic.

Table 9.1 Defining the metabolic syndrome

NCEP definition
At least three of the following factors:

- Fasting plasma glucose ≥110 mg/dl
- Abdominal obesity: waist girth >102 cm (definition 1) or >94 cm (definition 2)
- Serum triglycerides ≥150 mg/dl
- Serum HDL cholesterol <40 mg/dl
- BP ≥130/85 mmHg or medication

Modified WHO definition

- Hyperinsulinaemia (upper quartile of the non-diabetic population) or fasting glucose ≥110 mg/dl

and at least two of the following:

- Abdominal obesity: waist to hip ratio >0.90, or body mass index ≥30 (definition 1), or waist girth >94 cm
- Dyslipidaemia: serum triglycerides ≥150 mg/dl or HDL cholesterol <35 mg/dl
- Hypertension: BP ≥140/90 mmHg or medication

Source: Laaksonen *et al.* (2002).

The authors assessed the sensitivity and specificity of the definitions of the metabolic syndrome for prevalent and incident DM in a Finnish population-based cohort of middle-aged men ($n = 1005$) followed for 4 years since the late 1980s. Four definitions based on the WHO and NCEP recommendations were compared |1,2|.

All definitions identified persons at high risk for developing diabetes during the 4-year follow-up (odds ratios = 5.0–8.8). The WHO definition including waist–hip ratio >0.90 or body mass index 30 kg/m^2 was the most sensitive (0.83 and 0.67) and least specific (0.78 and 0.80) in detecting the 47 prevalent and 51 incident cases of diabetes. The NCEP definition in which adiposity was defined as waist girth >102 cm detected only 61% of prevalent and 41% of incident diabetes, although it was the most specific (0.89 and 0.90).

The WHO and NCEP definitions of the metabolic syndrome appear valid, identifying those with a five- to ninefold increased likelihood of developing diabetes during follow-up in this population-based cohort of middle-aged men. The modified WHO definition based on waist–hip ratio >0.90 was the most sensitive in detecting prevalent and incident diabetes and had good specificity. The NCEP definition in which adiposity was defined as waist girth >102 cm was the most specific, but it did not detect most cases of incident diabetes. Defining adiposity as waist circumference >94 cm improves the sensitivity of the NCEP definition.

The metabolic syndrome and total and cardiovascular disease mortality in middle-aged men.
Lakka HM, Laaksonen DE, Lakka TA, *et al. JAMA* 2002; **288**(21): 2709–16.

BACKGROUND. The metabolic syndrome, a concurrence of disturbed glucose and insulin metabolism, overweight and abdominal fat distribution, mild dyslipidaemia and hypertension, is associated with subsequent development of type 2 DM and CVD. Despite its high prevalence, little is known of the prospective association of the metabolic syndrome with cardiovascular and overall mortality.

INTERPRETATION. CVD and all-cause mortality are increased in men with the metabolic syndrome, even in the absence of baseline CVD and diabetes. Early identification, treatment and prevention of the metabolic syndrome present a major challenge for health care professionals facing an epidemic of overweight individuals and sedentary life-style.

Comment

The objective of this study was to assess the association of the metabolic syndrome with cardiovascular and overall mortality using recently proposed definitions and factor analysis. To do this, they used data from the Kuopio Heart Disease Risk Factor Study, a prospective cohort study of 1209 Finnish men who were aged 42–60 years of age at baseline (1984–89) and were free of CVD, cancer or diabetes and who were followed through 1998. The main outcome measured were death due to CHD, CVD

Table 9.2 Relative risk of CHD death associated with the metabolic syndrome

Definition	Relative risk	95% CI
NCEP definition 1	2.9	1.2–7.2
NCEP definition 2	4.2	1.6–10.8
WHO definition 1	2.9	1.2–6.8
WHO definition 2	3.3	1.4–7.7

Source: Lakka *et al.* (2002).

and any cause among men with vs without the metabolic syndrome, using four definitions based on the NCEP and the WHO, as the definitions of the metabolic syndrome and cut-offs for the various components have varied widely (as shown in previous paper, see above).

The data showed that the prevalence of the metabolic syndrome in this group ranged from 8.8% to 14.3%, depending on the definition used. Over 11.4 years of follow-up, 109 deaths occurred, 46 of these from CVD and 27 from CHD. Men with the metabolic syndrome were three to four times more likely to die of CHD, after adjustment for other cardiovascular risk factors, than those without the syndrome, using all four definitions. Metabolic syndrome defined by the two WHO definitions was associated with higher relative risks of both CVD mortality (2.6–3.0) and all-cause mortality (1.9–2.1), but the two NCEP definitions predicted these two outcomes less consistently. Factor analysis using 13 of the variables associated with metabolic or cardiovascular risk suggested that the metabolic syndrome explains 18% of total variance in mortality risk.

Recent studies such as the Finnish Diabetes Prevention Study and the US Diabetes Prevention Program suggest even modest life-style changes can affect the risk for diabetes in individuals with glucose intolerance, and physical activity, weight loss and diet have been shown to affect favourably components of the metabolic syndrome. One of these reports comes from this study cohort by Lakka *et al.*, where it was observed that men who had regular moderate, and especially vigorous, physical activity were less likely to develop the metabolic syndrome over follow-up, but no randomized data are available.

Middle-aged men with the metabolic syndrome as defined by the NCEP and WHO have an increased cardiovascular and overall mortality, even when initially without diabetes and CVD. Thus early identification, treatment and prevention of the metabolic syndrome present a major challenge for physicians and public health policy makers facing an epidemic of overweight individuals and sedentary life-style.

Components of the 'metabolic syndrome' and incidence of type 2 diabetes.

Hanson RL, Imperatore G, Bennett PH, Knowler WC. *Diabetes* 2002; **51**(10): 3120–7.

BACKGROUND. Type 2 diabetes and CVD have many risk factors in common, and many of these risk factors are highly correlated with one another. The relationships among these risk factors may be attributable to a small number of physiological phenomena, perhaps even a single phenomenon. The combination of hypertension, dyslipidaemia, insulin resistance, hyperinsulinaemia, glucose intolerance and obesity, particularly central obesity, has been termed the 'metabolic syndrome'. It has been proposed that this syndrome is a powerful determinant of diabetes and CVD. There are few prospective data, however, on the extent to which this syndrome or its constituent components predict incidence of type 2 diabetes.

INTERPRETATION. Identification of four unique factors with different associations with incidence of diabetes suggests that the correlations among these variables reflect distinct metabolic processes, about which substantial information may be lost in the attempt to combine them into a single entity.

Comment

In this study, a large prospective database collected from the Pima Indian population (a well known American Indian population with high prevalence of type 2 diabetes and obesity) were analysed with the objectives to identify major factors that determine 'metabolic syndrome' (defined either by WHO or NCEP criteria), and to examine the relations of these factors to incidence of type 2 DM.

A total of 1918 Pima Indians were included. Data were analysed using factor analysis, which is a mathematical tool by which a large number of interrelated variables can be condensed to a smaller set of 'uncorrelated factors' that represent distinct attributes that account for a large proportion of the variance in the original variables. Prospective epidemiological studies of factor 'scores' from these analyses can further determine relations between components of the metabolic syndrome and incidence of diabetes. The original 10 variables included are: fasting and 2-hour plasma glucose concentrations, fasting and 2-hour serum insulin concentrations, systolic and diastolic BP, body weight, waist circumference, serum triglyceride, and HDL cholesterol concentrations. Because many of these variables change dramatically as children mature, analyses were restricted to individuals who were ≥20 years of age.

In the present study, factor analysis identified four factors that accounted for 79% of the variance in the original 10 variables. Each of these factors reflected a proposed component of the metabolic syndrome: insulinaemia, body size, BP and lipid metabolism. The insulinaemia factor was strongly associated with diabetes incidence (incidence rate ratio [IRR] for a 1 SD difference in factor scores = 1.81, *P* <0.01). The

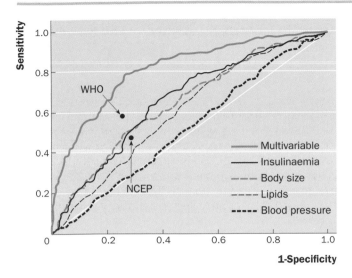

Fig. 9.2 ROC curves for prediction of development of diabetes. Curves are plotted for each of the four factors identified by factor analysis and for an optimally predictive multivariable score derived from all 10 original variables. Areas under the ROC curves (±SEs) are 0.81 ± 0.022 for the multivariable score, 0.66 ± 0.026 for insulinaemia, 0.65 ± 0.027 for body size, 0.60 ± 0.027 for lipids, and 0.52 ± 0.027 for BP. Predictive properties for metabolic syndrome defined by WHO and NCEP criteria are also shown. Source: Hanson *et al.* (2002).

body size and lipids factors also significantly predicted diabetes (IRR 1.52 and 1.37, respectively, $P <0.01$ for both), whereas the BP factor did not (IRR 1.11, $P = 0.20$).

The present analyses show that, among the Pimas, hyperinsulinaemia and obesity are strong risk factors for type 2 diabetes. The combination of hypertriglyceridaemia and low HDL cholesterol is a more modest, but still significant, risk factor, whereas high BP is only weakly, if at all, associated with diabetes incidence. Furthermore, in receiver operating characteristic (ROC) curves analyses the insulinaemia, body size and lipid factors were all significantly more strongly predictive of diabetes than the BP factor. These findings suggest that the different physiological processes associated with various components of the metabolic syndrome contain unique information about diabetes risk. In addition, the analyses also indicated that WHO criteria were much more strongly associated with diabetes incidence than NCEP criteria. This difference was due to the greater weight given to hyperglycaemia/insulin resistance in the WHO criteria than with the NCEP criteria, which essentially give the individual components equal weight.

As pointed by the authors, previous studies have used factor analyses for the same purpose and in general have provided consistent results, including the present study, suggesting that relationships among the variables typically proposed as constituting the metabolic syndrome are best explained as resulting from multiple physiological processes. Ultimately, an attempt to reduce these to a single entity will result in a substantial loss of information about these metabolic processes.

Conclusion

In a public health perspective these data, from both observational and intervention studies, underline the high prevalence and importance of the metabolic syndrome in the development of CVDs. They give strong support to the urgent need to implement health measures, such as increased exercise and healthy diet. Body weight reduction increases insulin sensitivity and improves both blood glucose and BP control. Because the BP targets are difficult to achieve in these patients, weight reduction, physical exercise, and a combination of several antihypertensive and antidiabetic agents are usually necessary.

References

1. World Health Organization. Definition, Diagnosis and Classification of Diabetes Mellitus and its Complications: Report of a WHO Consultation. Part 1: Diagnosis and Classification of Diabetes Mellitus. Geneva, World Health Org., 1999. Available from http://whqlib.who.int/hq/1999/WHO NCD NCS 99.2.pdf.
2. Expert Panel on Detection Evaluation and Treatment of High Blood Cholesterol in Adults. Executive summary of the third report of the National Cholesterol Education Program (NCEP) Expert Panel on Detection Evaluation and Treatment of High Blood Cholesterol in Adults (Adult Treatment Panel III). *J Am Med Assoc* 2001; **285**: 2486–97.

10

Hypertension and ethnicity

Introduction

There are well-described ethnic variations in the incidence, pathophysiology and management of hypertensive disease, which is particularly pertinent to the black or Afro-Caribbean populations in Africa, North America, the Caribbean and Europe. Our understanding of the underlying pathophysiology of hypertensive disease and the optimal treatment of hypertension in non-Caucasian patients continues to evolve, especially with the introduction of new antihypertensive agents and the need for prognostic data in this ethnic population. Nevertheless, it has been our perception that there continues to be some uncertainty over the optimal management of such patients. Indeed, the lack of large, long-term prospective randomized trials with hard outcome data has made it difficult to ascertain the precise benefits for the different antihypertensive agents in non-Caucasian patients. There is also the difficulty of defining (say) a 'pure' black (or white) population, as many subgroups within a particular ethnic group may exist.

Ethnic differences in blood pressure and the prevalence of hypertension in England.
Lane D, Beevers DG, Lip GYH. *J Hum Hypertens* 2002; **16**(4): 267–73.

BACKGROUND. **Since the first studies that demonstrated clear blood pressure (BP) differences between African-Americans and white-Americans, virtually every population-based study conducted in the USA has reported higher mean BPs at all ages, with a 1.5–2-fold greater prevalence of hypertension, among African-Americans. However, the data regarding elevated BP and a greater prevalence of hypertension among ethnic groups in the UK are not as consistent as data from the USA.**

INTERPRETATION. This study, in a UK population of Caucasians found that the prevalence of hypertension and mean BPs were higher among Afro-Caribbeans compared with Caucasians. South-Asian men had similar rates of hypertension and mean BPs to Caucasians.

Comment

The objective of this study was to examine the prevalence of hypertension and mean BPs among Afro-Caribbeans and South-Asians in England compared with Caucasians.

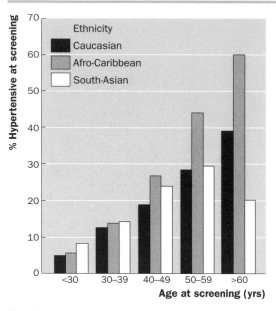

Fig. 10.1 Prevalence of hypertension in men by age and ethnic group. Source: Lane *et al.* (2002).

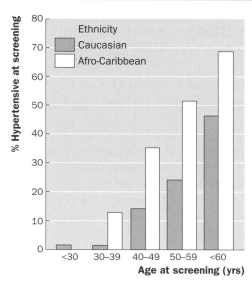

Fig. 10.2 Prevalence of hypertension in women by age and ethnic group. Source: Lane *et al.* (2002).

Data from the Birmingham Factory Screen, Birmingham INTERSALT (INTER-national study of SALT and blood pressure) volunteers, and four West Midlands churches were combined into a single database ($n = 2853$), as all three studies employed identical methods. The cohort comprised 2169 (76%) Caucasians (71% men), 453 (16%) Afro-Caribbean (60% men) and 231 (8%) South-Asian men. The overall prevalence of hypertension (>160/95 mmHg or taking antihypertensives) was greater in both Afro-Caribbean men (31%) and women (34%) (both P <0.001), compared with Caucasians (19% and 13% respectively), while South-Asian men had a similar overall prevalence to Caucasians (16%). Compared with Caucasians, Afro-Caribbeans had significantly higher mean systolic BP (SBP), with higher mean diastolic BPs (DBPs) evident among Afro-Caribbean women. After adjustment for age, body mass index (BMI), smoking and weekly alcohol intake, the odds ratios (95% confidence interval [CI]) for being hypertensive were 1.56 (1.14–2.13; $P = 0.005$) and 2.40 (1.51–3.81; $P = 0.0002$) for Afro-Caribbean men and women, respectively and 1.31 (0.88–1.97; $P = 0.19$) for South-Asian men, compared with Caucasians.

Thus, the prevalence of hypertension and mean BPs are higher among Afro-Caribbeans compared with Caucasians. South-Asian men had similar rates of hypertension and mean BPs to Caucasians.

Ethnic differences in coronary atherosclerosis.
Budoff MJ, Yang TP, Shavelle RM, Lamont DH, Brundage BH. *J Am Coll Cardiol* 2002; **39**(3): 408–12.

BACKGROUND. The study was done to evaluate whether ethnic differences exist in the prevalence of coronary artery calcification (CAC), and to determine whether differences in calcification correlate with the degree of coronary obstruction. Electron beam tomography (EBT) can be used to quantitate the amount of CAC and assist in prognostication of future cardiac events. It is unclear whether ethnic differences in coronary mortality are related to differences in the prevalence of coronary obstruction and CAC.

INTERPRETATION. As compared with white people, black and Hispanic people had a significantly lower prevalence of CAC and obstructive coronary disease. Ethnic differences in risk-factor profiles do not explain these differences. This study demonstrated that white people have a higher atherosclerotic burden than black and Hispanic people, independent of risk-factor differences among symptomatic patients referred for angiography.

Comment

Coronary artery disease (CAD) is a major cause of mortality and morbidity in all ethnic and racial subsets. Identification of those subjects with a very high probability of suffering coronary death and/or myocardial infarction, therefore, is of great interest, particularly because coronary disease is an increasingly treatable pathological entity in both its early and later stages. Both EBT and measurement of CAC have been found useful as sensitive markers of atherosclerosis and are currently used as methods for early detection of coronary disease.

However, prevalence of coronary disease varies among different ethnicities, as evident in the UK. This variability may be due in part to ethnic differences in the prevalence of coronary atherosclerosis and its risk factors. Indeed, despite an increased prevalence of both hypertension and diabetes, the overall risk of CAD in the black male population, in Europe, in the Caribbean and to a lesser extent in North America, is lower than in white males. By contrast, Indo-Asians have an excess prevalence of CAD. This contrast may be due to a multitude of reasons, although many of the traditional risk factors do not fully explain the ethnic differences in cardiovascular disease (CVD) and stroke. One reason, however, may be the more favourable lipid profiles, seen particularly in black males, with higher high-density lipoprotein cholesterol levels and lower plasma triglycerides. In contrast, the increased frequency of cerebrovascular disease, renal complications and cardiac hypertrophy in black people may be related to a higher incidence of severe hypertension, including malignant hypertension.

This study reports substantial ethnic differences in prevalence of both CAC and angiographic stenosis. In white people ($n = 453$), prevalence of CAC (score >0) was 84%, and significant obstruction on angiogram was 71%. Compared with white people, black people ($n = 108$) had a significantly lower prevalence of CAC (62%, $P <0.001$) and angiographic disease (49%, $P <0.01$). Hispanics ($n = 177$) also had a lower prevalence of CAC (71%, $P <0.001$) and angiographic obstruction (58%, $P <0.01$). Asians ($n = 44$) were not significantly different in regard to CAC (73%, $P = 0.06$) or angiographic stenosis (64%, $P = 0.30$). These ethnic differences remained after controlling for age, gender and cardiac risk factors.

Thus, in this symptomatic population, white people and Asian-Americans had a higher burden of atherosclerosis, both angiographically and by EBT, when compared with black people and Hispanics. The sensitivity and specificity of EBT in detecting significant angiographic obstruction did not differ among different ethnic groups despite a different prevalence in CAC. The EBT-detected CAC correlated well with extent and prevalence of angiographic CAD across all ethnicities, demonstrating a considerable similarity in calcifying stenotic lesions.

Insulin sensitivity and blood pressure in black and white children.

Cruz ML, Huang TT, Johnson MS, Gower BA, Goran MI. *Hypertension* 2002; **40**: 18–22.

BACKGROUND. The aims of the present study were (i) to establish if BP in pre-pubertal children was associated with fasting insulin, insulin sensitivity and the acute insulin response, and if this relationship was independent of total body fat and lean mass, and (ii) to establish if BP was different between white and black children, and if any

difference was explained by body composition, insulin sensitivity and acute insulin response.

INTERPRETATION. The relationship between insulin sensitivity and SBP was evident early in life. Black ethnicity and low insulin sensitivity contribute independently to higher BP in children.

Comment

In adults, hypertension has been associated with insulin resistance and hyperinsulin-aemia, all of which are components of the insulin resistance syndrome. Insulin resistance and the compensatory hyperinsulinaemia may even play a causal role in the development of hypertension. Insulin resistance and hyperinsulinaemia appear to develop in obese children at an early age, as does the relationship between fasting insulin and BP, which appears to be independent of adiposity. However, it is less clear if a relationship between insulin sensitivity and BP exists in children. In a small group of pre-pubertal white children, only DBP appeared to be correlated with insulin sensitivity after adjusting for percentage of body fat.

The relationship between insulin resistance and hypertension has also been found in black adults. However, the age at which ethnic differences in BP emerge has not been clearly delineated. The Coronary Artery Risk Development in Young Adults (CARDIA) study has documented significant differences in BP between black people and white people in the young adult age group. The results of studies in school-age children and adolescents have been mixed, with some showing higher BP in black children compared with white children, and others reporting no differences.

In the present study, insulin sensitivity and the acute insulin response were established by the minimal model and body composition by dual-energy X-ray absorptiometry. BP was recorded in the supine position. Body composition, fasting insulin ($P < 0.01$) and the acute insulin response ($P < 0.05$) were positively related to SBP but not to DBP, and insulin sensitivity ($P < 0.001$) was negatively related to SBP but not to DBP. Insulin sensitivity was negatively associated with SBP and DBP after adjustment for body composition ($P < 0.01$). Black children had higher SBP (110 ± 9.2 vs 105 ± 8.5 mmHg, $P = 0.01$) and DBP (59 ± 7.0 vs 54 ± 8.0 mmHg, $P < 0.01$) than did white children. Thus, the ethnic difference in BP was not explained by body composition, fasting insulin, acute insulin response or insulin sensitivity.

Reactivity as a predictor of subsequent blood pressure: racial differences in the Coronary Artery Risk Development in Young Adults (CARDIA) study.

Knox SS, Hausdorff J, Markovitz JH; Coronary Artery Risk Development in Young Adults Study. *Hypertension* 2002; **40**: 914–19.

BACKGROUND. **The goal of the present study was to investigate whether cardiovascular reactivity to mental stress predicted subsequent ambulatory BP** differently in race/gender subgroups. Ambulatory BP was chosen because it better reflects BP variation and levels throughout the day than clinical measurements made at a single point in time. A second objective was to test whether previously reported higher night-time BP in black people would be verified in a young, healthy cohort.

INTERPRETATION. Hyperresponsivity to stress may be a risk factor for subsequent BP elevation in black people and may be one pathway leading to the higher prevalence of hypertension in black people than in white people.

Comment

In this study, cardiovascular laboratory reactivity was examined in subjects 20–33 years old, and ambulatory BP and heart rate were measured 3 years later. Average ambulatory pressure during a 24-hour period was regressed separately on stress reactivity and standard covariate risk factors in each race/gender subgroup. Black people had higher BP and heart rates than white people, men had a higher BP than women, and women had higher heart rates than men. After controlling for age, baseline systolic pressure, familial history of hypertension, smoking, alcohol consumption, BMI and exercise, SBP reactivity to star tracing and cold pressor stress were significantly associated with systolic ambulatory pressure in black men and women 3 years later (partial $r = 0.24$–0.37). Heart rate reactivity to video challenge and star tracing were also significantly predictive of subsequent ambulatory heart rate in black people. Diastolic star tracing reactivity was significantly associated with subsequent ambulatory BP in black women ($r = 0.23$), and diastolic reactivity to video and star tracing were significantly predictive of ambulatory diastolic pressure in white men ($r = 0.39$).

BP responsiveness to mental stress has been reported to be a significant predictor of exercise-induced myocardial ischaemia and carotid artery atherosclerosis. Although it has also been reported to predict stable hypertension in borderline-hypertensive individuals, its utility as a prognostic measure has been questioned, and data concerning the association between stress reactivity and ambulatory BP have been equivocal. A number of these studies are difficult to interpret because they were either based solely on correlations, only examined absolute levels during reactivity, or did not control for relevant covariates. There has been little research examining the effect of race and gender on the association between reactivity and subsequent ambulatory pressure, despite the fact that previous research has been fairly consistent in showing race as well as gender differences in reactivity and BP measured at a single sitting.

Reduced endothelium-dependent and -independent dilation of conductance arteries in African-Americans.

Campia U, Choucair WK, Bryant MB, Waclawiw MA, Cardillo C, Panza JA. *J Am Coll Cardiol* 2002; **40**(4): 754–60.

B A C K G R O U N D . Compared with Caucasians, African-Americans have a higher prevalence of CVD and its complications, which may be related to reduced nitric oxide-dependent and -independent vasodilation of the microvasculature. However, whether a similar impairment is also present at the level of the conductance arteries is unknown. The purpose of the present investigation, therefore, was to determine whether racial differences exist in the functional behaviour of conduit vessels.

I N T E R P R E T A T I O N . African-Americans show reduced responsiveness of conductance vessels to both endogenous and exogenous nitric oxide compared with Caucasian Americans. These findings expand our understanding of racial differences in vascular function and suggest a mechanistic explanation for the increased incidence and severity of CVD observed in African-Americans.

Comment

Several epidemiological studies have shown that atherosclerosis and its complications, the leading cause of death among adults in the USA, carry significantly higher morbidity and mortality in African-Americans compared with Caucasian Americans. These observations may be partly explained by a considerably higher prevalence, among African-Americans, of risk factors traditionally associated with atherosclerosis, such as essential hypertension, diabetes mellitus and tobacco use.

An increased cardiovascular reactivity to stress has been reported in young normotensive black people and has been considered to be a contributor to their greater prevalence of hypertension. Research has also focused on potential differences in arterial wall function between black people and white people and their impact on vascular homeostasis, with reduced nitric oxide-mediated vasodilation of forearm resistance vessels to mental stress and to endothelium-dependent and -independent pharmacological stimuli, indicating reduced vascular smooth muscle relaxation. This diminished response to vasodilators may result in a decreased pattern of haemodynamic reactivity leading, in the long term, to increased vascular tone and hypertension. However, because these phenomena refer to resistance vessels, they may not account for the increased predisposition of African-Americans for developing atherosclerosis in large conductance arteries.

Target organ damage: ethnicity differences are important

The presence of hypertensive target organ damage is an important prognostic factor. In particular, hypertensive left ventricular hypertrophy (LVH) substantially increases the risk of sudden death, myocardial infarction, stroke, atherosclerotic vascular disease and arrhythmias (ventricular and supraventricular). Thus, attention has been directed towards unravelling the pathophysiological contributors to target organ damage in hypertension.

One condition that has attracted much attention is the insulin resistance syndrome, which includes central obesity, hyperinsulinaemia, dyslipidaemia, hypertension, hypercoagulability, and an increased potential for developing atherosclerotic disease. Among hypertensives, both renal disease and cardiac disease have been related to the insulin resistance syndrome. Indeed, there is the possibility that insulin resistance and hyperinsulinaemia may contribute to elevated arterial pressure in patients with essential hypertension.

Several studies suggest that insulin resistance and/or hyperinsulinaemia also contribute to concentric LVH and diastolic dysfunction in normotensives and hypertensives. Ethnic differences in CVD are increasingly important considerations, and (in the UK, at least) black people are at higher risk of hypertension and hypertension-related target organ disease than white people. Hypertensive black people have a greater rate of decline of renal function over time than do white people, and black men have a fourfold higher incidence of age-adjusted end-stage renal disease than white men. In addition, LV mass and the prevalence of LVH are greater among hypertensive black people than among white people. Hypertensive black people also have an increased prevalence of concentric remodelling and concentric hypertrophy of the left ventricle.

Left ventricular systolic dysfunction in a biracial sample of hypertensive adults. The Hypertension Genetic Epidemiology Network (HyperGEN) Study.
Devereux RB, Bella JN, Palmieri V, et al. Hypertension 2001; **38**: 417–23.

BACKGROUND. The proportion of cases of clinical congestive heart failure (CHF) that are due to LV systolic dysfunction compared with LV diastolic dysfunction, valvular heart disease, or other causes is not well established. Furthermore, few data are available on the combined prevalence of symptomatic and asymptomatic LV systolic dysfunction in population samples, especially of high-risk groups such as black people.

INTERPRETATION. In a population-based sample of hypertensive patients, LV systolic dysfunction was related to male gender, black race, diabetes and elevated uric acid levels, as well as higher ventricular mass and lower relative wall thickness.

Comment

This study evaluated the clinical variables and echocardiographic data of 2086 participants in the Hypertension Genetic Epidemiology Network (HyperGEN). The purpose was to assess comprehensively the prevalence and correlates of LV systolic dysfunction in hypertensive patients in a biracial population-based sample of relatively mild and more severe LV systolic dysfunction. Multivariate analyses reveal significant associations, independent of previous myocardial infarction or overt CHF, of LV systolic dysfunction with male gender, higher BMI, and black race. Taken together with recent evidence of higher mortality in black than white patients with LV dysfunction, this report supports a disproportionate burden from CHF in black people. In addition, the analyses identified a previously unrecognized, weak association independent of diuretic use between severe LV dysfunction and higher uric acid levels.

Predictors of target organ damage in hypertensive blacks and whites.

El-Gharbawy AH, Kotchen JM, Grim CE, *et al. Hypertension* 2001a; **38**: 761–6.

BACKGROUND. The insulin resistance syndrome is a complex phenotype. The relationship of insulin resistance and/or hyperinsulinaemia to hypertension or to the development of hypertension is conflicting. Among hypertensives, both renal disease and cardiac disease have been related to the insulin resistance syndrome. Black people are at greater risk for developing hypertension-related target organ disease than white people.

INTERPRETATION. In black people, microalbumin excretion was related to insulin resistance. These observations are consistent with the hypothesis that there is a genetic contribution to cardiac hypertrophy, glomerular hyperfiltration and sodium retention in black people with essential hypertension.

Comment

The purpose of this study was to evaluate the relationship between the anthropomorphic and metabolic components of the insulin resistance syndrome and both BP and BP-related target organ damage in black people and in white non-diabetic French Canadians with essential hypertension.

El-Gharbawy *et al.* report in this study where in black people, microalbumin excretion was related to insulin resistance, consistent with the hypothesis that there is a genetic contribution to cardiac hypertrophy, glomerular hyperfiltration and sodium retention in black people with essential hypertension. In their study of 82 black and 63 white French Canadian patients, black patients had an attenuated nighttime reduction in BP ($P <0.02$), increased cardiac dimensions ($P <0.001$), greater microalbumin excretion ($P <0.05$), increased inulin clearance (indicative of glomerular hyperfiltration; $P <0.001$) and decreased lithium clearance (indicative of increased sodium reabsorption in the proximal tubule; $P <0.001$). BP levels were not related to insulin resistance; although in black people, the night-time reduction in SBP was inversely related to fasting plasma insulin ($r = -0.18$, $P <0.04$). In a stepwise multivariate analysis (including BP levels and components of the insulin resistance syndrome as independent variables), race was the strongest predictor of LV mass ($r = 0.53$, $P <0.000$), relative wall thickness ($r = 0.49$, $P <0.000$), and both inulin ($r = 0.53$, $P <0.000$) and lithium ($r = 0.41$, $P <0.000$) clearances. Night-time SBP was also a significant determinant of concentric LVH ($r = 0.37$, $P <0.000$).

In summary, comparing black and white patients with essential hypertension, black race was a stronger predictor of cardiac size and inulin and lithium clearances (indicative of glomerular hyperfiltration) than either BP or any of the components of the insulin resistance syndrome. In addition, BP was associated with concentric LVH in both patient groups, and in black people, microalbumin excretion and glomerular hyperfiltration were also related to the insulin resistance syndrome. However, it is also of note that unlike several previous prospective cohort studies, there was no significant association of BP level (by 24-hour BP monitoring under controlled conditions) with plasma insulin and the possibility that environmental factors (e.g. diet) may also contribute to these cardiac and renal differences in the two patient groups cannot be excluded.

Arterial pressure, left ventricular mass, and aldosterone in essential hypertension.
El-Gharbawy AH, Nadig VS, Kotchen JM, *et al. Hypertension* 2001b; **37**(3): 845–50.

B A C K G R O U N D . Aldosterone may play a part in cardiac hypertrophy independent of its effect on BP. Within the myocardium, aldosterone acts via mineralocorticoid receptors to enhance extracellular matrix and collagen deposition. Pathological patterns of LV geometry have also been associated with elevations of plasma aldosterone concentrations in patients with essential hypertension. Black people have a higher prevalence of hypertension, salt-sensitive hypertension, LVH especially concentric LV remodelling.

I N T E R P R E T A T I O N . These results are consistent with the hypothesis that aldosterone contributes to elevated arterial pressure in obese black American and obese white French Canadian patients with essential hypertension and to the attenuated nocturnal decline of BP and LVH in obese, hypertensive black Americans.

Comment

The purpose of the present study was to evaluate the relationship of aldosterone to both BP and LV geometry in both black and white patients with essential hypertension. The studied subjects consisted of black American ($n = 109$) and white French Canadian ($n = 73$) patients with essential hypertension. The data confirm

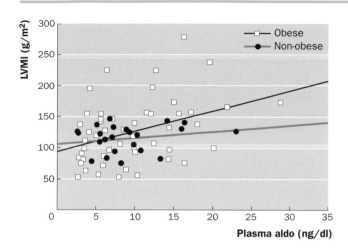

Fig. 10.3 Correlations of LV mass index (LVMI) with standing plasma aldosterone (Aldo) in obese and non-obese black Americans. For the obese, $r = 0.39$ ($P <0.003$), and for the non-obese, $r = 0.21$ ($P = 0.36$). Source: El-Gharbawy *et al.* (2001b).

that black hypertensives have relatively high plasma aldosterone concentrations in relation to low plasma renin activity, compared with white hypertensives. Serum potassium concentrations were also lower in the black American patients. Night-time BPs were correlated with plasma aldosterone in both obese black American and obese French Canadian patients. In addition, LV size and geometry were correlated with plasma aldosterone in the obese black Americans but not in the obese white French Canadians. These observations suggest that adiposity and race modify the relationship of aldosterone with both BP and LV mass. These factors should be taken into account in data analysis of future studies.

Ethnic differences in carotid and left ventricular hypertrophy.

Stanton AV, Mayet J, Chapman N, Foale RA, Hughes AD, Thom SA.
J Hypertens 2002; **20**(3): 539–43.

BACKGROUND. Afro-Caribbean subjects have a higher prevalence of hypertension, a lower prevalence of ischaemic heart disease and a higher premature mortality compared with white Europeans. LVH is also more prevalent in Afro-Caribbeans even at similar levels of BP. It is widely believed that carotid artery intima-media thickening (IMT) represents an early marker for the development of atheroma, and carotid IMT and LVH are associated in white populations. Whether the relationship between carotid IMT and LVH is similar in black subjects is unknown.

INTERPRETATION. Afro-Caribbean subjects with similar BPs have similar mean carotid and femoral IMTs compared with white Europeans, in spite of marked differences in LV mass index. Whether this reflects a discrepancy in the degree of cardiovascular risk for similar levels of the LV mass index or whether this is a reflection of an altered pattern of target organ damage associated with hypertension in Afro-Caribbean subjects is unclear.

Comment

In this study 38 subjects were studied using carotid and femoral ultrasonography and echocardiography; 19 Afro-Caribbean and 19 white European subjects were matched for age, sex and mean 24-hour SBP. The Afro-Caribbean group had a significantly greater LV mass index compared with the white European: 136.4 ± 6.1 vs 112.4 ± 6.2 g/m^2, $P < 0.01$. However, carotid IMT, carotid diameter, femoral IMT and femoral diameter were similar between the groups: 0.75 ± 0.02 vs 0.77 ± 0.04 mm, 6.54 ± 0.15 vs 6.56 ± 0.16 mm, 0.66 ± 0.03 vs 0.68 ± 0.03 mm and 8.40 ± 0.33 vs 8.25 ± 0.23 mm, respectively.

Thus, Afro-Caribbean subjects with similar BPs have similar mean carotid and femoral IMTs compared with white Europeans, in spite of marked differences in LV mass index. Whether this reflects a discrepancy in the degree of cardiovascular risk for similar levels of LV mass index in black and white subjects or whether this is a reflection of an altered pattern of target organ damage associated with hypertension in Afro-Caribbean subjects is unclear. A long-term prospective study assessing the association of carotid and LV structure with cardiovascular end-points in different ethnic populations is required to address this issue properly.

Growth of left ventricular mass in African-American and European American youth.

Dekkers C, Treiber FA, Kapuku G, Van Den Oord EJ, Snieder H. *Hypertension* 2002; **39**: 943–51.

BACKGROUND. Increased LV mass has been established as a strong independent risk factor for cardiovascular morbidity (e.g. arrhythmia, CHF and myocardial infarction) and mortality. As the pathogenesis of CVDs has its origin in childhood, moderators of LV mass growth need to be evaluated during this time period. Increased LV mass may contribute to the much higher prevalence of cardiovascular morbidity and mortality in African-Americans, compared with European Americans. It is not clear to what extent these variables account for LV mass variability over time.

INTERPRETATION. The results of the present study suggest that increased LV mass in boys and African-Americans has its origin in late childhood. Apart from these ethnicity and gender effects, individual differences in cardiac growth can mainly be explained by body growth and increases in general adiposity.

Comment

LV mass is known to increase with body growth, i.e. height and weight, from childhood to adulthood, with body growth accounting for less variability of LV mass with increasing age. Cross-sectional paediatric and adult studies have shown greater LV mass in males and African-Americans compared with females and European Americans, respectively, and these studies have shown positive associations of LV mass with several anthropometric and haemodynamic variables in youths and adults.

The number of longitudinal studies on LV mass growth and moderators of LV mass changes in youths and young adults is limited, and none have comprehensively evaluated LV mass in a multiethnic population over a longer period of time from childhood through young adulthood.

In the present study individual growth curves across age of LV mass were created for 687 African-American and European American males and females with a maximum of 10 annual assessments (age 8.2–27.5 years). African-Americans and males had significantly greater LV mass ($P < 0.001$) than did European Americans and females, respectively. Males also showed a larger rate of change in LV mass than did girls ($P < 0.001$). The ethnicity and gender effects on LV mass only became apparent in early adolescence, and they persisted when controlling for socio-economic status and anthropometric and haemodynamic variables. BMI and height were the strongest anthropometric predictors, and pulse pressure was the strongest haemodynamic predictor of LV mass. Although significant, the contribution of pulse pressure to the prediction of LV mass was small, once BMI and height were entered into the model. Thus increased LV mass in boys and African-Americans has its origin in late childhood—some individual differences in cardiac growth can also be explained by body growth and increases in general adiposity.

Left ventricular mass and arterial compliance: relation to coronary heart disease and its risk factors in South Indian adults.

Kumaran K, Fall CHD, Martyn CN, Vijayakumar M, Stein CE, Shier R. *Int J Cardiol* 2002; **83**: 1–9.

BACKGROUND. Rates of coronary heart disease (CHD) in India are rising, and are now similar to those in Western countries. The prevalence of conventional CHD risk factors such as hypercholesterolaemia, hypertension, smoking and obesity, tend to be lower in Indian than Western populations, and fail to explain these high rates of disease. Increased LV mass and decreased arterial compliance predict a higher risk of CHD in Western populations, but there are no published data from India.

INTERPRETATION. The mean LV mass in the Indian population was lower compared with Western populations, though as in the West, increased LV mass was associated with an increased risk of CHD. Greater LV mass and reduced arterial compliance are associated with higher levels of many known CHD risk factors especially with those that form the insulin resistance syndrome.

Comment

CHD rates in India are rising and projected statistics show that CHD will be the leading cause of mortality by 2015. People of Indian origin living outside India have higher rates than indigenous populations. These findings are not completely explained by the prevalence of classical CHD risk factors such as high total cholesterol concentrations, hypertension and obesity, or life-style factors, such as high saturated fat intake and smoking, all of which tend to be lower in South Asian Indian populations than Western populations. However, CHD in Indians has been associated with features of the insulin resistance syndrome. This still does not account for all of the elevated risk of CHD in Indians compared with Western populations.

Relationship between treatment-induced changes in left ventricular mass and blood pressure in black African hypertensive patients: results of the Baragwanath trial.

Skudicky D, Sareli P, Libhaber E, *et al. Circulation* 2002; **105**: 830–6.

B A C K G R O U N D . The Baragwanath Hypertension Study was a single-centre, randomized trial that compared several drug classes to initiate treatment in black African patients with sustained hypertension confirmed by ambulatory BP monitoring. The present analysis compared what extent changes in conventional and automated BP readings at the clinic and in the ambulatory BP predicted regression of LV mass index in response to antihypertensive treatment in previously untreated or treated patients with sustained hypertension.

I N T E R P R E T A T I O N . In previously untreated patients with sustained hypertension followed at a single center, reductions in clinic and ambulatory systolic pressure in response to antihypertensive treatment equally predicted the regression in LV mass index.

Comment

Left ventricular hypertrophy is a strong and independent predictor of cardiovascular morbidity and mortality both in hypertensive patients and in the general population. It is associated with a higher risk of myocardial infarction, stroke, sudden death, and death from any cause. Furthermore, echocardiographically determined LV mass confers prognostic information beyond that provided by traditional risk factors, including hypertension. Controversy still exists with regard to what type of BP measurement (conventional, automated or ambulatory) correlates better with changes in LV mass induced by antihypertensive treatment. Most previous studies did not exclude previously treated or white-coat hypertensive patients or were multicentric, which makes clinic measurements of BP more difficult to standardize.

This study found significant and positive correlations between the changes in LV mass index and all types of SBP in response to treatment in previously untreated patients, whereas in previously treated patients these correlations were non-significant.

Furthermore, in untreated patients, regression of LV mass index was not significantly better correlated with the reduction in 24-hour, daytime or night-time systolic pressure than with the decrease in the conventional systolic pressure.

Renal perfusion in blacks: alterations caused by insuppressibility of intrarenal renin with salt.
Price DA, Fisher ND, Lansang MC, Stevanovic R, Williams GH, Hollenberg NK.
Hypertension 2002; **40**: 186–9.

BACKGROUND. **An increased intrarenal renin–angiotensin system activity may be responsible for the reduction in renal plasma flow (RPF) in apparently healthy black people in comparison with healthy white people during high salt balance.**

INTERPRETATION. The intrarenal tissue renin system is more active in black people than white people on a typical (high salt) diet and that the difference reflects primarily incomplete tissue renin suppression with an increase in salt intake. The mechanism involved may contribute to the increased susceptibility to renal injury in black people.

Comment
The striking increase in risk of nephropathy in black people has focused attention on the determinants of renal perfusion and function in this ethnic group. To ascertain

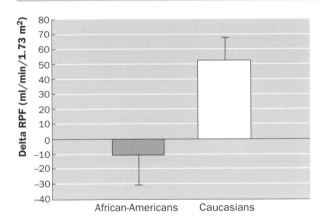

Fig. 10.4 Change in RPF response to increase salt in African-Americans and Caucasians. Change in RPF response when going from low to high salt balance in the two groups is shown. In blacks, RPF does not change in response to high salt diet (–0.7 ± 17.5 mL/min per 1.73 m^2). In whites, RPF increased significantly in response to an increase in salt ($P = 0.05$). Change in RPF from low to high salt state was significantly different in the two groups ($P = 0.01$). $P = 0.01$, difference in RPF from LS to HS in African-Americans vs Caucasians. Source: Price *et al.* (2002).

whether these differences only exist in the high salt state, Price *et al.* measured in 19 healthy black people and 22 healthy white people para-aminohippurate and inulin clearances as an indication of RPF and glomerular filtration rate, respectively, on both high (200 mmol/day) and low (10 mmol/day) salt balance in random order. A subset of 11 black people and 12 white people additionally received an angiotensin II infusion while in low salt balance (3 ng/kg per minute for 45 min) and captopril to assess differences in RPF response to a converting enzyme inhibitor. The 19 white people had significantly higher RPF when compared with black people ($P = 0.033$) when studied on high salt. However, during low salt balance, the RPFs were comparable in the two groups. Plasma renin activity was similar in the two groups on both diets. In the subset that received angiotensin II and captopril while in low salt balance, the renal vascular response was not different in white people and black people. These data therefore provide additional support for the concept that the intrarenal tissue renin system is more active in black people than white people on a typical (high salt) diet and that the difference reflects primarily incomplete tissue renin suppression with an increase in salt intake. The mechanism involved may contribute to the increased susceptibility to renal injury in black people.

Successful blood pressure control in the African-American Study of Kidney Disease and Hypertension.

Wright JT Jr, Agodoa L, Contreras G, *et al.*; African-American Study of Kidney Disease and Hypertension Study Group. *Arch Intern Med* 2002; **162**: 1636–43.

BACKGROUND. The African-American Study of Kidney Disease and Hypertension (AASK) was a trial to evaluate the effect of BP and choice of antihypertensive drug on the rate of decline of renal function.

INTERPRETATION. The BP goals set and achieved in AASK participants clearly demonstrate that adequate BP control can be achieved even in hypertensive populations whose BP is the most difficult to control.

Comment

AASK is multi-centre, randomized, double-masked trial to determine the effect of lower BP levels and choice of initial antihypertensive drug selection on the rate of decline of glomerular filtration rate assessed by iothalamate clearance. The AASK participants are randomized to an antihypertensive regimen initiated with either an angiotensin-converting enzyme inhibitor (ramipril), a dihydropyridine calcium channel blocker (amlodipine besylate), or a sustained-release beta-blocker (metoprolol succinate). In addition, patients were randomized to one of two BP goals based on mean arterial BP (MAP), either 102–107 mmHg (inclusive), approximating the usual level of BP control of 140/90 mmHg, or to 92 mmHg or less, approximating the lower goal of less than 125/75 mmHg. This substudy found that in participants randomized to the low MAP goal, the percentage of participants who achieved a BP of less than 140/90 mmHg increased from a baseline of 20.0% to 78.9% by 14 months after randomization. For usual MAP goal participants, the corresponding percentages increased from 21.5% to 41.8%. The difference in median levels of MAP between the two MAP goal groups increased and remained at approximately 12 mmHg. BP reduction was similar regardless of age, sex, BMI, education, insurance or employment status, income or marital status. Thus adequate BP control can be achieved even in hypertensive populations whose BP is the most difficult to control.

Urinary protein and essential hypertension in black and in white people.

Chelliah R, Sagnella GA, Markandu ND, MacGregor GA. *Hypertension* 2002; **39**: 1064–70.

BACKGROUND. The objectives of this work were to examine the association between urinary protein and BP and to compare the pattern of urinary protein excretion with essential hypertension in people of European origin (white people) and in people of African or African-Caribbean origin (black people) living in south-west London, UK.

INTERPRETATION. In the groups as a whole, there were no significant differences in urinary albumin and in total urinary protein excretion between black people and white people. The increase in protein excretion in essential hypertension could be due, at least in part, to an increase in glomerular protein ultrafiltration.

Comment

Microalbuminuria, defined as urinary albumin excretion of 30–300 mg/24 h, is a well-recognized major risk factor for the development of overt proteinuria, nephropathy, and vascular disease in people with diabetes mellitus. However, it is now apparent that an increase in urinary albumin excretion is also associated with an increased risk of CVD independent of the presence of diabetes.

Microalbuminuria is also associated with essential hypertension, ranging from 5% to 37%. Importantly, not every study has demonstrated a direct association with BP levels. Nevertheless, the presence of microalbuminuria and proteinuria in people with essential hypertension is an independent risk factor for end-organ damage and renal failure. Microalbuminuria in black people may reflect a greater susceptibility to renal damage from relatively smaller increases in BP. Although in normal people albumin is the major urinary protein excreted, it is not clear whether increased albumin excretion in people with essential hypertension is also associated with raised excretion of other proteins. This is important because the pattern of protein excretion may provide further insight into the renal defects leading to increased protein excretion.

In this study, there were no significant differences in total urinary protein excretion between black people and white people (geometric means [95% CI]: 94.0 [85.9–102.9] mg/24 h for black people [n = 151] and 102.1 [96.1–108.4] mg/24 h for white people [n = 219]). There were also no significant differences between black people and white people in urinary albumin (6.5 [4.9–8.5] mg/24 h for black people [n = 97] and 7.1 [5.6–9.0] mg/24 h for white people [n = 123]). In both groups, those with essential hypertension displayed a significantly raised urinary protein excretion (1.21-fold higher for black people and 1.19-fold higher for white people) and albumin excretion (1.69-fold higher for black people and 2.40-fold higher for white people). Urinary transferrin excretion measured in a subgroup of 67 subjects was also raised in those with essential hypertension (3.22-fold higher in black people and 2.76-fold higher in white people). Examination of urinary proteins by sodium dodecyl sulphate–polyacrylamide gel electrophoresis did not identify any pattern consistent with a reduction in renal tubular protein reabsorption in those with essential hypertension. Thus the increase in protein excretion in essential hypertension could be due, at least in part, to an increase in glomerular protein ultrafiltration.

Conclusion

Racial/ethnic differences in CVD outcomes are a pressing public health concern. Evaluation is often difficult as to what extent biological (include genetic), dietary and/or social inequality factors contribute to these differences. However, such information can be valuable for local and national policy makers in targeting resources and in designing effective strategies for the elimination of racial and ethnic disparities in morbidity and mortality.

11

Relationship between hypertensive cardiac and extracardiac target organ damage

Introduction

The adverse effects of systemic hypertension on target organs are widespread and thus lead to a varying degree of macrovascular and microvascular damage. The relationships of blood pressure (BP) with various indexes of target organ damage (TOD) are complex and have not been well described. With the increased availability of ambulatory and home BP measurements, these relationships have become more conveniently assessed and compared with that of office BP measurements. Indeed, a positive correlation has been shown between various BP components (24-hour, daytime, night-time, systolic BP [SBP] and diastolic BP) and microalbuminuria or increased left ventricular (LV) mass. Furthermore, the relationship between micro-albuminuria and atherosclerotic processes are also tightly related and increased urinary albumin excretion has been considered a marker of prevalent subclinical atherosclerosis. Indeed, patients who have elevated urinary albumin excretion are more likely to exhibit increased LV mass and LV hypertrophy (LVH), demonstrating more carotid plaque or intima-media thickness and retinal major vascular changes. Such a relationship is particularly strong for coronary artery disease as micro-albuminuria has been shown to be the most potent independent determinant of ischaemic heart disease especially among the hypertensive or borderline hypertensive subjects.

By establishing such complex relationships this may enable physicians to make an early prediction of impending TOD and thus more aggressive management before such damage sets in. Indeed, many studies have shown microalbuminuria to be an early predictor of cardiovascular morbidity and mortality. Furthermore, an abnormally high LV mass, detected by either standard electrocardiography (ECG) or echocardiography, has been shown to be associated with increased cardiovascular morbidity and mortality. The following articles will demonstrate some of the relationships between increased LVH or LV mass and albuminuria.

High prevalence of cardiac and extracardiac target organ damage in refractory hypertension.

Cuspidi C, Macca G, Sampieri L, et al. J Hypertens 2001; **19**(11): 2063–70.

BACKGROUND. TOD in chronically treated hypertensives is related to effective BP control. The aim of this study was to evaluate the prevalence of cardiac and extracardiac TOD in patients with refractory hypertension (RH) compared with well-controlled treated hypertensives.

INTERPRETATION. The study suggests that RH is a clinical condition associated with a high prevalence of TOD at cardiac, macrovascular and microvascular level and consequently with high absolute cardiovascular risk, which needs a particularly intensive therapeutic approach aimed to normalize BP levels and to induce TOD regression.

Comment

This study further reaffirmed the well-established relationship of BP control and TOD. The study included 54 consecutive middle-aged patients with RH (57 ± 10 years), selected according to World Health Organization/International Society of Hypertension guidelines definition, and 51 essential hypertensives with satisfactory BP control obtained by association therapy. As expected the RH group had higher clinic BP, higher prevalences of LVH, carotid intima-media thickening and carotid plaques as well as a more advanced retinal involvement (grade II and III) and a greater albumin urinary excretion compared with treated hypertensives.

Left ventricular concentric remodelling and extracardiac target organ damage in essential hypertension.

Cuspidi C, Macca G, Michev I, et al. J Hum Hypertens 2002; **16**(6): 385–90.

BACKGROUND. LV concentric remodelling is an adaptive change in cardiac geometry frequently observed in arterial hypertension. This study was addressed to investigate the extent of extracardiac TOD in patients with LV concentric remodelling.

INTERPRETATION. In hypertensive patients with similar BP and LV mass index levels, LV concentric remodelling is not associated with more prominent TOD.

Table 11.1 Extracardiac target organ damage in patients with normal geometry and with LC concentric remodelling

	Normal geometry (n = 31)	LV concentric remodelling (n = 31)	P
Carotid arteries			
CCA IMT (mm)	0.7 ± 0.02	0.7 ± 0.02	NS
CCA diameter (mm)	6.2 ± 0.9	6.2 ± 0.8	NS
RWT	0.23 ± 0.04	0.23 ± 0.05	NS
Prevalence of thickening (%)	22.5	25.8	NS
Prevalence of plaques (%)	35.4	35.4	NS
Retinal changes			
KWB I (%)	19.3	22.5	NS
KWB II (%)	32.5	32.5	NS
Renal involvement			
Mean UAE (mg/24 h)	9 ± 9	14 ± 12	NS
Prevalence of microalbuminuria (%)	3.2	6.4	NS

CCA = common carotid artery; RWT = relative wall thickness; KWB = Keith Wagener Barker; NS = not significant.
Source: Cuspidi *et al.* (2002).

Correlation between silent cerebral white matter lesions and left ventricular mass and geometry in essential hypertension.

Sierra C, de la Sierra A, Pare JC, Gomez-Angelats E, Coca A. *Am J Hypertens* 2002; **15**(6): 507–12.

BACKGROUND. **It has been proposed that concentric LVH is related to a worse degree of TOD in hypertensives with this feature than in those without. Moreover, the presence of cerebral white matter lesions (WMLs) is considered to be an early marker of brain damage in essential hypertension.**

INTERPRETATION. There is a close association between cerebral WMLs and concentric LVH in asymptomatic middle-aged hypertensive patients, independent of BP values.

Comment

The presence of cerebral WMLs in hypertensive patients is indicative of early cerebral damage. Indeed, the presence of WMLs is an important predictor for the development of stroke. The objective of this study was to investigate the relationship between the presence of silent WMLs in brain magnetic resonance imaging and echocardiographically determined LV mass and geometry in never-treated middle-aged patients with uncomplicated essential hypertension. The study included 62 patients (39 men,

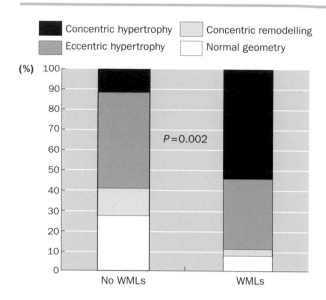

Fig. 11.1 Relationship between the presence of cerebral WMLs and different patterns of LV morphology in asymptomatic hypertensive patients. Source: Sierra *et al.* (2002).

mean age 54.4 ± 3.2 years), all underwent brain magnetic resonance imaging and were classified into two groups according to the presence or absence of WMLs. Importantly, patients with diabetes, alcohol abuse or other established risk factors for the development of silent cerebrovascular damage were excluded. The results showed that patients with WMLs had significantly higher LV wall thickness, LV mass index and RWT (relative wall thickness) when compared with hypertensive patients without WMLs. Furthermore, as many as 23 of 26 hypertensive patients with WMLs showed echocardiographic criteria for LVH that was significantly higher than that observed in hypertensive patients without WMLs (21 of 36; $P = 0.01$). Concentric hypertrophy (LVH and RWT 0.45) was present in 14 hypertensive patients with WMLs and in only four patients without WMLs ($P = 0.002$). The latter finding supports the notion that concentric hypertrophy is related to a worse degree of TOD in hypertensive patients with this feature.

The mechanism of the link between LV mass and geometry and WMLs is not clear and remains speculative at this time. LVH and WMLs share common risk factors, such as hypertension, that might promote atherosclerosis. However, concentric LVH was found to be associated with WMLs after adjusting for BP values, suggesting a different pathogenic cause.

Association of left ventricular hypertrophy with metabolic risk factors: the HyperGEN study.

de Simone G, Palmieri V, Bella JN, et al. J Hypertens 2002; **20**(2): 323–31.

B A C K G R O U N D . To determine whether combinations of metabolic risk factors (obesity, diabetes and hypercholesterolaemia) influence the magnitude of LV mass and prevalence of LVH.

I N T E R P R E T A T I O N . The progressive addition of metabolic risk factors, including central obesity, diabetes and hypercholesterolaemia is associated with higher LV mass normalized by height$^{2.7}$, independently of hypertension and other important biological covariates. Obesity played a major part in this association. This finding indicates that LV mass is a potentially useful bioassay of strategies of global cardiovascular prevention.

Comment

There is increasing evidence that the variability of LV mass is only partially related to the levels of arterial pressure, suggesting that its magnitude can also be influenced by stimuli other than arterial pressure, such as metabolic risk factors.

This is a large cross-sectional study with an objective to determine whether combinations of metabolic risk factors (obesity, diabetes and hypercholesterolaemia) influence the magnitude of LV mass and prevalence of LVH. A total of 1627 hypertensive (85.9% treated, 1036 women, 1041 African-Americans) and 342 normotensive (180 women, 183 African-Americans) participants in the Hypertension Genetic Epidemiology Network (HyperGEN) Study, without prevalent cardiovascular disease, were studied. Several indices were recorded including LV mass corrected for height$^{2.7}$ or fat-free mass or body surface area and the ratio of stroke volume to pulse pressure as a percentage of predicted (as a crude estimate of arterial compliance), and were analysed in relation to obesity (by body mass index), central fat distribution (by waist circumference), diabetes (by American Diabetes Association criteria) and hypercholesterolaemia.

The results were not unexpected. They found obesity, hypercholesterolaemia and diabetes were more frequent among hypertensives than normotensives (all $P < 0.001$). After controlling for other biological important covariates age, sex, race and type and combination of antihypertensive medication LV mass/height$^{2.7}$, but not LV mass/fat-free mass and LV mass/body surface area, increased with the number of metabolic risk factors, both in normotensive and hypertensive subjects. Prevalence of LVH was predicted by older age, hypertension, central fat distribution, black race and independently increased with the number of associated metabolic risk factors ($P < 0.0001$).

Obesity, especially central fat distribution obesity is the most important metabolic risk factor in contributing to the magnitude of LV mass. This can be demonstrated in hypertensive patients as well as, to a lesser extent, in normotensive individuals.

Certainly, the study would be more interesting if a subset of patients also have insulin-resistance status established as this is particularly relevant to patients with central obesity who are at higher risk for type 2 diabetes.

Urine albumin/creatinine ratio and echocardiographic left ventricular structure and function in hypertensive patients with electrocardiographic left ventricular hypertrophy: the LIFE study. Losartan Intervention for Endpoint Reduction.

Wachtell K, Palmieri V, Olsen MH, *et al. Am Heart J* 2002; **143**(2): 319–26.

BACKGROUND. Albuminuria, reflecting systemic microvascular damage, and LV geometric abnormalities have both been shown to predict increased cardiovascular morbidity and mortality. However, the relationship between these markers of cardiovascular damage has not been evaluated in a large hypertensive population.

INTERPRETATION. In hypertensive patients with electrocardiographic LVH, abnormal LV geometry and high LV mass are associated with high urine albumin/creatinine ratio (UACR) independent of age, SBP, diabetes and race, suggesting parallel cardiac and microvascular damage.

Comment

This study adds to the existing literatures that LVH or increased LV mass is significantly associated with microalbuminuria and vice versa. A continuous relationship between albumin excretion rate, LV mass and ambulatory BP load has been demonstrated in newly diagnosed patients with essential hypertension and suggest the occurrence of early effects on target organs. Thus, it is really unsurprising that increased LV mass or microalbuminuria have been consistently shown in various studies as an important predictor for cardiovascular morbidity and mortality, even in the general population without overt cardiovascular disease. This probably is a reflection of underlying subclinical atherovascular disease in these patients. Indeed, in this study, patients with eccentric or concentric LVH had both higher prevalences of microalbuminuria (average 26–30% vs 9%, P <0.001) and macroalbuminuria (6–7% vs < 1%, P <0.001). Furthermore, patients with microalbuminuria and macroalbuminuria had a significantly higher LV mass and lower endocardial and midwall fractional shortening. Moreover, patients with abnormal diastolic LV filling parameters had a significantly increased prevalence of microalbuminuria. In univariate analyses, UACR correlated positively to LV mass, SBP, age and pulse pressure/ stroke volume and negatively to relative wall thickness and endocardial and midwall shortening but not to diastolic filling parameters. In multiple regression analysis, higher UACR was associated with higher LV mass independently of older age, higher systolic pressure, black race and diabetes.

Microalbuminuria in hypertensive patients with electrocardiographic left ventricular hypertrophy: the LIFE study.

Wachtell K, Olsen MH, Dahlof B, *et al. J Hypertens* 2002; **20**(3): 405–12.

BACKGROUND. LVH and albuminuria have both been shown to predict increased cardiovascular morbidity and mortality. However, the relationship between these markers of cardiac and renal glomerular damage has not been evaluated in a large hypertensive population with TOD.

INTERPRETATION. In patients with moderately severe hypertension, LVH on two consecutive ECGs is associated with increased prevalences of microalbuminuria and macroalbuminuria compared with patients without persistent ECG LVH. High albumin excretion was related to LVH independent of age, BP, diabetes, race, serum creatinine or smoking, suggesting parallel cardiac damage and albuminuria.

Comment

The present study was undertaken to determine whether albuminuria is associated with persistent ECG LVH, independent of established risk factors for cardiac hypertrophy, in a large hypertensive population with LVH who were free of overt renal failure. The study included 8029 patients, mean age 66 years, with stage II–III hypertension and LVH on a screening ECG. The clinic BPs were between 160–200/95–115 mmHg and plasma creatinine <160 mmol/l. Renal glomerular permeability was evaluated by UACR (mg/mmol). Microalbuminuria was found in 23% and macroalbuminuria in 4% of patients.

Unsurprisingly, microalbuminuria was more prevalent in patients of African-American (35%), Hispanic (37%) and Asian (36%) ethnicity, heavy smokers (32%), diabetics (36%) and in patients with ECG LVH by both Sokolow–Lyon voltage criteria and Cornell voltage-duration product ECG criteria (29%). Urine albumin/creatinine was also positively related to Sokolow–Lyon voltage criteria and Cornell voltage-duration product criteria. In multiple regression analysis, higher UACR was independently associated with older age, diabetes, higher BP, serum creatinine, smoking and LVH. Patients smoking >20 cigarettes/day had a 1.6-fold higher prevalence of microalbuminuria and a 3.7-fold higher prevalence of macroalbuminuria than never-smokers. ECG LVH by Cornell voltage-duration product or Sokolow–Lyon criteria was associated with a 1.6-fold increased prevalence of microalbuminuria and a 2.6-fold increase risk of macroalbuminuria compared with no LVH on the second ECG.

A blood pressure independent association between glomerular albumin leakage and electrocardiographic left ventricular hypertrophy. The LIFE Study. Losartan Intervention For Endpoint reduction.

Olsen MH, Wachtell K, Borch-Johnsen K, *et al. J Hum Hypertens* 2002; **16**(8): 591–5.

BACKGROUND. In the Losartan Intervention For Endpoint reduction (LIFE) study LVH was associated with increased UACR at baseline. To evaluate whether this association was due only to parallel BP-induced changes, this study re-examined the patients after 1 year of antihypertensive treatment to investigate whether changes in LVH and UACR were related independently of changes in BP.

INTERPRETATION. The data suggest that the relationship between LVH and glomerular albumin leakage is not just due to parallel BP-induced changes. As glomerular albumin leakage may represent generalized vascular damage we hypothesize a vascular relationship between cardiac and glomerular damage.

Does treatment of non-malignant hypertension reduce the incidence of renal dysfunction? A meta-analysis of ten randomized, controlled trials.

Hsu CY. *J Hum Hypertens* 2001; **15**(2): 99–106.

BACKGROUND. It remains controversial whether non-malignant 'benign' hypertension causes renal dysfunction. The effect of lowering BP on the incidence of renal dysfunction among patients with non-malignant hypertension is not clear. This meta-analysis was conducted to determine whether antihypertensive drug therapy reduces the incidence of renal dysfunction in patients with non-malignant hypertension.

INTERPRETATION. Among patients with non-malignant hypertension enrolled in randomized trials, treated patients did not have a lower risk of renal dysfunction. The 95% confidence interval suggests that a 25% or more true protective effect of antihypertensive drugs is unlikely.

Comment

While it is well established that malignant hypertension damage the kidneys, it remains unclear whether treating patients with non-malignant 'benign' hypertension would prevent renal dysfunction in long-term. This meta-analysis included 10 randomized controlled trials of antihypertensive drug therapy, involving a total of 26 521 individuals with non-malignant hypertension (equivalent to 114 000 person-years) but with normal baseline renal function. As expected, treated patients had lower BP and fewer cardiovascular events. However, patients randomized to anti-hypertensive therapy (or more intensive therapy) did not have a significant reduction in their risk of developing renal dysfunction (relative risk = 0.97; 95% confidence interval 0.78–1.21; $P = 0.77$). While the majority of us agree that lowering BP in patients with hypertension would lead to a reduction of both cardiac and cerebrovascular events, many of us would also expect a reduction in the risk of renal dysfunction. The conclusion of this study that BP lowering had no evident renoprotective effect in the studied population is certainly a surprise to many of us at first glance. As usual, the interpretation of any conclusion generated from any meta-analyses should be done with caution, as patients' inclusion/exclusion criteria could be significantly different. Furthermore, it is of note that the trials included in the analysis had no renal end-points as primary outcomes, such as doubling of serum creatinine or time to dialysis, and thus lower the power to detect any renal events. Quite rightly, however, the author recognized the importance of treating BP in these patients as there are clear 'non-renal benefits' with BP lowering.

Conclusion

LVH by echocardiography has proved to be a strong independent predictor of cardiovascular morbidity and mortality in hypertensive patients. Patients with LVH or increased LV mass often have extracardiac TOD, such as elevated urinary albumin excretion, and are more likely to exhibit carotid plaque or intima-media thickness and retinal major vascular changes. Furthermore, patients with a concentric hypertrophy geometry appear to carry the highest risk, while an eccentric hypertrophy geometry carries an intermediate risk for TOD. It has been shown that hypertensive patients with concentric LVH have the greater peripheral vascular remodelling as well as other extracardiac TOD, such as more advanced retinopathy and nephropathy [1].

Increased urinary albumin excretion has been related to several unfavourable metabolic and non-metabolic risk factors and subclinical hypertensive organ damage. Long-term longitudinal studies have confirmed the unfavourable prognostic significance of microalbuminuria in hypertensive patients. Microalbuminuria is a specific, integrated marker of cardiovascular risk and TOD in hypertension and one can be used as an identifier of patients at higher global risk.

Reference

1. Shigematsu Y, Hamada M, Ohtsuka T, Hashida H, Ikeda S, Kuwahara T, Hara Y, Kodama K, Hiwada K. Left ventricular geometry as an independent predictor for extracardiac target organ damage in essential hypertension. *Am J Hypertens* 1998; **11**: 1171–7.

12

Diastolic dysfunction and left ventricular hypertrophy

Introduction

Patients with hypertension with increased left ventricular (LV) mass are susceptible to diastolic heart failure because of decreased LV relaxation and compliance during diastole (i.e. unable to increase their end-diastolic volume), particularly when these patients are subjected to haemodynamic stress or increased workload such as exercise. Consequently, a cascade begins, in which the LV end-diastolic pressure rises, left atrial pressure increases, and pulmonary oedema develops. Thus, early identification by detection of LV diastolic dysfunction or inappropriate increase of LV mass in the early phase of disease in those at risk, e.g. Afro-Caribbean is highly desirable before LV decompensation set in.

Echocardiographic detection of LV diastolic dysfunction (principally Doppler imaging studies of mitral inflow) has been hampered by difficulties in interpretation of the results as it varies with different loading conditions, heart rate and systolic function. Newer measures that are load-independent, such as tissue Doppler imaging, have improved the non-invasive assessment of LV diastolic function in the research setting, but further study is needed to determine their accuracy and usefulness for clinical practice. Similarly, LV mass also varies according to individuals' age, sex, build, and possibly ethnicity. Most clinical echocardiographic laboratories do not routinely evaluate LV diastolic function or mass, because such an assessment requires a detailed echocardiographic examination that is technically demanding, time consuming, and above all, lacks standardization. Given the difficulties of the current techniques available, it is not surprising that some experts have viewed the occurrence of isolated diastolic heart failure sceptically. Indeed, there are many other possible reasons that may account for patient's symptoms of 'heart failure' in the presence of true LV hypertrophy (LVH).

Early signs of cardiac involvement in hypertension.
Palatini P, Frigo G, Vriz O, *et al. Am Heart J* 2001; **142**(6): 1016–23.

BACKGROUND. Whether abnormalities of diastolic function are the earliest cardiac change in hypertension is still a matter for dispute. The aim of this study was to assess whether LV diastolic dysfunction is an early sign of cardiac involvement in hypertension.

INTERPRETATION. Earliest signs of cardiac involvement in hypertension are LV structural abnormalities. Left ventricular diastolic function is only marginally affected, even when multiple parameters of LV filling are taken into account.

Comment

Several reports have documented reduced LV filling rate as an early sign of cardiac involvement in hypertension occurring before LV mass increases. Such early cardiac abnormalities might be useful for recognizing hypertensive patients who are at greater risk, hence, allow early identification of patients who require antihypertensive therapy. The present study investigates whether various LV filling parameters and their combination could detect early abnormalities of diastolic function in a large cohort of young subjects with never treated borderline to mild hypertension from the Hypertension and Ambulatory Recording Venetia Study (HARVEST). The study showed that in the early stage of hypertension increased blood pressure (BP) and the initial structural LV changes only marginally influence diastolic function studied with Doppler assessment of transmitral flow. Doppler parameters also seem to be heavily dependent on age within a group of young subjects. However, A-wave peak velocity appears to be the most sensitive one for assessing diastolic function.

Diastolic dysfunction precedes myocardial hypertrophy in the development of hypertension.
Aeschbacher BC, Hutter D, Fuhrer J, Weidmann P, Delacretaz E, Allemann Y.
Am J Hypertens 2001; **14**(2): 106–13.

BACKGROUND. LVH and impaired diastolic function may occur early in systemic hypertension, but longitudinal studies are missing.

INTERPRETATION. Over a 5-year follow-up, initially lean, normotensive, young men with a moderate genetic risk for hypertension, developed Doppler echocardiographic alterations of LV diastolic function compared with matched offspring of normotensive (ONorm) parents. These alterations were more pronounced in the offspring of hypertensive (OHyp) parents who developed mild hypertension and occurred without a distinct rise in LV mass.

Comment

Offspring of hypertensive parents are at increased genetic risk for developing systemic hypertension. Impaired diastolic function and increased LV mass may occur very early in the development of essential hypertension. This is the first longitudinal study investigating the changes of LV structure and function over time in initially normotensive male offspring of OHyp and ONorm parents. Echocardiographic data (including pulmonary vein flow pattern and septal myocardial Doppler imaging) at baseline and after 5 years were compared between the two groups. At 5 years, compared with matched ONorm, OHyp developed Doppler echocardiographic signs of diastolic dysfunction without a significant increase in LV mass. Pulmonary vein flow is increasingly used in the non-invasive assessment of LV diastolic function. There was a significantly increased pulmonary vein reverse A wave duration in the OHyp. The results suggest that alterations of diastolic function may precede a significant increase in LV mass in subjects at risk of essential hypertension and corroborate the results of cross-sectional studies conducted in offspring of hypertensive parents. However, the sample size in this study is relatively small and the clinical relevance of the findings is unknown.

Changes in diastolic left ventricular filling after one year of antihypertensive treatment. The Losartan Intervention For Endpoint Reduction in Hypertension (LIFE) Study.
Wachtell K, Bella JN, Rokkedal J, *et al. Circulation* 2002; **105**(9): 1071–6.

BACKGROUND. It is well established that hypertensive patients with LVH have impaired diastolic filling. However, the impact of antihypertensive treatment and LV mass reduction on LV diastolic filling remains unclear.

INTERPRETATION. Antihypertensive therapy resulting in a reduction of LV mass or relative wall thickness regression is associated with significant improvement of diastolic filling parameters related to active relaxation and passive chamber stiffness compared with patients without regression, independent of BP reduction; however, abnormalities of diastolic LV filling remain common.

Comment

The first assessment of the relation of changes in LV geometry to changes in diastolic LV function during antihypertensive treatment in a large series in hypertensive patients with electrocardiographically (ECG) verified LVH. The improvement of diastolic dysfunction may contribute to the ability of BP reduction to prevent congestive heart failure (CHF) and highlights the role of antihypertensive therapy in primary prevention of CHF in hypertensive patients with LVH. However, the investigators cannot yet determine which BP lowering strategy, losartan or the atenolol-based regimen, had the greatest effect on BP, or on LV filling parameters as treatment was blinded.

Prognostic significance of left ventricular diastolic dysfunction in essential hypertension.
Schillaci G, Pasqualini L, Verdecchia P, *et al. J Am Coll Cardiol* 2002; **39**(12): 2005–11.

BACKGROUND. Alterations in LV diastolic function are frequent in patients with hypertension, even in the absence of LVH, but their prognostic significance has never been investigated.

INTERPRETATION. Impaired LV early diastolic relaxation, detected by pulsed Doppler echocardiography, identifies hypertensive patients at increased cardiovascular risk. Such association is independent of LV mass and ambulatory BP.

Comment

This large prospective study included 1839 Italian never-treated hypertensive patients (50 ± 12 years, 53% men, BP 156/98 mmHg) without previous cardiovascular events at baseline and who underwent conventional Doppler echocardiography and 24-hour BP monitoring before therapy. Patients were followed up for 11 years (mean 4.4 years). During follow-up, there were 164 major cardiovascular events (2.04 per 100 patient-years). The results showed that the age- and heart rate-adjusted E/A ratio was predictive of subsequent cardiovascular morbid events. This remained significant after correction for the influence of several traditional risk factors, including age, gender, diabetes, cigarette smoking, LV mass, serum cholesterol level and 24-hour ambulatory and office visit BP.

As pointed out by the authors, there were several limitations with their study and should be interpreted with caution. Their data were obtained in initially untreated Caucasian patients, and thus the results may not be extrapolated to different ethnic groups or to patients on antihypertensive treatment. Furthermore, the PIUMA (Progetto Ipertensione Umbria Monitoraggio Ambulatoriale) database does not include information on BP control during follow-up in the whole population; this information was available in ~30% of the study patients. Another limitation, inherent to observational cohort studies, is the lack of control over occasional changes in the antihypertensive regimen over time.

Left ventricular diastolic function in physiologic and pathologic hypertrophy.
Schannwell CM, Schneppenheim M, Plehn G, Marx R, Strauer BE. *Am J Hypertens* 2002; **15**(6): 513–17.

BACKGROUND. Patients with hypertensive heart disease and LVH demonstrate an impaired LV diastolic filling pattern. The aim of this study was to find out whether physiological LVH induced by endurance training causes disturbances in LV systolic and diastolic filling.

INTERPRETATION. Doppler echocardiographic parameters of LV diastolic function can be of diagnostic importance for discrimination between pathological and physiological LVH.

Comment

This is a case–control study involving 49 athletes with LVH due to endurance training, 49 patients with LVH due to arterial hypertension, and 26 untrained healthy control subjects by conventional echocardiography. Rather surprisingly, all three study groups showed normal fractional shortening and mid-wall fractional shortening. However, as expected, LV mass index in subjects with LVH were higher than controls (athletes, 99 ± 10 g; hypertensive patients, 95 ± 11 g; controls: 52 ± 7 g; P <0.01 for athletes and hypertensive patients). Patients with arterial hypertension had a diastolic dysfunction consisting of a delayed relaxation pattern with reversed E/A ratio, whereas athletes had a normal LV diastolic filling pattern.

Thus, the authors advocated that Doppler echocardiographic parameters of LV diastolic function can be of diagnostic importance for discrimination between pathological and physiological LVH. The study would have been more interesting if tissue Doppler imaging was also compared.

Heart failure with a normal ejection fraction: is measurement of diastolic function necessary to make the diagnosis of diastolic heart failure?

Zile MR, Gaasch WH, Carroll JD, et al. Circulation 2001; **104**(7): 779–82.

BACKGROUND. The diagnosis of diastolic heart failure is generally made in patients who have the signs and symptoms of heart failure and a normal LV ejection fraction (LVEF). Whether the diagnosis also requires an objective measurement of parameters that reflect the diastolic properties of the ventricle has not been established.

INTERPRETATION. Objective measurement of LV diastolic function serves to confirm rather than establish the diagnosis of diastolic heart failure. The diagnosis of diastolic heart failure can be made without the measurement of parameters that reflect LV diastolic function.

Comment

Zile *et al.* hypothesized that the vast majority of patients with heart failure and a normal ejection fraction exhibit abnormal LV diastolic function. They tested this hypothesis by prospectively identifying 63 patients with a history of heart failure and an echocardiogram suggesting LVH and a normal ejection fraction; we then assessed LV diastolic function during cardiac catheterization. All 63 patients had standard haemodynamic measurements; 47 underwent detailed micromanometer and echocardiographic-Doppler studies. The LV end-diastolic pressure was >16 mmHg in 58 of the 63 patients; thus, 92% had elevated end-diastolic pressure (average, 24 ± 8 mmHg). The time constant of LV relaxation (average, 51 ± 15 ms) was abnormal in 79% of the patients. The E/A ratio was abnormal in 48% of the patients. The E-wave deceleration time (average, 349 ± 140 ms) was abnormal in 64% of the patients. One or more of the indexes of diastolic function were abnormal in every patient.

Coronary flow reserve and myocardial diastolic dysfunction in arterial hypertension.
Galderisi M, Cicala S, Caso P, *et al. Am J Cardiol* 2002; **90**(8): 860–4.

B ACKGROUND. In view of the fact that coronary blood flow occurs predominantly during diastole, it is conceivable that LV diastolic changes also play a part in coronary flow reserve (CFR) impairment in hypertensives. In contrast, myocardial ischaemia may produce LV diastolic alterations, even before the detection of wall motion and/or electrocardiographic ST segment changes. Elevations of LV end-diastolic pressure have long been recognized to occur during spontaneous or provoked ischaemia.

I NTERPRETATION. This study provides evidence of an independent association between CFR and myocardial diastolic function. In hypertensive patients without coronary artery stenosis, CFR alteration may be a determinant of myocardial diastolic dysfunction or diastolic impairment that should be taken into account as possibly contributing to coronary flow reduction.

Comment

The aim of this study was to assess the relation between coronary blood flow and LV myocardial diastolic dysfunction in arterial hypertension using both second-harmonic Doppler and colour tissue Doppler during dobutamine stress. CFR was estimated as the ratio of hyperaemic and baseline diastolic flow velocities. The study included 30 hypertensive patients who were free of coronary artery disease and pharmacological therapies. Hypertensives were divided into two groups according to CFR level, with the cut-off point for normal CFR ≥2. The main findings of the study are: (i) hypertensives with abnormal CFR have a lower tissue Doppler myocardial Em/Am ratio at baseline and particularly with high-dose dobutamine, and (ii) a strong positive association between the high-dose dobutamine Em/Am ratio and CFR is evident in all of the hypertensive patients, independent of clinical and echocardiographic variables.

The study is novel that as no association between CFR and Doppler-derived LV diastolic function has previously been found. Colour tissue Doppler provides additional information about myocardial function also during dobutamine stress while transmitral diastolic measurements were not significantly different in hypertensives with normal or altered CFR. This suggests that tissue Doppler imaging may provide a more reliable assessment of diastolic function in these patients. Indeed, a decrease in CFR in these patients especially those with LVH might be potentially responsible for LV diastolic failure, even in the absence of coronary artery disease.

Congestive heart failure and blood pressure: recent insights

Predictors of congestive heart failure in the elderly: the Cardiovascular Health Study.
Gottdiener JS, Arnold AM, Aurigemma GP, *et al. J Am Coll Cardiol* 2000; **35**: 1628–37.

BACKGROUND. The elderly constitute a growing proportion of patients admitted to hospital with CHF, and CHF is a leading source of morbidity and mortality in this group. Elderly patients differ from younger individuals diagnosed with CHF in terms of biological characteristics.

INTERPRETATION. The incidence of CHF is high in the elderly and is related mainly to age, gender, clinical and subclinical coronary heart disease, systolic BP (SBP) and inflammation. Despite the high relative risk of subnormal systolic LV function and atrial fibrillation, the actual population risk of these for CHF is small because of their relatively low prevalence in community-dwelling elderly people.

Comment

This study sought to characterize the predictors of incident CHF, as determined by central adjudication, in a community-based elderly population.

Hypertension has long been considered as a risk factor for the development of heart failure. In the Framingham study, hypertension was reported as an aetiological factor for heart failure in approximately 50% of cases. Nevertheless it is difficult to appreciate the discrepancy from other epidemiological studies, where ischaemic heart disease is the commonest cause of heart failure. It is possible that hypertension leads to heart failure by a number of mechanisms, including the development of coronary artery disease (and myocardial infarction) and arrhythmias (e.g. atrial fibrillation). It should also be remembered that alcohol can lead to both hypertension and heart failure.

In these data from the Cardiovascular Health Study, on 5625 non-institutionalized, community-dwelling individuals aged 65–100 years who were followed for an average of 5.5 years (median follow-up 6.3 years), 597 participants developed CHF. The incidence of CHF increased according to gender, with men almost twice as likely to develop CHF as women, and according to age, with the incidence of CHF increasing markedly as subjects got older. Furthermore, prevalent and incident atherosclerosis and elevated SBP were important considerations. Indeed, the use of diuretics, beta-blockers or other agents to control the SBP may help avert CHF.

The pathogenesis of acute pulmonary oedema associated with hypertension.

Gandhi SK, Powers JC, Nomeir AM, *et al. N Engl J Med* 2001; **344**: 17–22.

BACKGROUND. Patients with acute pulmonary oedema often have marked hypertension but, after reduction of the BP, have a normal LVEF (≥0.50). However, the pulmonary oedema may not have resulted from isolated diastolic dysfunction but, instead, may be due to transient systolic dysfunction, acute mitral regurgitation, or both.

INTERPRETATION. In patients with hypertensive pulmonary oedema, a normal ejection fraction after treatment suggests that the oedema was due to the exacerbation of diastolic dysfunction by hypertension—not to transient systolic dysfunction or mitral regurgitation.

Comment

Contrary to their hypothesis, the authors found that the LVEF and the extent of regional wall motion measured during the acute episode of hypertensive pulmonary oedema were similar to those measured after the resolution of the congestion, when BP was controlled. This finding is consistent with previous observations suggesting that in 40% or more of such patients, particularly elderly patients, heart failure is due to isolated diastolic (not systolic) dysfunction.

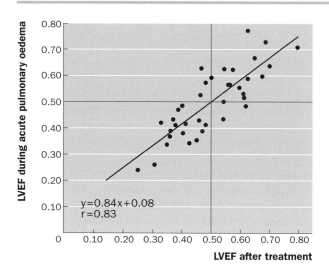

Fig. 12.1 LVEF during acute pulmonary oedema and one to three days later, after treatment. The solid line is the regression line. The dotted lines indicate normal values for the ejection fraction. Source: Gandhi *et al.* (2001).

Conclusion

Left ventricular diastolic dysfunction is a common cause of heart failure in hyper tensive patients with LVH. However, breathlessness in these patients may be due to LV systolic dysfunction as assessed by LV mid-wall mechanics despite 'supranormal' systolic performance assessed by traditional LV endocardial fractional shortening or ejection fraction. Furthermore, decreased coronary vasodilator reserve that is often observed in hypertensive patients with increased LV mass in the absence of coronary disease may also contribute to 'heart failure' symptoms. Conventional echocardio-graphic Doppler indices may be unreliable for assessing LV diastolic function, and newer methods hold some promise. Pulse Doppler tissue imaging is increasingly popular and has been advocated to complement the conventional method and pul-monary venous flow measurements.

13

Left ventricular hypertrophy: the most potent prognostic marker besides advanced age

Introduction

Left ventricular hypertrophy (LVH) significantly increases the risk of cardiovascular morbidity and mortality in hypertensive and non-hypertensive populations, independent of blood pressure (BP), in either population with or without cardiovascular disease. Indeed, it is the most potent prognostic marker beside advanced age. The incidence of hypertension increases with ageing, and ageing aggravates hypertensive changes. The mechanisms that underlie this risk are increasingly understood. Impairments in coronary circulation and thus reduced myocardial perfusion leading to ventricular fibrosis and impaired myocardial contractile function, and disturbances in cardiac electrophysiology contribute to such increased risk in LVH. Owing to its strong prognostic significance of LVH, normalization or regression of LV mass has emerged as one of the desirable goals of antihypertensive treatment. Indeed, prospective evidence is accumulating indicating that reduction in LV mass is associated with lower cardiovascular complications. Many studies have been published suggesting that regression is achievable using a variety of antihypertensive classes. The question remains whether certain agents or class of agents are more superior than the other to reduce LV mass and whether such agents are able to do so beyond that which can be achieved by its BP lowering effect.

The study and treatment of LVH, in particular the prognostic implications of changes in LV mass, require an accurate, safe and reproducible method of measurement. Twelve-lead electrocardiography (ECG) is the most accessible method clinically but lacks reproducibility. Echocardiographic assessment of LVH is currently the gold standard and affordable by most centres, though its use in large clinical trials is logistically difficult.

Left ventricular mass and cardiovascular morbidity in essential hypertension: the MAVI (MAssa Ventricolare sinistra nell'Ipertensione) study.

Verdecchia P, Carini G, Circo A, *et al.* *J Am Coll Cardiol* 2001; **38**(7): 1829–35.

BACKGROUND. Only a few single-centre studies support the prognostic value of LV mass in uncomplicated hypertension. This study investigated the prognostic value of LV mass at echocardiography in uncomplicated subjects with essential hypertension.

INTERPRETATION. The findings show a strong, continuous and independent relationship of LV mass to subsequent cardiovascular morbidity. This is the first study to extend such demonstration to a large nationwide multi-centre sample of uncomplicated subjects with essential hypertension.

Comment

This study showed a simple message: the left ventricle mass at echocardiography, independent of other factors, can help physicians predict cardiovascular events in patients who are hypertensive but have no history of cardiovascular problems. The study followed 1033 asymptomatic patients with essential hypertension (396 men, BP >140 mmHg systolic or 90 mmHg diastolic) aged >50 for a median 3 years. LVH was defined as an LV mass >125 g/m^2, a partition point supported by ample prognostic evidence. After adjustment for age, diabetes and smoking, there was an independent 37% increase in the risk of primary events for any 39 g (1 standard deviation) increase in LV mass and after further adjustment for serum creatinine concentration there was a 40% rise in the risk of total cardiovascular events. However, LVH at ECG did not achieve significance as a predictor of cardiovascular risk after controlling for LV mass. It is of note that renal function was normal in all subjects at entry into the study, the predictive value of creatinine may simply reflect continuous chronic insults of hypertension on the kidneys and therefore predict outcome also in non-renal target organs.

These findings support the view that both prevention of LVH development and regression of hypertrophy once established are key targets in the management of asymptomatic patients with essential hypertension.

Left ventricular hypertrophy as an independent predictor of acute cerebrovascular events in essential hypertension.

Verdecchia P, Porcellati C, Reboldi G, *et al. Circulation* 2001; **104**: 2039–44.

BACKGROUND. It is uncertain whether LVH confers an increased risk for cerebrovascular disease in apparently healthy patients with essential hypertension.

INTERPRETATION. In apparently healthy patients with essential hypertension, LVH diagnosed by ECG or echocardiography confers an excess risk for stroke and transient ischaemic attack independently of BP and other individual risk factors.

Comment

Cerebrovascular events are well-recognized consequences of elevated BP, which in turn may lead to LVH. It may be difficult to differentiate the relative role of elevated BP from a direct contribution of LVH to the increased risk of developing stroke. As pointed out by Devereux [1], long-term prognostic studies of stroke in populations with baseline measurements of both LV mass and ambulatory BP are needed to resolve this uncertainty. The present study consisted of a total 2363 initially untreated hypertensive patients (mean age 51 ± 12 years, 47% women) free of previous cardiovascular disease and followed up for up to 14 years (mean 5 years) has clearly answered the question above. By contrast, however, it is still unclear whether LVH regression will lead to a reduction of stroke risk.

Prognostic implications of the compensatory nature of left ventricular mass in arterial hypertension.

de Simone G, Palmieri V, Koren MJ, Mensah GA, Roman MJ, Devereux RB.
J Hypertension 2001; **19**: 119–25.

BACKGROUND. An increase in LV mass occurs in adults as a primary adaptive mechanism to compensate for increased cardiac workload produced by conditions causing volume and/or pressure overload. At some point in the evolution of this adaptation, the increase in LV mass becomes a potent marker of cardiovascular risk.

INTERPRETATION. In hypertensive patients, increase in LV mass beyond values required to compensate cardiac workload at a given body size and sex predicts cardiovascular risk independently of age and BP, in the whole population as well as in the subset of patients with LVH. Hypertensive patients with levels of LV mass lower than needed to compensate cardiac workload exhibit hyperdynamic circulatory status and the same risk pattern as patients with higher values of LV mass, possibly due to activation of the sympathetic system.

Comment

The purpose of this prospective longitudinal study was to test whether inappropriate echocardiographic LV mass (i.e. higher or lower than predicted by individual body size, sex and cardiac load [% LV mass]) is associated with an increased rate of cardiovascular events, and whether values of LV mass lower than appropriate confer protection. The association of increased LV mass with adverse cardiovascular events is not new. However, there are three interesting features of this study. First, the evaluation of LV mass in terms of its appropriateness (corrected for a given stroke work, gender and body size) increases our knowledge of pathophysiology of LV adaptation

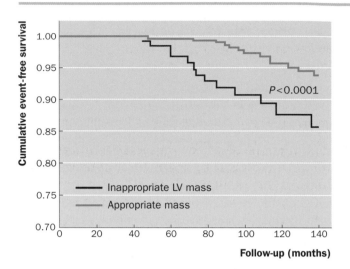

Fig. 13.1 Survival function for cardiovascular fatal and non-fatal events at mean of covariates in patients with appropriate (grey line) or inappropriate (black line) LV mass. Source: de Simone *et al.* (2001).

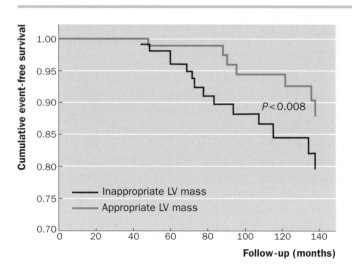

Fig. 13.2 Survival function for cardiovascular fatal and non-fatal events at mean of covariates in patients with LVH (based on normalization of LV mass for height$^{2.7}$) divided in relation to the presence of appropriate (grey line) or inappropriate (black line) LV mass. Source: de Simone *et al.* (2001).

in arterial hypertension. Secondly, its utility for prognostic stratification in cardio-vascular risk in selected populations might add important information to the traditional method of definition of LVH. Finally, demonstrated for the first time, values of LV mass lower than 'appropriately' predicted exhibit hyperdynamic circulatory status and the same cardiovascular risk pattern as patients with higher values of LV mass.

Left ventricular function and haemodynamic features of inappropriate left ventricular hypertrophy in patients with systemic hypertension: the LIFE study.

Palmieri V, Wachtell K, Gerdts E, *et al. Am Heart J* 2001; **141**(5): 784–91.

BACKGROUND. Predicted LV mass for sex, height$^{2.7}$, and haemodynamic load can be used as an intrapatient reference for the observed LV mass. The ratio of observed/predicted LV mass may allow more physiologically correct comparisons of LV geometry, systolic and diastolic functions, and haemodynamics among hypertensive patients.

INTERPRETATION. Among hypertensives with LVH, inappropriate LVH identified cardiac phenotypes with a high prevalence of myocardial systolic dysfunction.

Comment

LVH in arterial hypertension develops in response to an increased afterload, but underlying pathophysiological mechanisms are complex and include a variety of non-haemodynamic factors. Definition of LVH relies on partition values based on distributions in reference populations and does not account for appropriateness of LV mass to actual haemodynamic burden. Appropriateness of LV mass to loading condition and body size can be assessed by relating observed LV mass to levels predicted by an equation, including sex, body height, BP and echocardographic stroke volume. Therefore, predicted LV mass can be used as an intra-individual reference to define the appropriateness of actual LV mass, facilitating inter-individual comparisons. This study illustrated nicely the practicability of such method. They studied 659 participants in the LIFE (Losartan Intervention for Endpoint Reduction in Hypertension) study with both ECG and echocardiographic LVH (68% of the echocardiographic cohort) without previous myocardial infarction. LV mass was predicted by an equation, including sex, stroke work and height. Observed/predicted LV mass >128% defined inappropriate LVH. Relative wall thickness ≥0.43 defined concentric LV geometry. Systolic myocardial dysfunction was assessed by mid-wall mechanics and abnormal LV relaxation by isovolumic relaxation time. Accordingly, they were able to demonstrate the extent to which inappropriate/appropriate LV mass (concentric and eccentric hypertrophy) is related to LV dysfunction. As compared with appropriate LVH, inappropriate LVH is independently associated with

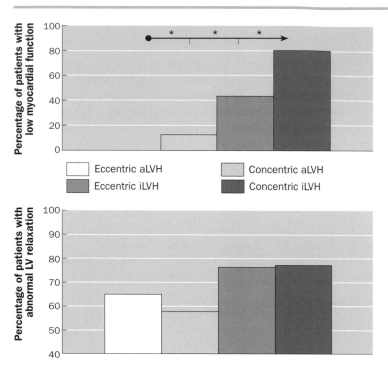

Fig. 13.3 Upper panel: bars represent percentage of patients with low myocardial function in relation to eccentric or concentric appropriate LVH/inappropriate LVH. *All *P* <0.01. Lower panel: bars represent percentage of patients with abnormal LV relaxation in relation to eccentric or concentric appropriate LVH/inappropriate LVH. *P* for trend = 0.03. Source: Palmieri *et al.* (2001).

higher prevalence of depressed systolic myocardial function, lower pump performance and abnormal diastolic relaxation, suggesting a more adverse cardiovascular risk profile. Again, long-term follow up data are eagerly awaited.

Relation of echocardiographic left ventricular mass and hypertrophy to persistent electrocardiographic left ventricular hypertropy in hypertensive patients: the LIFE study.

Okin PM, Devereux RB, Jern S, *et al. Am J Hypertens* 2001; **14**(8 Pt 1): 775–82.

B A C K G R O U N D . The LIFE trial used LVH on a screening ECG to identify patients at high risk for morbid events. Because of regression to the mean, not all patients who met screening criteria had persistent ECG LVH on the ECG performed at study baseline.

INTERPRETATION. Persistent ECG LVH between screening and LIFE study baseline identified patients with greater LV mass and a higher prevalence of ECG LVH, suggesting that these patients may be at higher risk for subsequent morbid and mortal events.

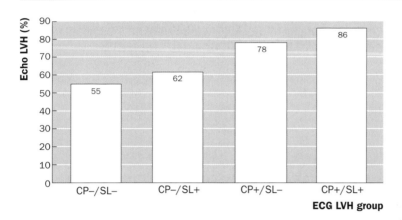

Fig. 13.4 Prevalence of echocardiographic LVH according to the persistence or resolution of ECG LVH by Cornell voltage-duration product criteria or Sokolow–Lyon voltage criteria. Source: Okin *et al.* (2001).

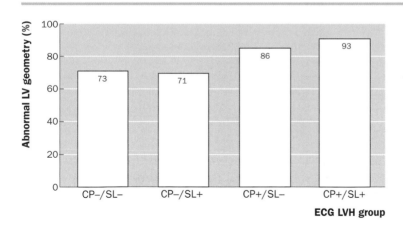

Fig. 13.5 Prevalence of abnormal LV geometry (concentric remodelling, eccentric hypertrophy or concentric hypertrophy) according to the persistence or resolution of ECG LVH by Cornell voltage-duration product or Sokolow–Lyon voltage criteria. Source: Okin *et al.* (2001).

Comment

In this study, about 75% of patients screened had persistent ECG LVH at baseline, and those with persistent ECG LVH by Cornell voltage-duration product or Sokolow–Lyon voltage criteria had a greater LV mass and a higher prevalence of ECG LVH compared with patients in whom ECG LVH was no longer manifest. Indeed, the presence of ECG LVH by both criteria had a more than fourfold higher risk of echocardiographic LVH compared with the absence of these criteria, even after factoring in the older age, higher SBP, and greater body mass index in these patients. Compared with Sokolow–Lyon voltage criteria, Cornell voltage-duration product had higher positive predictive value for detection of hypertrophy. On the other hand, it is also important to note that even patients in whom ECG LVH was not present on the second ECG had a >50% likelihood of having LVH by echocardiogram, further illustrating the clinical value of ECG methods for identifying hypertensive patients at high risk.

Echocardiographic left ventricular geometry in hypertensive patients with electrocardiographic left ventricular hypertrophy: The LIFE Study.

Devereux RB, Bella J, Boman K, et al. Blood Press 2001; **10**(2): 74–82.

B A C K G R O U N D . **The LIFE trial used LVH on a screening ECG to identify patients at high risk for morbid events. Because of regression to the mean, not all patients who met screening criteria had persistent ECG LVH on the ECG performed at study baseline.**

I N T E R P R E T A T I O N . Persistent ECG LVH between screening and LIFE study baseline identified patients with greater LV mass and a higher prevalence of echocardiographic LVH, suggesting that these patients may be at higher risk for subsequent morbid and mortal events.

Comment

This is another paper from the LIFE study re-enforcing the findings of Okin *et al.* (2001) above.

Effects of drug therapy on cardiac arrhythmias and ischaemia in hypertensives with LVH.

Novo S, Abrignani MG, Novo G, et al. Am J Hypertens 2001; **14**(7 Pt 1): 637–43.

B A C K G R O U N D . **LVH in hypertensive subjects is associated with an increased prevalence of ventricular arrhythmias. It has been suggested that antihypertensive treatment may reduce cardiac arrhythmias (CA), and that the mechanism may be related to the reduction in LV mass.**

INTERPRETATION. The present study shows that in hypertensive patients with LVH, antihypertensive treatment with atenolol, enalapril and verapamil slow-release reduces LVH and decreases the prevalence of CA and transient episodes of myocardial ischaemia (TEMI). Treatment with hydrochlorothiazide during the 6-month study did not alter LVH and did not appear to reduce CA and TEMI.

Comment

The aim of this randomized study was to assess the efficacy of four different frequently used antihypertensive drugs, enalapril, atenolol, verapamil slow-release and hydrochlorothiazide, to reduce LVH, CA and TEMI in hypertensive patients with LVH but without clinical history of CHD. All patients underwent echocardiography, ECG Holter monitoring, and exercise stress testing. As pointed out by the authors because the reduction in CA was similar with the three different drug classes, it is unlikely that the underlying mechanism is an antiarrhythmic-specific effect of one drug on the myocardium. However, it is more likely the effect common to all three drugs, to lower BP and to reduce LV mass, which may be implicated in the decrease of CA. Furthermore, the LV mass regression may restore the LVH-related perfusion imbalance and thus the reduction of TEMI. Quite rightly, the authors pointed out a few limitations of their study, and future study with a larger sample size and longer follow-up are needed.

Reference

1. Devereux RB. Therapeutic options in minimizing left ventricular hypertrophy. *Am Heart J* 2000; **139**(1 Pt 2): S9–14.

14

Left ventricular hypertrophy regression: from improved left ventricular function to increased survival

Introduction

Many studies have unequivocally demonstrated the risk associated with increased left ventricular (LV) mass or LV hypertrophy (LVH). Indeed, LVH is probably the most visible manifestation of hypertensive target organ damage. As reduction of LVH by antihypertensive treatment is associated with a substantial decrease in cardiovascular mortality and morbidity, regression of LVH is being considered as a possible intermediate end-point for clinical trials. However, it is of note that there are several differences between the so-called physiological LVH (as occurs in endurance athletes) from pathological LVH associated with hypertension. Pathological LVH is to a large extent, the result of excessive fibrosis and the loss of tissue homogeneity that accompanies hypertrophy of the myocytes and is characterized by impaired LV filling, reduced coronary reserve, increased ventricular electric activity, and decreased LV pump function. Indeed, the renin–angiotensin–aldosterone system has been linked to LVH and cardiac fibrosis. Drugs that block the production or action of aldosterone or angiotensin II lower blood pressure (BP), regress LVH and reduce cardiac fibrosis.

Notably, many pharmacological agents have been tested and claimed to be superior over one another in inducing LV mass regression. Even non-pharmacological measures too have been shown to be able to cause a clinically significant degree of LV regression. However, whether such therapeutic 'ability' to regress LV mass could result in long-term benefit is still a matter of debate, although the recently published Heart Outcomes Prevention Evaluation (HOPE) substudy (see below) has provided data on electrocardiographic (ECG) LVH regression using ramipril resulting in a reduction of the primary outcomes (cardiovascular death, myocardial infarction or stroke) and the prevention of congestive heart failure, intriguingly this was achieved with only a modest reduction of BP. However, whether this effect was specific to angiotensin-converting enzyme inhibitor (ACEI) or to any other agent that can achieve a similar degree of ECG LVH regression is still unknown. It should be noted that there were no strict ECG criteria for LVH on study entry into the HOPE trial and more importantly, there was no echocardiographic data to correlate the results with ECG LVH. The following articles will reinforce the viewpoints above.

Ventricular and myocardial function following treatment of hypertension.

Aurigemma GP, Williams D, Gaasch WH, Reda DJ, Materson BJ, Gottdiener JS. *Am J Cardiol* 2001; **87**(6): 732–6.

BACKGROUND. Antihypertensive therapy has been associated with reductions in LV mass and changes in LV geometry. Most clinical studies of cardiac function before and after LV mass regression have used indexes of LV chamber function; none have performed an analysis of LV mid-wall mechanics.

INTERPRETATION. Reductions in LV mass associated with antihypertensive therapy are generally not accompanied by a decrement in LV chamber or myocardial function. Improvement in mid-wall shortening is more closely related to normalization of LV geometry than to reduction in LV mass.

Comment

The aim of this study was to investigate LV contractile function after treatment of hypertension, with an emphasis on mid-wall mechanics. LV mid-wall fractional shortening, in relation to stress, may be impaired in hypertensive patients with a normal or supranormal LV ejection fraction. The findings suggest that geometric remodelling preserves chamber indexes of function (endocardial shortening or ejection fraction) in the face of reduced myocardial shortening; the dissociation between chamber and myocardial indexes is directly related to relative wall thickness (RWT). Furthermore, improvement or deterioration in the chamber or myocardial function was more closely related to changes in LV geometry than to changes in LV mass alone. In pressure overload hypertrophy or in subjects with high RWT, endocardial shortening may overestimate myocardial function. Moreover, previous studies have shown that depressed mid-wall fractional shortening predicts adverse outcome in hypertensive patients, especially in the subgroup with hypertrophy.

Left ventricular mass and systolic dysfunction in essential hypertension.

Schillaci G, Vaudo G, Pasqualini L, Reboldi G, Porcellati C, Verdecchia P. *J Hum Hypertens* 2002; **16**: 117–22.

BACKGROUND. A relation between LVH and depressed mid-wall systolic function has been described in hypertensive subjects. However, a strong confounding factor in this relation is concentric geometry, which is both a powerful determinant of depressed mid-wall systolic function and a correlate of LV mass in hypertension.

INTERPRETATION. The inverse association between LV mass and mid-wall systolic function is partly independent from the effect of RWT. LVH is a determinant of subclinical LV dysfunction independently of the concomitant changes in chamber geometry.

Comment

The conventional chamber function measurements using LV endocardial fractional shortening or ejection fraction often report a normal or 'supranormal' systolic performance in hypertensive patients even in the absence of significant LVH. A newer method expressed as mid-wall fractional shortening (LV mid-wall mechanics) has been developed that takes into consideration the non-uniform wall thickness that contracts radially and longitudinally, and the wall volume (myocardial mass) is assumed to be constant throughout the cardiac cycle. This model has been shown to reduce substantially the number of hypertensive patients with supranormal LV function and identified low LV myocardial performance in approximately one-sixth of the patients, especially in those with an abnormal LV geometry. Such a method eliminated the artefactual effect of the endocardial motion and thus thought to be more representative of LV systolic function in hypertension-induced hypertrophy. Hence, this would allow a better assessment for improved myocardial performance and/or LV mass reduction with antihypertensive therapy. Indeed, decreased mid-wall fractional shortening has been identified as an independent predictor of cardiovascular morbidity and mortality and has been associated with diminished contractile reserve, abnormal diastolic function, LVH and extracardiac target organ damage. Moreover, recent studies have also reported associations of low mid-wall fractional shortening with abnormal LV diastolic filling in selected hypertensive patients with normal LV fractional shortening.

The present study further supports the use of mid-wall fractional shortening (rather than endocardial fractional shortening) as a more physiological assessment of LV systolic function in the presence of LVH or abnormal LV geometry, particularly in the presence of concentric LV geometry. The Progetto Ipertensione Umbria Monitoraggio Ambulatoriale (PIUMA) Study is a prospective follow-up study of Caucasian adult patients with essential hypertension. The present study included a large sample of never-treated subjects ($n = 1827$, age 48 ± 12 years, men 58%), with uncomplicated hypertension. The purpose of this substudy was to evaluate the independent contribution of LV mass to depressed systolic function. It was found that RWT was the strongest determinant of low mid-wall fractional shortening ($r = -0.63$, $P < 0.0001$). In the present population of never-treated subjects with essential hypertension, however, there was an inverse correlation between LV mass and mid-wall systolic function ($r = -0.43$, $P < 0.0001$), which remained significant also after adjustment for the powerful confounding effect of concentric LV geometry (partial $r = -0.27$, $P < 0.0001$). For every given value of RWT, the proportion of subjects with subnormal afterload-corrected myocardial function was greater in the presence than in the absence of LVH. In the presence of an identical chamber geometry, mid-wall fractional shortening progressively decreases with increasing LV mass values. All subjects were free from concomitant overt cardiovascular disease and diabetes mellitus, which may have an independent influence on LV mass and function.

The present findings support the role of LVH as a determinant of depressed myocardial function in never-treated subjects with uncomplicated hypertension, but do not provide a mechanism to explain these results.

There is some evidence that regression of LVH induced by antihypertensive treatment is accompanied by an improvement in mid-wall systolic function, even in the absence of concomitant changes in LV geometry (see below).

Midwall mechanics are improved after regression of hypertensive left ventricular hypertrophy and normalization of chamber geometry.

Perlini S, Muiesan ML, Cuspidi C, *et al. Circulation* 2001; **103**(5): 678–83.

BACKGROUND. It is still unclear whether substantial regression of hypertensive LVH and normalization of chamber geometry are associated with improved LV myocardial function.

INTERPRETATION. Regression of concentric LVH is associated with an improvement of mid-wall systolic function, which is more dependent on the normalization of LV geometry than on the reduction in LV systolic stress.

Comment

Although there is good evidence for LVH regression in hypertensive patients treated with antihypertensive drugs, the results may be difficult to interpret as it is often difficult to separate the direct effects of individual pharmacological agents on hypertrophy from the BP reduction.

This study was performed on patients enrolled in the SAMPLE study (Study on Ambulatory Monitoring of Blood Pressure and Lisinopril Evaluation), a multi-centre trial involving 11 hypertension clinics in Italy. Two-dimensionally directed M-mode echocardiography was performed as follows: (i) after a 4-week placebo 'run-in' period; (ii) after 1 year of treatment with 20 mg/day lisinopril (alone or associated with 12.5–25 mg/day hydrochlorothiazide); and (iii) after a final 1-month placebo period to allow BP (24-hour average ambulatory monitoring) to return to pre-treatment levels. In the 152 hypertensive patients (with concentric LVH), the 12-month administration of an ACEI (plus, when needed, a diuretic) was accompanied by a clear-cut reduction in BP, which was associated with a reduced prevalence of LVH (−46%), LV geometric remodelling, and a reduction in the initially elevated LV mass index (−14%). The main finding of the study, however, is that while leaving systolic chamber function relatively unaffected, the 12-month treatment was accompanied by a significant improvement in LV mid-wall shortening, which was entirely maintained after the 1-month placebo period that followed the treatment, during which: (i) one-third of the regression of LVH was reversed; (ii) any direct cardiac effect of antihypertensive treatment was washed out; and (iii) BP was restored almost to the elevated pre-treatment values. This indicates that myocardial systolic function is improved by LVH regression and normalization of chamber geometry, independent of the drugs used to cause it or on the favourable consequences of a reduced LV afterload on the myocardium. This study was claimed to be the first unequivocal evidence of this phenomenon obtained in a large human database. Thus, the beneficial evidence of LVH regression in hypertension patients is growing stronger with the results of this study and this should be a logical aim of antihypertensive therapy, preferably with agent that blocks the angiotensin II effects.

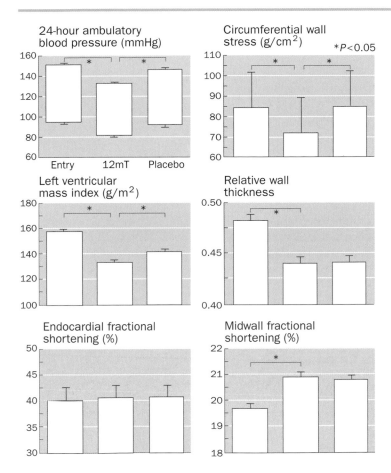

Fig. 14.1 Ambulatory BP, circumferential end-systolic wall stress, LV mass index, RWT, and endocardial and mid-wall fractional shortening at study entry (left bar), at end of the 12-month treatment period (middle bar), and after the final 4-week placebo period (right bar). Data are shown as mean ± SD. *$P <0.05$. Source: Perlini et al. (2001).

Effects of once-daily angiotensin-converting enzyme inhibition and calcium channel blockade-based antihypertensive treatment regimens on left ventricular hypertrophy and diastolic filling in hypertension. The Prospective Randomized Enalapril Study Evaluating Regression of Ventricular Enlargement (PRESERVE) Trial.

Devereux RB, Palmieri V, Sharpe N. *et al. Circulation* 2001; **104**: 1248–54.

BACKGROUND. The Prospective Randomized Enalapril Study Evaluating Regression of Ventricular Enlargement (PRESERVE) study was designed to test whether enalapril achieves greater LV mass reduction than does a nifedipine gastrointestinal treatment system by a prognostically meaningful degree on a population basis (10 g/m^2).

INTERPRETATION. Once-daily antihypertensive treatment with enalapril or long-acting nifedipine, plus adjunctive hydrochlorothiazide and atenolol when needed to control BP, both had moderately beneficial and statistically indistinguishable effects on regression of LVH.

Comment

Prevention or reversal of hypertensive LVH is widely accepted as a desirable treatment goal. However, despite numerous trials of pharmacological and non-pharmacological therapy, uncertainty persists about how best to regress hypertensive LVH. Most published studies have been relatively small and have had additional limitations, including short duration, lack of comparative agents, unblinded echo-cardiogram readings, and study populations without sexual and ethnic diversity. The PRESERVE trial provides the largest (with 303 patients) prospective, randomized, double-blind study to date comparing cardiac effects of ACE inhibition and calcium channel blockade in patients with hypertensive LVH. However, the study simply showed that after 1 year of either treatment regimens based on enalapril or the nifedipine–gastrointestinal treatment system in hypertensive patients with LVH, there was no statistically significant difference in the degree of LV mass regression and Doppler diastolic LV filling between the two groups. Few issues remained un-settled, for example, a similar degree of LV mass regression does not necessarily translate into similar clinical effects, and the results of this study may not be extrapo-lated to other ACEIs or calcium channel blockers, and more importantly, the clinical significance of LV regression on hard end-points remains uncertain.

Reduction of cardiovascular risk by regression of electrocardiographic markers of left ventricular hypertrophy by the angiotensin-converting enzyme inhibitor ramipril.

Mathew J, Sleight P, Lonn E, *et al. Circulation* 2001; **104**(14): 1615–21.

BACKGROUND. **ECG markers of LVH predict poor prognosis. We determined whether the ACEI ramipril prevents the development and causes regression of ECG-LVH and whether these changes are associated with improved prognosis independent of BP reduction.**

INTERPRETATION. The ACEI ramipril decreases the development and causes regression of ECG LVH independent of BP reduction, and these changes are associated with a reduced risk of death, myocardial infarction, stroke and congestive heart failure.

Comment

The results showed that ramipril prevented LVH, or caused a gradual regression of LVH, in 91.9% of patients, irrespective of their BP reduction. Intriguingly, 90.2% of patients assigned to placebo also had regression or prevention of LVH. Those who had regression/prevention of LVH had a lower risk of the pre-defined primary outcome compared with those who had development/persistence of LVH (12.3% vs 15.8%, $P = 0.006$) and of congestive heart failure (9.3% vs. 15.4%, $P < 0.0001$). Mathew *et al.* noted that the regression of LVH seen in the placebo arm could be

Table 14.1 LVH status in ramipril vs placebo patients

LVH status	Ramipril (n = 4135)	Placebo (n = 4146)	RR (95% CI) for ramipril/placebo
LVH development/persistence	336 (8.1%)	406 (9.8%)	0.83 (0.72–0.95)
LVH regression/prevention	3799 (91.9%)	3740 (90.2%)	1.02 (1.01–1.03)

Source: Mathew *et al.* (2001).

Table 14.2 LVH status and CV risk

Outcome	LVH regression/ prevention (n = 7539)	LVH development/ persistence (n = 742)	P value
Predefined primary outcome	925 (12.3%)	117 (15.8%)	0.006
CHF	697 (9.3%)	114 (15.4%)	<0.0001

Source: Mathew *et al.* (2001).

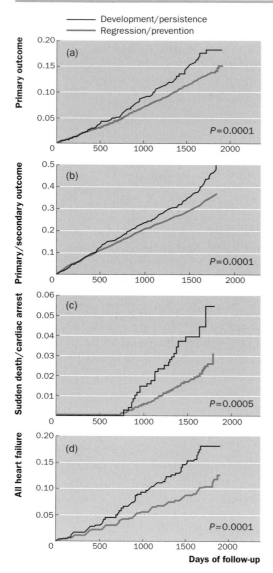

Fig. 14.2 Kaplan–Meier estimates of outcomes in patients who had regression/prevention vs development/persistence of ECG markers of LVH. (A) Primary outcome events (cardiovascular death, myocardial infarction or stroke). (B) Primary outcome events (cardiovascular death, myocardial infarction or stroke) plus secondary outcome events (revascularization, hospitalization for unstable angina, hospitalization for congestive heart failure, and complications of diabetes). (C) Unexpected (sudden) death or cardiac arrest. (D) All congestive heart failure whether hospitalized or not.
Source: Mathew *et al.* (2001).

related to a number of factors, including multiple risk factor modification in patients who participate in clinical trials, as well as the use of concomitant medications, including beta-blockers and other BP-lowering drugs. As previously suggested in our editorial commentary, ECG criteria in defining LVH, though readily available clinic-ally but not as ideal compared with echocardiography, could hopefully be better answered by the ongoing LIFE study. Furthermore, the benefit of LVH regression in Afro-Caribbean patients is still yet to be established.

Recovery of coronary function and morphology during regression of left ventricular hypertrophy.

Kingsbury M, Mahnke A, Turner M, Sheridan D. *Cardiovasc Res* 2002; **55**: 83–96.

BACKGROUND. Evidence that better cardiovascular outcome is accompanied by reversal of the pathophysiological features of LVH is unclear. In some studies coronary vascular remodelling and coronary reserve have been shown to improve, if not normalize, with regression of LVH, while others show no change in coronary reserve despite regression of LVH.

INTERPRETATION. LV haemodynamic unloading can result in complete normalization of LVH, coronary morphology and haemodynamic function. Although morphological and functional recovery were closely correlated, recovery of coronary morphology and function slightly preceded that of the myocardium in this aortic banded/debanded model.

Comment

The purpose of this study was to investigate changes in (guinea-pigs) myocardial and coronary morphology and systemic and coronary haemodynamics following the induction of LVH by aortic banding and during regression after a subsequent debanding. The degree of LVH, coronary haemodynamic function and contempor-aneous vessel morphology 42 days post-operation were measured. These animals were then debanded and the same parameters measured after 1, 3 and 6 weeks to assess haemodynamic and morphological changes as hypertrophy regressed. Band-ing resulted in an aortic pressure gradient of 41 ± 9 mmHg with concomitant increases in heart/body weight ratio (46%), myocyte size (26%) and a doubling of arteriolar wall thickness. At the same time, they observed a reduction in coronary reserve (38%) and significantly decreased maximal response to acetylcholine (70%), sodium nitroprusside (87%), adenosine (70%) and reactive hyperaemia (52%). Interestingly, 7 days after debanding systemic haemodynamics normalized, but there was only limited improvement in coronary structure and coronary function until 23 days after debanding, although systolic impedance to flow remained significantly increased. After 44 days, debanding resulted in complete cardiac morphological and functional recovery, including the systolic impediment to coronary flow. Thus, while recovery of coronary morphology and function slightly preceded that of the myocardium, surgical unloading resulted in full recovery of established LVH; furthermore, morphological and a functional recovery were closely correlated.

Although experimental animal models of hypertrophy are useful to study short-term pathophysiological changes following a surgically induced increase in afterload, which may be more relevant to an acute increase in aortic stenosis in humans, but not to that of human systemic hypertension. As in common with most models of LVH, the duration of hypertrophy is shorter than in human disease. As pointed out by the authors, the present findings do not address whether normalization of long-standing LVH can be achieved. Nevertheless it may be reasonable to hypothesize that with adequate treatment recent onset hypertrophy may be capable of full reversal.

Change of left ventricular geometric pattern after 1 year of antihypertensive treatment: the Losartan Intervention For Endpoint reduction in hypertension (LIFE) study.

Wachtell K, Dahlof B, Rokkedal J, *et al.*; Losartan Intervention For Endpoint reduction in hypertension. *Am Heart J* 2002; **144**(6): 1057–64.

BACKGROUND. Patients with hypertension have different types of LV geometry, but the impact of BP reduction on LV geometry change during antihypertensive treatment remains unclear.

INTERPRETATION. Antihypertensive treatment reduces LV mass and decreases the prevalence of LVH and concentric LV remodelling. Additional control of Doppler stroke volume potentiates the effect of BP reduction on LV mass regression independent of the BP reduction *per se*.

Comment

Using LV mass indexed for body size and RWT, LVH can be characterized by geometric subtypes (also see Chapter 16):

- concentric LVH: with increased RWT and LVH have been reported to have the highest incidence of cardiovascular events, including death
- eccentric LVH: with normal RWT and LVH; intermediate risk
- concentric LV remodelling: with increased RWT and normal LV mass; intermediate risk
- normal LV geometry: lowest risk.

In the LIFE Echocardiography Substudy, 963 patients with stage II–III hypertension were initially enrolled at baseline. However, data from 853 patients were available after 1 year of blinded treatment with either a losartan-base or atenolol-base regimen.

After 1 year of follow-up:

- baseline systolic/diastolic BP were reduced from 174 ± 20/95 ± 11 to 151 ± 19/84 ± 11 mmHg
- LV mass was reduced from 234 ± 56 to 207 ± 51 g
- RWT from 0.41 ± 0.07 to 0.38 ± 0.06
- prevalence of concentric LVH decreased from 24% to 6%
- eccentric LVH decreased from 46% to 37%
- concentric LV remodelling decreased from 10% to 6%
- normal geometry increased from 20% to 51%
- 73% of those with concentric LV remodelling at baseline shifted to normal geometric pattern
- only 7% of those with normal pattern at baseline shifted to concentric LV remodelling
- of patients with concentric LVH at baseline, 34% shifted to eccentric LVH
- only 3% with eccentric LVH at baseline had concentric LVH
- Doppler stroke volume reduction was a significant correlate of LV mass reduction ($\beta = 0.108$, $P < 0.001$) independent of BP, heart rate change, and assigned drug treatment.

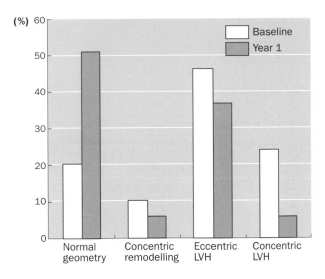

Fig. 14.3 Change in prevalence (%) of LV geometric patterns after 1 year of antihypertensive treatment. Source: Wachtell *et al.* (2002).

These findings indicate that abnormal LV geometries could be altered favourably by antihypertensive treatment and these changes may be independent of the BP reduction and treatment type *per se.*

Change in systolic left ventricular performance after 3 years of antihypertensive treatment: the Losartan Intervention for Endpoint (LIFE) Study.

Wachtell K, Palmieri V, Olsen MH, *et al. Circulation* 2002; **106**(2): 227–32.

BACKGROUND. One of the earlier echocardiographic substudies of LIFE has shown that hypertensive patients with LVH have decreased LV mid-wall mechanics, but the effect of antihypertensive therapy remains unclear.

INTERPRETATION. Antihypertensive therapy reduced LV mass and increased LV mid-wall shortening and contractility with a small decrease in LV chamber function and significant increase in stroke volume. Change in systolic LV performance was independently associated inversely with change in LV mass, RWT and BP, and directly with change in stroke volume.

Comment

Depressed systolic LV mid-wall function in patients with hypertensive LVH may play a key role in the development of heart failure and ultimately in hypertensive pulmonary oedema, which might be the cause of increased mortality found in these patients.

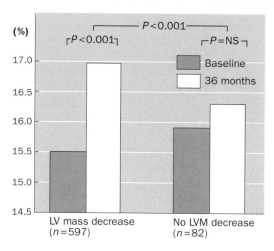

Fig. 14.4 Effect of LVH regression on mid-wall fractional shortening. Source: Wachtell *et al.* (2002).

Basically, this substudy has shown that 3 years of antihypertensive treatment in patients with LVH leads to mean BP reduction and LV mass regression of 15% and 17%, respectively, and myocardial systolic mid-wall contractility increased significantly despite small decreases in indices of LV chamber performance. These findings indicate that partial normalization of arterial pressure and LV geometry can result in the reversal of both the supranormal LV chamber function usually seen in hypertensive patients and the low function of the average myocardial fibres at the LV mid-wall that is even more common in hypertension. These may therefore contribute to additional reduction of morbidity and mortality associated with LVH regression.

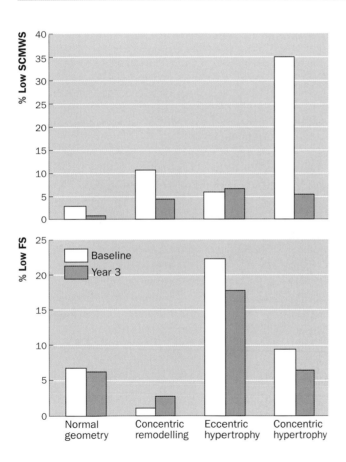

Fig. 14.5 Changes in the prevalence of LV chamber and myocardial contraction at baseline and after 3 years according to LV geometry pattern. FS, endocardial fractional shortening; SCMWS, stress-corrected midwall shortening. Source: Wachtell *et al.* (2002).

Losartan-dependent regression of myocardial fibrosis is associated with reduction of left ventricular chamber stiffness in hypertensive patients.

Diez J, Querejeta R, Lopez B, Gonzalez A, Larman M, Martinez Ubago JL.
Circulation 2002; **105**: 2512–17.

BACKGROUND. This study was designed to investigate whether myocardial collagen content is related to myocardial stiffness in patients with essential hypertension.

INTERPRETATION. There was a strong association between myocardial collagen content and LV chamber stiffness in patients with essential hypertension. The results also suggest that the ability of losartan to induce regression of severe myocardial fibrosis is associated with diminution of myocardial stiffness in hypertensive patients.

Comment

This study was designed to investigate whether myocardial collagen content is related to myocardial stiffness (KLV [left ventricular, LV, chamber stiffness, K_{LV}], assessed by deceleration time of the early mitral filling wave [T_{DEC}] as measured by Doppler echocardiography where KLV = [0.07: T_{DEC}]^2 mmHg/ml) in 34 patients with essential hypertension and whether 12 months treatment with losartan alter LV chamber stiffness and collagen volume fraction (measured from transvenous endomyocardial biopsies of the interventricular septum), serum concentrations of carboxy-terminal propeptide of procollagen type I and carboxy-terminal telopeptide of collagen type I, markers of collagen type I synthesis and degradation, respectively.

In summary, their findings are as follows: (i) a strong association exists between predominance of collagen type I synthesis over collagen type I degradation, exaggerated collagen accumulation in myocardial tissue, and abnormally high KLV in patients with essential hypertension; (ii) chronic angiotensin II receptor type 1 blockade with losartan is associated with reduction of both myocardial collagen content and KLV in a subgroup of patients with essential hypertension; and (iii) the efficacy of losartan in improving collagen type I metabolism predicts its capacity to regress myocardial fibrosis and reduce myocardial stiffness in hypertensive patients.

Indeed, myocardial fibrosis may play a crucial part in the compromise of diastolic function in patients with essential hypertension. This is further supported by the findings of this study that alterations of diastolic function were more prominent in patients with severe fibrosis than in patients with non-severe fibrosis. It would be interesting to incorporate tissue Doppler imaging in this study as a measure of LV diastolic filling and in relation to indices of myocardial fibrosis. It is interesting that losartan may induce regression of severe myocardial fibrosis parallel with a diminution of myocardial stiffness in hypertensive patients.

Further comment and conclusion

The LIFE Study (see Chapter 16) was specifically designed to investigate whether a 'clinically' meaningful LV mass reduction would follow by improving cardiovascular outcomes. However, the recently published results have raised more questions than answers. Despite losartan-based therapy reducing LVH more significantly ($P < 0.0001$) than atenolol-based antihypertensive therapy for a similar decrease in systolic and diastolic pressure, there was no difference in cardiac end-points, though there was a reduction in hospitalization for heart failure in the diabetic patients on losartan. The incidence of fatal and non-fatal myocardial infarction was similar and cardiovascular mortality was only non-significantly reduced in the losartan arm. There was also no significant reduction of myocardial infarction (odds ratio 0.87, 95% confidence interval 0.67–1.17) in the LIFE Echocardiography Substudy of 960 patients. On the other hand, fatal and non-fatal strokes were significantly reduced by >20% in the whole study population as well as in the echocardiography substudy. Such dissociation in cardiovascular benefits, cardiac vs cerebrovascular, is rather difficult to reconcile. The absence of any cardiac benefit in the presence of a well-documented LVH reduction remains baffling. The results may be interpreted in two or three ways. First, angiotensin receptor inhibitors may have a specific cerebro-vascular protective effect that does not share by other agents. Second, atenolol-based therapy is inferior to losartan-based therapy in preventing stroke but afforded similar cardiac protection as the latter. Third, losartan-based therapy reduced LV mass levels that may go beyond one that would be physiologically appropriate for the BP reduction. Indeed, as already pointed out, pathophysiological LVH encompasses both myocardial myocytes and fibrocytes, thus LVH regression may lead to LV mass reduction, but leave fibrotic tissue relatively unchanged. Such an inappropriate or unbalanced LVH reduction can lead to a preponderance of fibrosis in some patients, conceivably explaining the lack of cardiac benefits.

Certainly, more substudies/data from the LIFE Study will be released bit by bit over the next year or so, and in this regard, any differential effects between the two therapeutic regimens on LV geometry changes would be interesting.

15

Hormone replacement therapy and cardiovascular protection: Has the bubble burst?

Introduction

The evidence that oestrogen alone (oestrogen replacement therapy, ERT) or in combination with a progestin (hormone replacement therapy, HRT) may be beneficial in preventing cardiovascular disease (CVD) in post-menopausal women came from numerous large epidemiological observational studies over the past several decades. These strongly suggested that oestrogen has a cardioprotective effect. In addition, a lower incidence of coronary heart disease (CHD) in pre-menopausal women is believed to be due to a higher oestrogen level, and thus more 'cardioprotected', naturally. In contrast, post-menopausal women are particularly vulnerable to post-myocardial infarction (post-MI) morbidity and mortality in view of their age and generally widespread coronary artery disease (CAD) at the time of presentation. Improving the outcome as well as lowering the incidence of CHD by replacing oestrogen thus seems an attractive therapeutic approach. However, more robust evidence from several recent large prospective randomized placebo-controlled trials repeatedly provided disappointing results that HRT is neither beneficial in primary prevention nor secondary prevention of major cardiovascular events in this population. The data from these randomized trials contrasted sharply from those of promising prospective cohort studies and many mechanistic studies that have shown potential vascular benefits. Few arguments had been raised to try to explain the discrepancy. One of these arguments was the bias in patient selection theory that women on HRT might have been healthier and taken a greater interest in modifying cardiovascular risks—the 'healthy woman' hypothesis. Uncertainty also exists about the duration and optimal type of HRT regimen to use, because different oestrogens and progestins may have yielded different results.

There have been two well-known, prospective, randomized trials published in the past few years: the Estrogen Replacement and Atherosclerosis (ERA) trial in 2000 and the Heart and Estrogen/progestin Replacement Study (HERS) in 1998. The ERA trial investigated the effects of conjugated equine oestrogen (CEE) or CEE plus medroxyprogesterone acetate (MPA) on the progression of atherosclerosis. The HERS trial tested only the latter combination for the secondary prevention of heart disease in older women. The ERA study found no benefit of ERT or HRT for various angiographic outcomes. The HERS study found no benefit for HRT in the prevention of new CHD events. These two secondary prevention studies indicated that ERT or HRT may offer little or no benefit to older women with established CVD. However, it was thought that ERT may have beneficial cardiovascular effects in healthy post-menopausal women.

Disappointedly, the latest results from the primary prevention trial Women's Health Initiative (WHI) study (see below) has also reported that HRT (CCE plus MPA) provides no cardioprotective effect to women who were free of CHD initially. Indeed, an interim safety report released in 2000 showed that during the first 2 years of the study, there was a slightly greater incidence of cardiovascular events (coronary, stroke and thromboembolic) among women in the active HRT groups vs the placebo group. The Data and Safety Monitoring Board (DSMB) determined that this small increase in risk was not deemed a safety hazard and recommended that the study continue. The WHI study was not scheduled for completion until 2005. However, on 31 May 2002, after a mean of 5.2 years of follow-up, the DSMB recommended stopping the trial of oestrogen plus progestin vs placebo because the test statistic for invasive breast cancer exceeded the stopping boundary for this adverse effect and the global index statistic supported risks exceeding benefits. This report includes data on the major clinical outcomes through 30 April 2002. However, other clinical trials being conducted under the auspices of the WHI, including one comparing oestrogen alone vs placebo in women who have had a hysterectomy, are continuing.

Women's Health Initiative: End of the story of hormone replacement therapy for cardiovascular protection?

Risks and benefits of estrogen plus progestin in healthy post-menopausal women: Principal results from the Women's Health Initiative randomized controlled trial.
Writing Group for the Women's Health Initiative Investigators. *JAMA* 2002; **288**: 321–33.

BACKGROUND. Despite decades of accumulated observational evidence, the balance of risks and benefits for hormone use in healthy post-menopausal women remains uncertain. The objective is to assess the major health benefits and risks of the most commonly used combined hormone preparation in the USA.

INTERPRETATION. Overall health risks exceeded benefits from use of combined oestrogen plus progestin for an average 5.2-year follow-up among healthy post-menopausal US women. All-cause mortality was not affected during the trial. The risk–benefit profile found in this trial is not consistent with the requirements for a viable intervention for primary prevention of chronic diseases, and the results indicate that this regimen should not be initiated or continued for primary prevention of CHD.

Comment

The WHI, conducted by the National Institutes of Health in the USA, is a randomized trial involving approximately 30 000 women (aged 50–79 years) recruited by 40 US clinical centres in 1993–98, to receive either combined continuous oestrogen (0.625 mg CEE) and progestogen (MPA) or placebo (women who have had a hysterectomy receive oestrogen alone or placebo) to evaluate the impact of HRT in the primary prevention of CHD over a duration of 8.5 years. This paper reports the oestrogen plus progestin component of the trial, which involved 16 608 postmenopausal women with an intact uterus at baseline: 8506 on HRT and 8102 on placebo.

After 5.2 of the planned 8.5 years of follow-up, the trial was halted because the data revealed an increased risk for invasive breast cancer, CHD events (non-fatal MI or CHD death), stroke and pulmonary embolism (PE) among actively treated

Table 15.1 HRT vs placebo in the WHI: hazard ratios for major clinical outcomes

Outcome	Cases	Hazard ratio	95% CI
CHD	286	1.29	1.02–1.63
Breast cancer	290	1.26	1.00–1.59
Stroke	212	1.41	1.07–1.85
PE	101	2.13	1.39–3.25
Colorectal cancer	112	0.63	0.43–0.92
Endometrial cancer	47	0.83	0.47–1.47
Hip fracture	106	0.66	0.45–0.98
Death due to other causes	331	0.92	0.74–1.14

Source: Women's Health Initiative Investigators (2002).

Table 15.2 HRT vs placebo in the WHI: hazard ratios for composite outcomes

Composite outcome	Hazard ratio	95% CI
Total CVD (arterial plus venous disease)	1.22	1.09–1.36
Total cancer	1.03	0.90–1.17
Combined fractures	0.76	0.69–0.85
Total mortality	0.98	0.82–1.18
Global index	1.15	1.03–1.28

Source: Women's Health Initiative Investigators (2002)

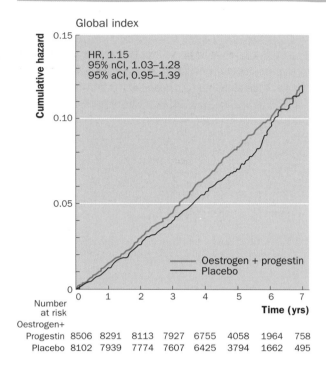

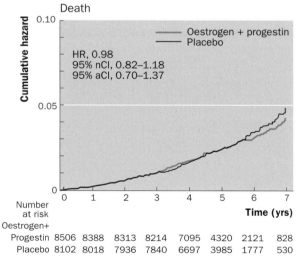

Fig. 15.1 Kaplan–Meier estimates of cumulative hazards for global index and death. HR indicates hazard ratio; nCI, nominal confidence interval; and aCI, adjusted confidence interval. Source: Women's Health Initiative Investigators (2002).

women. All-cause mortality rates did not differ between groups, and colorectal cancer and hip-fracture rates were found to be lower with active treatment than with placebo. However, using a global index, the risks were judged to outweigh some benefit seen with HRT in reduced fractures and colorectal cancers.

Absolute excess risks per 10 000 person-years attributable to the combination therapy were seven more CHD events, eight more strokes, eight more PEs, and eight more invasive breast cancers, while absolute risk reductions per 10 000 person-years were six fewer colorectal cancers and five fewer hip fractures. The absolute excess risk of events included in the global index was 19 per 10 000 person-years.

Indeed, on the basis of the HERS study, which showed an increased risk of CHD events with this same combination among older post-menopausal women with established heart disease, the American Heart Association (AHA; see below, Hulley *et al.* 2002) had recommended against starting HRT for secondary prevention but had made no firm recommendation on primary prevention pending findings from this study.

In view of the substantial risk for CHD events, stroke, PE and breast cancer associated with long-term HRT, the combined post-menopausal hormones CEE, 0.625 mg/day, plus MPA, 2.5 mg/day, should not be initiated or continued long term for the primary prevention of CHD. Along with the results from HERS II and from other studies, these data are part of a large body of evidence showing that HRT is associated with a significantly increased cardiovascular risk in post-menopausal women with and without CHD. Combination HRT should no longer be viewed as a therapy to prevent heart disease. The WHI trial comparing oestrogen alone with placebo among women without a uterus is still ongoing and results would be expected in 2005.

The WHI investigators stated, however, that their findings do not necessarily apply to short-term use of oestrogen plus progestin for the treatment of menopausal symptoms such as hot flushes, which was not specifically addressed by their study, and where the risk–benefit ratio may still be favourable. HRT is very effective in treating perimenopausal vasomotor symptoms, which could occur in up to 85% of women. Women taking the hormone combination for this purpose should discuss with their physicians whether to continue. This will depend on their overall health status and their duration of hormone use. In addition, the substantial risks for CVD and breast cancer must be weighed against the benefit for fracture in selecting from the available agents to prevent osteoporosis.

The results from this paper have enormous public health implications and to hundreds of millions of women world-wide on this particular type of HRT, which in fact is one of the most commonly used HRT in the USA, second only to ERT.

Non-cardiovascular disease outcomes during 6.8 years of hormone therapy: Heart and Estrogen/Progestin Replacement Study Follow-up (HERS II).

Hulley S, Furberg C, Barrett-Connor E, *et al. JAMA* 2002; **288**: 58–66.

BACKGROUND. The HERS study was a randomized trial of oestrogen plus progestin therapy after menopause. The purpose of this analysis was to examine the effect of long-term post-menopausal hormone therapy on common non-CVD outcomes.

INTERPRETATION. Treatment for 6.8 years with oestrogen plus progestin in older women with coronary disease increased the rates of venous thromboembolism and biliary tract surgery. Trends in other disease outcomes were not favourable and should be assessed in larger trials and in broader populations.

Cardiovascular disease outcomes during 6.8 years of hormone therapy: Heart and Estrogen/Progestin Replacement Study Follow-up (HERS II).

Grady D, Herrington D, Bittner V, *et al. JAMA* 2002; **288**: 49–57.

BACKGROUND. The HERS study found no overall reduction in risk of CHD events among post-menopausal women with CHD. However, in the hormone group, findings did suggest a higher risk of CHD events during the first year, and a decreased risk during years 3–5.

INTERPRETATION. Lower rates of CHD events among women in the hormone group in the final years of HERS did not persist during additional years of follow-up. After 6.8 years, hormone therapy did not reduce risk of cardiovascular events in women with CHD. Post-menopausal hormone therapy should not be used to reduce risk for CHD events in women with CHD.

Comment

The objective of the original HERS paper was to determine if oestrogen plus progestin therapy alters the risk for CHD events in post-menopausal women with established coronary disease. The data showed HRT use was associated with an increase in CHD events in the first year. The data also demonstrated no protective effect of HRT on the risk of stroke or transient ischaemic attack among post-menopausal women with established heart disease. HERS was the first randomized trial to show no overall effect of HRT treatment in 2763 women (average age of 67 years), who were randomly assigned to take CEE plus progestin, or placebo over 4.1 years of follow up. There was an apparent early increase in risk with treatment compared with placebo, followed later by a protective effect during years 3–5.

The objective of the present re-analysis of the HERS is to determine if the risk reduction observed in the later years of HERS persisted and resulted in an overall reduced risk of CHD events with additional years of follow-up. The HERS II study is an open-label follow-up of women in the HERS study, who largely followed this advice and either stayed on HRT or did not start. The proportion of women with at least 80% adherence to treatment declined from 81% at year 1 to 45% at year 6 in the HRT group. In the placebo group, 80% adherence to HRT was 0% at year 1 and 8% at year 6. A total of 2321 women from HERS, 93% of survivors, agreed to participate in HERS II.

The results are unsurprising, and show that the apparent trend toward benefit in the rate of CVD events seen at 4.1 years did not persist over time. The total number of events at 6.8 years showed no hint of benefit from therapy. They found no significant differences in the rate of CHD events between the groups in the number of primary outcome events (290 with HRT, 293 with placebo) or in any of the secondary outcomes. There were, however, harms associated with HRT, including a significantly increased risk of venous thromboembolic events, and the need for biliary tract surgery for gallbladder disease.

Three of the 73 women with thromboembolism died within 30 days from PE.

These findings lend support to recent recommendations that post-menopausal hormone therapy should not be used for the purpose of reducing risk for CHD events in women with CHD. For both primary and secondary prevention of CHD, it is prudent to use strategies that are of proven benefit and that do not harm patients. In all women, these strategies include life-style approaches, such as smoking avoidance, proper nutrition and regular exercise. Lipid-lowering and blood pressure

Table 15.3 Relative hazard of CHD events with HRT vs placebo in HERS and HERS II

Studies	Unadjusted relative hazard	95% CI
HERS	0.99	0.81–1.22
HERS II	1.00	0.77–1.29
Overall	0.99	0.84–1.17

Source: Grady *et al.* (2002).

Table 15.4 Risk of venous thromboembolism with HRT vs placebo in HERS and HERS II

Study	Relative hazard	95% CI
HERS	2.66	1.41–5.04
HERS II	1.40	0.64–3.05
Overall	2.08	1.28–3.40

Source: Grady *et al.* (2002).

Table 15.5 Overall risk of non-cardiovascular outcomes in HERS and HERS II

Outcome	Relative hazard	95% CI
Biliary tract surgery	1.48	1.12–1.95
Any cancer	1.19	0.95–1.50
Any fracture	1.04	0.87–1.25
Total mortality	1.10	0.92–1.31

Source: Grady *et al.* (2002).

(BP) control with pharmacotherapy are indicated in women who do not meet target lipid or BP levels with life-style interventions. For women with CHD, aspirin, beta-blockers and angiotensin-converting enzyme inhibitors should be considered. Widespread under-use of established preventive therapies has been documented in women. These interventions should be emphasized in clinical practice.

Hormone replacement therapy effects: potential benefit in women with diabetes? More questions than answers

Current use of unopposed estrogen and estrogen plus progestin and the risk of acute myocardial infarction among women with diabetes: The Northern California Kaiser Permanente Diabetes Registry, 1995–1998.
Ferrara A, Quesenberry CP, Karter AJ, *et al.* *Circulation* 2003 Jan; **107**(1): 43–8.

BACKGROUND. Little is known about HRT and risk for MI in diabetic women. This analysis examined associations of current HRT, oestrogen dosage and time since HRT initiation with risk of acute MI in diabetic women.

INTERPRETATION. In women without a recent MI, use of oestrogen plus progestin was associated with a decreased risk of MI. However, HRT was associated with an increased risk of MI in women with history of a recent MI. Data from clinical trials in diabetic women are needed.

Comment

This paper is yet another example of *observational data* that has associated the use of HRT with potential risk reduction of CHD events. This is in spite of robust evidence from randomized controlled trials that have proved the presumed cardiovascular benefits of HRT derived from numerous epidemiological data it has in fact caused more harm, more than anyone would have expected. To analyse a huge database such as that in this paper and attempt to find meaningful associations that neither prove causality nor reversible effect is to raise more questions than answers. There is a vast amount of data already suggesting that diabetes is more a CVD state than an endocrine disorder, and that the cardiovascular risk associated with diabetes may be equivalent to a non-diabetic who had suffered an MI.

HERS I and II have convincingly showed HRT use in these patients with established vascular disease increase CHD and venous thromboembolic events, as well as non-cardiovascular morbidity. This new observational data suggest a possible cardiovascular benefit for women with diabetes from HRT, as long as they had not already had a recent MI, where the risk apparently increased with HRT exposure. Quite rightly, the authors acknowledged that association 'does not prove causality', and that data from clinical trials are needed to understand the possible risks and benefits of treatment in this population. Indeed, given what we already know about the harmful cardiovascular effects associated with HRT use, further clinical trials will be unlikely. We could only retrospectively analyse subgroups of data or carry out *post-hoc* analysis from ongoing prospective studies such as the Raloxifene Use for the Heart (RUTH) study. The RUTH study is an ongoing randomized trial of 10 000 women evaluating whether selective oestrogen-receptor modulators (SERMs), such as raloxifene reduces the risk for heart disease and for breast cancer, which includes a large sample of women with diabetes. This should add to our knowledge of the magnitude of the effect of the risks and benefits of HRT in women with diabetes.

In this study, Ferrara *et al.* used the large and comprehensive Northern California Kaiser Permanente Diabetes Registry, drawn from the Kaiser Permanente Medical Care Program of Northern California, a group practice health plan providing medical services to some 2.7 million members. The registry includes about 25 000 women with diabetes aged 50 and over, 580 of whom have had a previous MI. The women were surveyed for demographic data, information on their diabetes, including age at diagnosis, and alcohol consumption and other related information; they were followed from 1995 until the first incidence of acute MI, death not related to acute MI, departure from the health plan, or until December 1998, whichever came first.

Table 15.6 Relative hazard for MI associated with HRT in women with diabetes and no previous MI

HRT use	Relative hazard for MI	95% CI
Current HRT use	0.84	0.72–0.98
Current use of unopposed oestrogen	0.88	0.73–1.05
Current use of oestrogen plus progestin	0.77	0.61–0.97

Source: Ferrara *et al.* (2003).

Table 15.7 Relative hazard for MI associated with HRT use in women with diabetes and a previous MI

HRT use	Relative hazard for MI	95% CI
Current HRT use	1.78	1.06–2.98
Current HRT use <1 year	3.84	1.60–9.20

Source: Ferrara *et al.* (2003).

The system's computerized pharmacy system allowed the researchers to assess baseline use of lipid-lowering therapy as well as HRT use, including all prescriptions, whether they were pills or patches, and the dose used in each prescription.

Among the 24 420 women without an MI at baseline, 2526 women were using unopposed oestrogen and 2088 were taking oestrogen plus progestin. Over 3 years of follow-up, 256 had a fatal MI and 854 a non-fatal MI. After adjustment for cardiovascular risk factors, current HRT use was associated with a reduced risk of MI, whether women were taking unopposed oestrogen or oestrogen plus progestin.

A reduction in MI risk was associated with low and medium doses of HRT but not with a high dose (>0.625 mg of CEE). Current use for less than a year was not associated with a protective effect, but after 1 year, the relative hazard with current use was 0.81 (95% CI 0.66–1.00). Among the 580 women who had had a previous MI at baseline, 89 had a recurrent MI during follow-up. In this group, HRT use was associated with a greater risk of MI, particularly in the first year, where the increased risk reached almost fourfold.

Indeed, as pointed out by the accompanying editorial in the issue of the journal this paper appeared in |1|, one of the most pressing issues now is to understand how 'results from observational studies and randomized clinical trials of HRT could produce such radically different results. The study by Ferrara *et al.* provides yet another illustration of this awkward reality.' The 'healthy women hypothesis' is still the most favourable explanation for such a discrepancy. However, one could not dismiss lightly the many mechanistic studies that have shown that oestrogen can have favourable effects on lipids, endothelial function and other aspects of vascular biology.

Hormone replacement therapy and cardiovascular disease. A statement for healthcare professionals from the American Heart Association.

Mosca L, Herrington DM, Mendelsohn ME, *et al. Circulation* 2001; **104**: 499–503.

B a c k g r o u n d . **For more than 50 million American women, and millions of women in other countries who are over the age of 50 years, the decision whether or not to use**

ERT for chronic disease prevention is often a difficult one. The purpose of this advisory was to summarize the currently available data concerning potential CVD benefits and risks associated with ERT/HRT and to provide updated clinical recommendations regarding its use in the secondary and primary prevention of CVD.

INTERPRETATION. HRT should not be initiated for the secondary prevention of CVD. Firm clinical recommendations for primary prevention await the results of ongoing randomized clinical trials.

Comment

For secondary prevention of CHD in women, the AHA recommends against initiating HRT based on studies that have shown no benefit and early harm. For patients with CHD already on HRT, the decision to continue or stop HRT should be based on established non-coronary risks and benefits and patient preference. There are insufficient data to suggest that HRT should be initiated for the sole purpose of primary prevention of CHD. When current HRT users suffer adverse cardiovascular events, consider stopping HRT altogether or consider anticoagulation to minimize thromboembolic events in the setting of immobilization. Although data from ongoing, randomized clinical trials are forthcoming, current data are insufficient to support initiating HRT solely for primary prevention in women without CVD.

The new AHA guidelines recommend placing significant weight on the non-cardiac benefits and risks of HRT, it is important to become familiar with these

Table 15.8 Summary recommendations for HRT* and CVD

Secondary prevention
- HRT should not be initiated for the secondary prevention of CVD
- The decision to continue or stop HRT in women with CVD who have been undergoing long-term HRT should be based on established non-coronary benefits and risks and patient preference
- If a woman develops an acute CVD event or is immobilized while undergoing HRT, it is prudent to consider discontinuance of the HRT or to consider VTE prophylaxis while she is hospitalized to minimize risk of VTE (venous thromboembolism) associated with immobilization. Reinstitution of HRT should be based on established non-coronary benefits and risks, as well as patient preference

Primary prevention
- Firm clinical recommendations for primary prevention await the results of ongoing randomized clinical trials
- There are insufficient data to suggest that HRT should be initiated for the sole purpose of primary prevention of CVD
- Initiation and continuation of HRT should be based on established non-coronary benefits and risks, possible coronary benefits and risks, and patient preference

*The majority of data available to make clinical recommendations are based on standard doses of oral CEE/MPA. Evidence is insufficient to determine whether different preparations, routes of delivery, doses or different progestins have a more favourable or more adverse effect on clinical CVD end-points.
Source: Mosca *et al.* (2001).

non-cardiac effects. The focus should be on optimizing the implementation of underutilized yet proven therapies including life-style and pharmacological interventions that are definitively known to reduce CVD, such as aspirin, statins and anti-hypertensives.

Hormone replacement therapy: no symptoms, no benefit

Quality-of-life and depressive symptoms in post-menopausal women after receiving hormone therapy: results from the Heart and Estrogen/Progestin Replacement Study (HERS) trial.

Hlatky MA, Boothroyd D, Vittinghoff E, Sharp P, Whooley MA; Heart and Estrogen/Progestin Replacement Study (HERS) Research Group. *JAMA* 2002; **287**(5): 591–7.

BACKGROUND. Post-menopausal hormone therapy is commonly used by women for disease prevention, but its effects on quality of life (QoL) have not been well documented. The purpose of this study is to determine the effect on QoL of oestrogen plus progestin therapy used as secondary prevention in women with CAD.

INTERPRETATION. Hormone therapy has mixed effects on QoL among older women. The effects of hormone therapy depend on the presence of menopausal symptoms; women without flushing had greater declines in physical measures, while women with flushing had improvements in emotional measures of QoL.

Comment

Safeguarding the health of an individual means not only ensuring his/her physical but also his/her psychological well-being. We now know that combined HRT does more harm than good in women with or without underlying CHD. However, peri/post-menopausal symptoms could be unpleasant and to some, they may even render disability. These symptoms are more frequent during the first years of menopause, and include mood alterations, sleeplessness, hot flushes and sweats, sexual dysfunction, the impact of which may be noteworthy on the QoL. It has long been established that HRT is extremely effective in alleviating these symptoms and thus restoring normal functional activities. Millions of women obviously still take HRT for these indications. QoL is often important to consider in HRT use, yet HRT's effects on QoL have not been documented well. The study by Hlatky and colleagues is important because of its large sample size and the paucity of existing research on health-related QoL in post-menopausal women, especially as it pertains to HRT.

Because it is well known that the severity of symptoms responsive to therapy affects QoL measures after treatment, and that therapy for asymptomatic conditions such as hypertension tends to decrease QoL, they stratified study subjects by the presence or absence of flushing at baseline, as the symptom most likely to be responsive to treatment.

Various aspects of HRT-related QoL were assessed in the HERS trial. Physical activity was measured by the Duke Activity Status Index, energy/fatigue and mental health were measured using RAND scales, and depressive symptom scores were based on the Burnam screening scale. During 3 years of follow-up, scores for physical function, mental health and energy/fatigue declined significantly across patients, regardless of HRT status and there were large differences in QoL according to clinical characteristics. In general, QoL scores were lower among women who were older, diabetic, hypertensive or who had angina or heart failure. Hormone replacement particularly in older women had overall significant negative effects on physical function, but it improved depressive symptoms compared with women who received placebo.

Where HRT use seemed to make the most difference was among women who had flushing (15.7%). In this subgroup, HRT recipients had better mental health and fewer depressive symptoms than did placebo recipients. Among women without flushing (84.3%), HRT users had worse physical function and more fatigue than placebo recipients did.

Table 15.9 HERS: QoL scores in all patients

Symptoms	Change in score from baseline to 36 months	P value
Physical function	−3.8	<0.001
Mental health	−0.6	0.05
Energy/fatigue	−3.8	<0.001
Depressive symptoms	—	NS

NS, not significant.
Source: Hlatky et al. (2002).

Table 15.10 HERS: Women with flushing assigned to HRT vs placebo

Symptoms	Flushing + HRT	Flushing + placebo	P value
Mental health	+2.6	−0.3	0.04
Depressive symptoms	−0.5	+0.007	0.01

Source: Hlatky et al. (2002).

Table 15.11 HERS: Women without flushing symptoms assigned to HRT vs placebo

Symptoms	No flushing + HRT	No flushing + placebo	P value
Physical function	−4.2	−3.3	0.04
Energy/fatigue	−4.6	−3.1	0.03

Source: Hlatky *et al.* (2002).

These mixed results suggest that hormone therapy does not have a general benefit for post-menopausal women with heart disease; rather, it improves QoL only for women with menopausal symptoms. Decision making about HRT should be based on non-coronary benefits and risks, and these mixed QoL data obviously do not change that. As the editorialists note |2|, the contribution of this report then is to establish that women without vasomotor symptoms at baseline experienced a decrease in physical function and no improvements in mental health with HRT. Presence or absence of hot flushing seemed to be the defining factor in improvement of depressive symptoms.

It should also be noted that participants in this study had a mean age of 67 years, whereas the detrimental effects of menopause are known to occur within the first few years after cessation of menses. Hlatky and colleagues noted that women with flushing who improved on hormone therapy tended to be much younger. Although not specifically addressed by the investigators, the greater decline in physical function among women treated with hormone therapy compared with placebo may well have been due to the increased rates of cardiovascular events associated with hormone therapy, especially in the first year of the HERS trial. Further studies are still needed to determine HRT effects on QoL and CHD risk in younger women without CHD.

Genotype may dictate responsiveness to hormone replacement therapy?

Estrogen-receptor polymorphisms and effects of estrogen replacement on high-density lipoprotein cholesterol in women with coronary disease.
Herrington DM, Howard TD, Hawkins GA, *et al. N Engl J Med* 2002; **346**: 967–74.

B A C K G R O U N D . Sequence variants in the gene encoding oestrogen receptor (ER−) may modify the effects of HRT on levels of high-density lipoprotein (HDL) cholesterol and other outcomes related to oestrogen treatment in post-menopausal women.

INTERPRETATION. Post-menopausal women with coronary disease who have the ER– IVS1–401 C/C genotype, or several other closely related genotypes, have an augmented response of HDL cholesterol to HRT.

Comment

Given the disappointing growing list of 'bad news' for HRT/ERT as already discussed, this study may perhaps shed some light to the HRT enthusiasts as women may be individually targeted to gain the most 'benefit' from HRT/ERT (hopefully also avoiding the associated non-cardiovascular adverse effects) simply by genetic profiling.

Indeed, this new analysis of data from the ERA trial has shown one polymorphism of the ERα-gene (encode for oestrogen receptor 1, ESR1) that was associated with twice the increase in HDL in response to ERT as that seen in women with other genotypes. And, low HDL is a known independent risk factor for CVD.

The authors examined the association between 10 ESR1 variants and changes in HDL and other lipids levels in 309 post-menopausal women with CHD who were randomized to oral CCE, oestrogen plus progestin, or placebo. Mean follow-up was 3.2 years. After adjustment for age, race, diabetes status, body mass index, smoking status, alcohol intake and exercise frequency, they found that women with one of these genotypes, IVS1-401C/C, had twice the increase in HDL in response to HRT seen in other women: 13.1 mg/dl compared with 6.0 mg/dl. Treatment–genotype interactions were statistically significant ($P = 0.04$). Women with this genotype showed the increased pattern of HDL response regardless of race or ethnicity, or whether they were receiving oestrogen alone or oestrogen plus progestin, and the association was greater for women who were compliant with therapy. Similar patterns of response were seen for three other polymorphisms closely linked to the IVS1-401C/C site.

The data have clearly showed that polymorphisms in the ESR1 gene can apparently account for the change in HDL levels to HRT treatment. The mechanism of this effect is unclear, and whether these dramatic increases in HDL will translate into similarly dramatic reductions in risk for CHD is also not known but the findings suggest that genotype may eventually be used to aid decision making about HRT. Obviously, blood drawn from other large studies such as the HERS and WHI could also be analysed in the same way, and should help to confirm this 'unexpected' interesting observation.

Hormone replacement therapy: 'bad news' for cardiovascular protection

 Oestrogen therapy for prevention of reinfarction in post-menopausal women: a randomized placebo controlled trial.
Cherry N, Gilmour K, Hannaford P, *et al.* and The ESPRIT team. *Lancet* 2002 Dec 21–28; **360**(9350): 1996–7.

BACKGROUND. Results of observational studies suggest that HRT could reduce the risk of CHD, but those of randomized trials do not indicate a lower risk in women who use oestrogen plus progestagen. The aim of this study was to ascertain whether or not unopposed oestrogen reduces the risk of further cardiac events in post-menopausal women who survive a first MI.

INTERPRETATION. Oestradiol valerate does not reduce the overall risk of further cardiac events in post-menopausal women who have survived an MI.

Comment

The oEStrogen in the Prevention of ReInfarction Trial (ESPRIT) was conducted at 35 hospitals in England and Wales where 1017 women 50–69 years of age who had survived a first MI were randomized to 2 mg 17-β oestradiol or placebo daily for 2 years. Unlike the HERS trial that used combined HRT (CCE + MAP), ESPRIT was designed to assess specifically the effect of unopposed oestradiol valerate on risk of recurrent CHD event or death. ESPRIT excludes women >69 years of age, who are at higher risk of major cardiovascular events and make up a large proportion of admissions for MI. Primary outcomes were reinfarction or cardiac death, and all-cause mortality. Secondary outcomes were uterine bleeding, endometrial cancer, stroke or other embolic events, and fractures. The results from ESPRIT are of immense interest as the WHI trial component comparing CCE alone vs placebo in healthy post-menopausal women who have had a hysterectomy is still ongoing.

After 24 months of follow-up, the results indicate that oral oestradiol alone offers no protection against reinfarction or cardiac death between the two trial arms in post-menopausal women with established CHD. All-cause mortality was not statistically different between the two groups, nor was the incidence of strokes and other embolic events, fractures or breast cancer. No instances of endometrial cancer were reported for either group; the low number of cancers and deaths generally likely reflects the short follow-up period. Vaginal bleeding was common among trial participants taking the study drug (56% among women taking oestradiol who had not had a hysterectomy, compared with 7% among non-hysterectomized women on

Table 15.12 ESPRIT outcomes

End-point	Oestradiol (n = 513)	Placebo (n = 504)	Risk ratio (95% CI)	P
Reinfarction or cardiac death	62	61	0.99 (0.7–1.4)	0.97
Cardiac death	21	30	0.58 (0.39–1.19)	0.17
All-cause death	32	39	0.79 (0.5–1.27)	0.34
Stroke	10	6	1.64 (0.6–0.47)	0.45
Transient ischaemic attack	15	13	1.13 (0.54–2.36)	0.85
PE	3	3	0.98 (0.2–4.84)	1.0
Breast cancer	4	4	0.98 (0.25–3.91)	1.0
Fracture	11	18	0.6 (0.29–1.26)	0.19

Source: Cherry *et al.* (2002).

placebo). This bleeding was blamed for the poor compliance in the active treatment arm: only 43% of women on oestradiol were still taking their medication at 24 months, compared with 63% of women on placebo.

The authors stated that the emerging evidence supports the idea that oral oestrogen with or without MPA is unlikely to offer cardiovascular benefit, at least in the first several years after starting the therapy. Thus, ESPRIT provides insufficient evidence of benefit to alter current guidance against the use of HRT for the secondary prevention of CVD. As stated by the accompanying editorialist |3|, for now, research should focus more on avoiding cardiovascular risk than finding benefit. Hormones for coronary disease prevention have come full circle.

Women's International Study of Long Duration Estrogen after Menopause (WISDOM): no wisdom continuing ... after the Women's Health Initiative

The Medical Research Council's WISDOM is a large primary prevention study in which 34 000 post-menopausal women (22 000 from the UK, Australia and New Zealand), 50–69 years of age, randomized (similar to WHI) to either HRT oestrogen plus progestin vs placebo; or in women without a uterus to oestrogen alone or placebo. The trial began recruiting in 1999 and was due to end in 2016. However, after the negative results from the WHI were announced, an International Independent Committee (IIC) was appointed to review its results to date; the committee has recently recommended a halt to WISDOM because the trial is considered 'unlikely to provide substantial evidence to influence clinical practice in the next 10 years', a new release from the MRC notes.

Effects of hormone replacement therapy and antioxidant vitamin supplements on coronary atherosclerosis in post-menopausal women: a randomized controlled trial.

Waters DD, Alderman EL, Hsia J, *et al. JAMA* 2002; **288**(19): 2432–40.

BACKGROUND. HRT and antioxidant vitamins are widely used for secondary prevention in post-menopausal women with coronary disease, but no clinical trials have demonstrated benefit to support their use.

INTERPRETATION. In post-menopausal women with coronary disease, neither HRT nor antioxidant vitamin supplements provide cardiovascular benefit. Instead, a potential for harm was suggested with each treatment.

Comment

The objective of the Women's Angiographic Vitamin and Estrogen (WAVE) Trial was to determine whether HRT (CEE with or without MPA, depending on whether or not the participant had an intact uterus) or antioxidant vitamin supplements (E + C), alone vs. placebo or in combination, influence the progression of CAD in post-menopausal women, as measured by serial quantitative coronary angiography. The trial was a double-blind randomize, 2 × 2 factorial design involved 423 post-menopausal women with at least one 15–75% coronary stenosis at baseline coronary angiography and was conducted from July 1997 to January 2002 in seven clinical centres in the USA and Canada. The primary outcome in this angiographic trial was the annualized mean change in minimum lumen diameter (MLD) between a baseline and follow-up angiogram, with all qualifying coronary lesions averaged for each patient. Patients with intercurrent death or MI were imputed the worst rank of angiographic outcome.

Table 15.13 Coronary progression: annualized mean (SD) change in MLD with HRT vs placebo

Measure	HRT	Placebo	P
Mean (SD) change in MLD (mm/y)	0.047 (0.15)	0.024 (0.15)	0.17

Source: Waters *et al.* (2002).

Table 15.14 Coronary progression: annualized mean (SD) change in MLD with antioxidant vitamins vs placebo

Measure	Antioxidants	Placebo	P
Mean (SD) change in MLD (mm/y)	0.044 (0.15)	0.028 (0.15)	0.32

Source: Waters *et al.* (2002).

Once again, after a mean of 2.8 years the results were disappointing—neither HRT nor antioxidant vitamin supplements slowed the progression of atherosclerosis; in fact, more progression and more cardiovascular events were actually seen among treated women in both arms of the trial.

When patient death and MI was included, the primary outcome showed an increased risk for women in the HRT group ($P = 0.045$) and suggested an increased risk in the antioxidant vitamin group ($P = 0.09$).

Patients randomized to both HRT and antioxidant vitamins actually had the highest number of deaths compared with those women who were randomized to placebo for both treatments. The fact that there was a trend toward more deaths found in patients on vitamin supplements compared with placebo was difficult to reconcile.

In the Women's Estrogen for Stroke Trial (WEST), an increase in stroke with HRT was seen during the first 6 months of treatment [4]. In HERS and WHI, women assigned to receive HRT also experienced an early increased risk of acute coronary events. These increases in risk early after initiation of HRT may account for the adverse effect of HRT in WAVE, as the mean duration of follow-up was 2.8 years. In the only previous coronary angiographic trial of HRT, the Estrogen Replacement and Atherosclerosis Trial, among the 248 women who underwent follow-up angiography, MLD over the 3.2 years of follow-up worsened by 0.09 (0.02) mm in both the placebo and unopposed oestrogen groups, and by 0.12 (0.02) mm in the combined HRT group [5]. These rates of progression were not reported as annual changes in MLD and are similar to the progression rates in WAVE.

In view of these data, the WAVE trial does not support the use of HRT or antioxidant vitamin supplements to post-menopausal women for secondary prevention of CHD.

Table 15.15 WAVE: Death, and death, MI and stroke with HRT vs placebo

Outcome	HRT	Placebo	Hazard ratio (95% CI)
Death (*n*)	14	8	1.8 (0.75–4.3)
Death, non-fatal MI, stroke (*n*)	26	15	1.9 (0.97–3.6)

Source: Waters *et al.* (2002).

Table 15.16 WAVE: Death, and death, MI and stroke with antioxidant vitamins vs placebo

Outcome	Vitamins	Placebo	Hazard ratio (95% CI)
Death (*n*)	16	6	2.8 (1.1–7.2)
Death, non-fatal MI, stroke (*n*)	26	18	1.5 (0.80–2.9)

Source: Waters *et al.* (2002).

Selective oestrogen receptor modulator may reduce cardiovascular risk

Raloxifene and cardiovascular events in osteoporotic post-menopausal women: four-year results from the MORE (Multiple Outcomes of Raloxifene Evaluation) randomized trial.
Barrett-Connor E, Grady D, Sashegyi A, *et al. JAMA* 2002; **287**(7): 847–57.

BACKGROUND. Raloxifene, a selective ER modulator, improves cardiovascular risk factors, but its effect on cardiovascular events is unknown. The objective of this was to determine the effect of raloxifene on cardiovascular events in osteoporotic post-menopausal women.

INTERPRETATION. Raloxifene therapy for 4 years did not significantly affect the risk of cardiovascular events in the overall cohort but did significantly reduce the risk of cardiovascular events in the subset of women with increased cardiovascular risk. There was no evidence that raloxifene caused an early increase in the risk of cardiovascular events. Before raloxifene is used for the prevention of cardiovascular events, these findings require confirmation in trials with evaluation of cardiovascular outcomes as the primary objective.

Comment

The Multiple Outcomes of Raloxifene Evaluation (MORE) trial was a double blind, placebo-controlled trial designed to determine the effect of raloxifene, a SERM, on bone mineral density and vertebral fractures in 7705 post-menopausal women (mean age 67 years) with osteoporosis. Raloxifene reduced the risk of osteoporotic vertebral fractures and newly diagnosed breast cancer without increasing the risk of endo-metrial cancer but increased the risk of venous thromboembolic events to an extent similar to that of HRT and tamoxifen. Patients were randomly assigned to receive raloxifene, 60 mg/day (n = 2557), or 120 mg/day (n = 2572), or placebo (n = 2576) for 4 years.

This paper describes the results of a *post hoc* analysis of the MORE data on cardio-vascular events. In the overall population, raloxifene did not significantly reduce the risk of cardiovascular events (including coronary and cerebrovascular events). Similar results were obtained when coronary and cerebrovascular events were analysed separately. However, treatment with raloxifene did significantly lower the risk of cardiovascular events in the subset of 1035 women with increased cardiovascular risk at baseline. There was a roughly 40% reduction in all events and a 62% reduction in stroke. The authors noted that the event rate Kaplan–Meier curves in the high-risk subset started to diverge after about 1 year and continued to diverge through 4 years, with fewer events in the raloxifene group vs. placebo. Importantly, there was no evidence that raloxifene treatment was associated with an early increase in cardio-vascular morbidity or mortality in the overall cohort, among women at high risk for or among women with established CHD, compared with placebo (relative risk, 0.60; 95% CI, 0.38–0.95 for both raloxifene groups).

Why raloxifene might behave differently from HRT is a matter of speculation, but it has similar effects in terms of provoking deep venous thrombosis, lowers low-density lipoprotein but not as much as HRT, has similar favourable effects on vascular function but no effect on C reactive protein, while HRT increases C reactive protein by about 80%.

However, it should be noted that women enrolled in the MORE trial were selected for increased risk for osteoporotic fracture rather than for an increased risk of CVD; thus, the overall study cohort was predominantly women without established CHD, all had osteoporosis and were at relatively low risk for cardiovascular events. Further-more, because of the *post hoc* nature of these analyses and the relatively small number of events involved, the possibility that the significant risk reduction with raloxifene observed in the high-risk subset was a chance finding cannot be discounted. In addi-tion, the effects observed with raloxifene 120 mg/day were less consistent compared with raloxifene 60 mg/day. The analysis was further limited by the fact that cardio-vascular events were assessed by self-report and complete supporting evidence for adjudication of events was not available in many cases.

As in other HRT studies, these findings from the MORE trial must be confirmed by an adequately powered, randomized trial with cardiovascular events as pre-defined outcomes before raloxifene can be used for the prevention of cardiovascular events.

Table 15.17 MORE 4-year results: overall cohort

Treatment group	Cardiovascular events	Relative risk	95% CI
Placebo	3.7%	–	–
Raloxifene 60 mg	3.2%	0.86	0.64–1.15
Raloxifene 120 mg	3.7%	0.98	0.74–1.30

Source: Barrett-Connor *et al.* (2001).

Table 15.18 Subset of women at increased cardiovascular risk at baseline (*n* = 1035)

Treatment group	Cardiovascular events	Relative risk	95% CI
Placebo	12.9%	–	–
Raloxifene 60 mg	7.8%	0.60	0.38–0.95
Raloxifene 120 mg	7.8%	0.60	0.38–0.95

Source: Barrett-Connor *et al.* (2001).

The RUTH trial, which involved 10 101 post-menopausal women with established heart disease or with multiple risk factors for heart disease randomized to either raloxifen or placebo, will certainly provide more clues. RUTH will look at the effect of raloxifen on a composite cardiovascular end-point that includes acute coronary syndromes and coronary death, and stroke as secondary end-point, but results will not be available for several years.

Third US Preventive Services Task Force recommendations on hormone replacement therapy and the prevention of chronic diseases

Post-menopausal hormone replacement therapy and the primary prevention of cardiovascular disease.
Humphrey LL, Chan BKS, Sox HC. *Ann Intern Med* 2002; **137**: 273–84.

BACKGROUND. To evaluate the value of HRT in the primary prevention of CVD and CAD.

INTERPRETATION. This meta-analysis differs from previous meta-analyses by evaluating potential explanatory variables of the relationship between HRT, CVD and CAD. The adjusted meta-analysis is consistent with recent randomized trials that have shown no benefit in the secondary or primary prevention of CVD events. A valid answer to the role of HRT in the primary prevention of CVD will best come from randomized controlled trials.

Comment

The authors conducted this systematic review and meta-analysis to examine the value of HRT for the primary prevention of CVD. They were particularly interested in whether bias might explain discordant results between recent trials and the observational literature. Their review is one of several that will serve as background for the Third US Preventive Services Task Force (USPSTF III) recommendations on HRT and the prevention of chronic diseases.

Their primary analysis compared event rates in patients with 'any HRT use' (current, past or ever use) with those who had 'never' used HRT. The study also compared event rates in 'current', 'past' or 'ever' HRT use groups with 'never' use to evaluate further variable findings among the studies. All relative risk estimates are compared with never use. The authors limited their review and meta-analyses to studies of good or fair quality based on pre-established criteria. In addition, they evaluated CVD and CAD separately when the data allowed, and conducted separate analyses of incidence and mortality for each outcome.

Earlier data on HRT and the primary prevention of CVD showing benefit to users are not supported by newer studies or by this analysis. The major points from these

Table 15.19 Meta-analysis summary table

Variable	Relative risk according to measure of hormone replacement therapy (95% CI)*			
	Current	Past	Ever	Any*
Mortality				
Total cardiovascular disease	0.64 (0.44–0.93)	0.79 (0.52–1.09)	0.81 (0.58–1.13)	0.75 (0.42–1.23)
Coronary artery disease	0.62 (0.40–0.90)	0.76 (0.53–1.02)	0.81 (0.37–1.60)	0.74 (0.36–1.45)
Incidence				
Total cardiovascular disease	1.27 (0.80–2.00)	1.26 (0.79–2.08)	1.35 (0.92–2.00)	1.28 (0.86–2.00)
coronary artery disease	0.80 (0.68–0.95)	0.89 (0.75–1.05)	0.91 (0.67–1.33)	0.88 (0.64–1.21)
Summary estimate	0.97 (0.82–1.16)	1.07 (0.90–1.27)	1.11 (0.84–1.53)	1.04 (0.79–1.44)

* 'Current', 'past', and 'ever' use are categories used in the individual studies. 'Any use' is a category created for this meta-analysis combining data from studies evaluating ever and never use of HRT with data from studies evaluating current, past, or never use (current + past + ever use).
Source: Humphrey et al. (2002).

review and meta-analyses are as follows: (i) no significant association was identified between past, ever, or any use of HRT and CVD or CAD death; (ii) HRT use did not reduce CVD incidence and, in fact, suggests a small increase in risk; and (iii) HRT showed no benefit in preventing CAD among the studies that adjusted for major CAD risk factors and socio-economic status or education and showed reduced risk among studies that did not adjust for these factors, suggesting confounding.

One of the most important findings of this review and analysis is how different evaluation and statistical control of CAD risk factors affect summary estimates. This is highlighted in this meta-analysis, which showed markedly different relative risks depending on the inclusion or exclusion of socio-economic status or education as predictor variables in a study's multivariable analysis. These findings suggest confounding, which is important because lower socio-economic status is a strong risk factor for CVD and CAD, as well as for most other poor outcomes. In addition, women using HRT tend to have higher socio-economic status, which may explain their better outcomes. Similarly, none of the studies with adjustment for alcohol use or exercise, both known to be more common in women who use HRT, showed benefit with HRT use.

Their review also supports the 'healthy women hypothesis' in explaining the discrepancies of results between prospective cohort studies and randomized clinical trials. Women who use HRT tend to be more affluent, leaner and more educated, tend to exercise more often, and tend to drink more alcohol. Women who take HRT also have different health characteristics before menopause. Women prescribed HRT have access to health care and are therefore more likely to be receiving treatment for other CVD–CAD risk factors, such as high cholesterol levels or high BP, which would lower their risk. Another aspect of healthy user bias is that women often discontinue HRT when they become ill. A more subtle bias, which may be apparent to practising physicians, is a tendency to offer and prescribe HRT to women who are perceived as being in better overall 'health', even in the absence of defined CVD or CAD risk factors.

Because of the limitations of observational studies, randomized, controlled trials are the best way to evaluate the relationship between HRT and CVD or CAD. Primary prevention of CVD and CAD in women should focus on proven strategies to reduce CVD and CAD risk. On the basis of current evidence, the authors do not advise consideration of CVD prevention when discussing HRT use with women.

Post-menopausal hormone replacement therapy for primary prevention of chronic conditions: recommendations and rationale.

US Preventive Services Task Force. *Ann Intern Med* 2002; **137**: 834–9.

B ACKGROUND. This statement summarizes the USPSTF recommendations for use of HRT for the primary prevention of chronic conditions in post-menopausal women and updates the 1996 USPSTF recommendations on this topic.

INTERPRETATION. The USPSTF concludes that the evidence is insufficient to recommend for or against the use of unopposed oestrogen for the prevention of chronic conditions in post-menopausal women who have had a hysterectomy. This is a grade I recommendation.

Comment

This updated 2002 USPSTF recommends against HRT use for prevention of chronic conditions. Such recommendation was based on the conclusion drawn from the review and meta-analyses by Humphrey *et al.* (2002) as already discussed above.

The USPSTF says it found fair to good evidence that the combination of oestrogen and progestin has both benefits and harms. Benefits include increased bone mineral density (good evidence), reduced risk for fracture (fair to good evidence) and reduced risk for colorectal cancer (fair evidence). Harms include increased risk for breast cancer (good evidence), venous thromboembolism (good evidence), CHD (fair to good evidence), stroke (fair evidence) and cholecystitis (fair evidence). Evidence was insufficient to assess the effects of HRT on other outcomes, such as dementia and cognitive function, ovarian cancer, mortality from breast cancer or CVD, or all-cause mortality.

The USPSTF did not evaluate the use of HRT to treat symptoms of menopause, such as vasomotor symptoms (hot flashes) or urogenital symptoms. The balance of benefits and harms for an individual woman will be influenced by her personal preferences, individual risks for specific chronic diseases, and the presence of menopausal symptoms.

These new guidelines are similar to those from other organizations, several of which have already revised their recommendations in light of the findings from recently reported clinical trials. The American College of Obstetricians and Gynecologists and the North American Menopause Society now recommend against the use of HRT for the primary or secondary prevention of CVD and recommend caution in using HRT solely to prevent osteoporosis, suggesting that alternative therapies should also be considered. Both organizations consider HRT an acceptable treatment option for menopausal symptoms but caution against the prolonged use of HRT for the relief of symptoms. The AHA also now recommends against the use of HRT for primary or secondary prevention of CVD.

Abnormal vascular function and hypertension in mice deficient in oestrogen receptor β.

Zhu Y, Bian Z, Lu P, *et al. Science* 2002; **295**: 505–8.

BACKGROUND. Blood vessels express ERs, but their role in cardiovascular physiology is not well understood.

INTERPRETATION. The study show that vascular smooth muscle cells and blood vessels from ERβ-deficient mice exhibit multiple functional abnormalities. In wild-type mouse blood vessels, oestrogen attenuates vasoconstriction by an ERβ-mediated increase in inducible nitric oxide (NO) synthase expression. In contrast, oestrogen augments vasoconstriction in blood vessels from ERβ-deficient mice. Vascular smooth muscle cells isolated from ERβ-deficient mice show multiple abnormalities of ion channel function. Furthermore, ERβ-deficient mice develop sustained systolic and diastolic hypertension as they age. These data support an essential role for ERβ in the regulation of vascular function and BP.

Comment

Oestrogens are known to influence gene expression, growth and cellular differentiation in target tissues by activating one or both of two ERs, ERα and ERβ. These receptors are found in many tissues, including breast and female reproductive organs as well as bone, liver, brain and cardiovascular system in both sexes. Specifically, ERα and ERβ are expressed in vascular endothelial and smooth muscle cells, and in myocardial cells, and could regulate the expression of a number of vasodilator and vasoconstrictor proteins, including multiple components of the renin–angiotensin system. Oestrogen also enhances production of NO by endothelial cells by increasing endothelial NO synthase (eNOS) activity or expression of the eNOS gene, or both. *In vivo*, oestrogen enhances vasodilatation in both primates and humans with normal and abnormal endothelial function.

To examine the role of ERs in vascular physiology, the existence of an oestrogen effect on vasoconstriction was explored in vessels from wild-type mice. The investigators were able to demonstrate that these mice exhibited chronic systolic and diastolic hypertension when their ERβ gene was knocked out. They postulated that multiple ERβ-regulated gene products may contribute to the abnormal vascular contraction, ion channel dysfunction and hypertension observed in these ERβ knocked-out mice. Vascular smooth muscle cells from this strain of mice showed abnormal function. These findings also support the concept that the transcription factor ERβ controls expression of genes critical to normal vascular physiology in both males and females. They hypothesized that gene targets of ERβ in relevant target tissues may provide insights into the pathophysiology and treatment of hypertension.

These results provide strong evidence of physiological roles for oestrogen and ERs in regulating vascular tone, at least in mice. Hence, it is conceivable that BP may

Table 15.20 Hormone replacement therapy and CHD prevention

- Observational and case–control studies: suggested coronary prevention
- Secondary prevention clinical trial (e.g. HERS): early harm, no long-term benefit
- Primary prevention clinical trial (e.g. WHI): excess cardiovascular events
- Secondary stroke prevention (e.g. WEST): no benefit

Source: Skegg CG. *Lancet* 2001; **358**: 1195–6.

be influenced by abnormalities of these ERs. A growing number of studies have documented physiological actions of oestrogen in organs that never were thought to be 'sex-hormone responsive'. We likely soon will see a group of new SERMs (or 'designer oestrogens') such as raloxifen that are designed to prevent or treat not only breast, bone and reproductive organ diseases but other diseases as well.

Conclusion

From Table 15.20, it is clear that HRT has no role in CVD prevention. From the clear benefit reported from various large-scale epidemiological studies to the contra-dictory results that are consistently shown in several randomized clinical trials, the bubble is finally burst!

References

1. Herrington DM. Hormone replacement therapy and heart disease: replacing dogma with data. *Circulation* 2003 Jan 7; **107**(1): 2–4.
2. Rexrode KM, Manson JE. Post-menopausal hormone therapy and quality of life: no cause for celebration. *JAMA* 2002 Feb 6; **287**(5): 641–2.
3. Rossouw JE. Hormones for coronary disease-full circle. *Lancet* 2002 Dec 21–28; **360**(9350): 1996–7.
4. Viscoli CM, Brass LM, Kernan WN, Sarrel PM, Suisa S, Horowitz RI. A clinical trial of estrogen replacement therapy after ischemic stroke. *N Engl J Med* 2001; **345**: 1243–9.
5. Herrington DM, Reboussin DM, Brosnihan KB, Sharp PC, Shumaker SA, Snyder TE, Furberg CD, Kowalchuk GJ, Stuckey TD, Rogers WJ, Givens DH, Waters D. Effects of estrogen replacement on the progression of coronary-artery atherosclerosis. *N Engl J Med* 2000 Aug; **343**(8): 522–9.

Part IV

Pharmacological

16

Recent clinical trials and substudies: LIFE, ALLHAT, BHF/MRC HPS, etc. . . .

Introduction

It is no longer a question of 'should we treat' hypertension, but 'how to treat' and 'who to treat'. However, a recurrent argument is that new antihypertensive agents are simply expensive ways of lowering blood pressure (BP) with limited evidence of a beneficial effect on prognosis—the job can equally be done by 'old' drugs, such as the thiazide diuretics and beta-blockers, which have withstood the test of time and outcome trials. This is despite some recent views that it is time 'to call a halt' to beta-blocker use in hypertension |**1**|.

The new agents have also been subject to some concern. Examples include the possibility that the alpha-blocker, doxazosin, may be associated with an excess of heart failure (HF) admissions and cardiovascular events in the ALLHAT (Antihypertensive and Lipid Lowering to prevent Heart Attack Trial) study |**2**|, and calcium antagonist usage being involved in an excess of myocardial events |**3**|. However, we have also had some meta-analyses, with comparisons between new drug classes, such as angiotensin-converting enzyme (ACE) inhibitors (ACEI) |**4**| and calcium antagonists |**5,6**|, vs traditional regimens based on older drugs, which have showed no significant difference between the treatment arms. Hence, the rationale of large megatrials, such as ALLHAT and ASCOT (Anglo Scandinavian Cardiac Outcomes Trial), which are supposed to determine the differences, if any, between 'old' and 'new' antihypertensive agents. In reality, such comparisons do pose some difficulties as more than 50% of hypertensives require at least two drugs, and one-third require more than two drugs, and thus it would be difficult to dissect out a beneficial or adverse effect of a particular drug class over another.

Comparisons between the angiotensin receptor blocker (ARB) class of drugs with older agents are only just emerging. Indeed, recent outcome data provided good evidence for ARBs in delaying the progression of diabetic nephropathy |**7**|. However, the ARBs finally come of age, with the presentation of the Losartan Intervention for Endpoint Reduction in Hypertension (LIFE) trial in 'high-risk' hypertensive patients, which showed that treatment with losartan reduced the incidence of stroke by 25% compared with beta-blocker therapy with atenolol |**8,9**|.

Interesting points include the similar reduction in myocardial infarction (MI) by both losartan and atenolol (the latter usually regarded as protective against MI). The possibility also arises that losartan could have a significant effect on stroke over and above BP reduction is in keeping with observations from the Heart Outcomes Prevention Evaluation (HOPE) trial |10|, which suggested that ACEI protected against stroke beyond reducing BP. Nevertheless, scrutiny of a HOPE substudy using ambulatory BP monitoring does show that ramipril (which was given at night in the study) did result in a marked reduction in nocturnal BP |11|, although 'office' BP readings did not show a marked fall, leading to the suggestion that the marked reduction in mortality and morbidity in the 'high-risk' HOPE study population was due to effects beyond that expected from BP lowering alone |12|.

This therefore leads to even more questions on the mechanism(s) leading to the beneficial effect(s) of losartan in LIFE. The renin–angiotensin–aldosterone system (RAAS) may well be 'the root of all evil' in cardiovascular disease (CVD), and blockade of angiotensin by losartan, or for that matter, any ARB or ACEI would suffice. We are still debating the observations from the PROGRESS study (Perindopril Protection Against Stroke Study), that treatment with perindopril and perindopril-indapamide resulted in significant reductions in BP among patients with previous cerebrovascular disease, but the beneficial effect on mortality and morbidity was only seen in the patients treated in combination with indapamide |13,14|. The CAPPP (Captopril Prevention Project) study |4|, despite its methodological problems, also suggested an excess of strokes among patients taking the ACEI, captopril.

Other aspects, such as regression of left ventricular (LV) hypertrophy (LVH), need to be explored. Indeed, losartan did result in greater LVH regression than atenolol, but even after adjusting for LVH effects, only a third of the difference in benefit could be explained by this. There may also be some benefical effects of renin–angiotensin blockade on the prothrombotic state in hypertension |15|, although one study in mild hypertensives could not confirm this |16|. There is also increasing evidence that angiogenesis is pathophysiologically related to hypertension |17|, and treatment with losartan may influence this |18|. Another mechanism to consider may be the effect of losartan on uric acid |19|, and indeed serum uric acid concentrations were significantly lower in those treated with losartan compared with atenolol. Nevertheless, it would be rather difficult to translate the small difference in uric acid levels between the losartan and atenolol groups to the differences in clinical end-points seen. Would there be an interaction between the ARBs and antiplatelet agents, such as aspirin, as seen with the ACEI |20|? We also need to see data on ARBs (and most of the other drug classes) in hypertensives from different ethnic groups. In particular, BP and prognostic data on Afro-Caribbeans and Indo-Asians, would be very interesting and relevant to the world-wide community. Would a 'double-wammy' of combined use of ACEIs and ARBs work even better? Some would suggest that the combination ACEI–ARB therapy would be the regimen of choice, at least in HF or diabetes |21|.

[A more detailed (and entertaining) version of this Introduction has been published in the *Journal of Human Hypertension* 2002; **16**: 289–91—the above is reproduced with permission.]

The Losartan Intervention For Endpoint reduction (LIFE) in Hypertension study: rationale, design, and methods.

Dahlof B, Devereux R, de Faire U, *et al.* The LIFE Study Group. *Am J Hypertens* 1997; **10**: 705–13.

BACKGROUND. **The treatment of hypertension mainly with diuretics and beta-blockers reduces cardiovascular mortality and morbidity, largely due to a decreased incidence of stroke, whereas the beneficial effects of antihypertensive therapy on the occurrence of coronary events have been less than expected from epidemiological studies. Furthermore, treated hypertensive patients still have a higher cardiovascular complication rate, compared with matched normotensives. This is particularly evident in patients with LVH, a major independent risk indicator for CVD. In addition to elevating BP, angiotensin II (Ang II) exerts an important influence on cardiac structure and function, stimulating cell proliferation and growth. Thus, to reduce further morbidity and mortality when treating hypertensive patients, it may be important to block effectively the effects of Ang II. This can be achieved directly at the Ang II receptor level by losartan, the first of a new class of antihypertensive agents. It therefore seems pertinent to investigate whether selective Ang II receptor blockade with losartan not only lowers BP but also reduces LVH more effectively than current therapy, and thus improves prognosis.**

INTERPRETATION. The LIFE study is a double-blind, prospective, parallel group study designed to compare the effects of losartan with those of the beta-blocker atenolol on the reduction of cardiovascular morbidity and mortality in approximately 8300 hypertensive patients (initial sitting diastolic BP [DBP] 95–115 mmHg or systolic BP [SBP] 160–200 mmHg) with electrocardiographically documented LVH. The study, which will continue for at least 4 years and until 1040 patients experience one primary end-point, has been designed with a statistical power that will detect a difference of at least 15% between groups in the incidence of combined cardiovascular morbidity and mortality. It is also the first prospective study with adequate power to link reversal of LVH to reduction in major cardiovascular events. The rationale of the study, which will involve more than 800 clinical centres in Scandinavia, the UK and USA, is discussed, and the major features of its design and general organization are described. On 30 April 1997, when inclusion was stopped, 9218 patients had been randomized.

Cardiovascular morbidity and mortality in the Losartan Intervention for Endpoint reduction in hypertension study (LIFE): a randomized trial against atenolol.

Dahlof B, Devereux RB, Kjeldsen SE, *et al.*; The LIFE Study Group. *Lancet* 2002; **359**: 995–1003.

BACKGROUND. **BP reduction achieved with beta-blockers and diuretics is the best recorded intervention to date for the prevention of cardiovascular morbidity and death in**

patients with hypertension. LVH is a strong independent indicator of risk of cardiovascular morbidity and death. The study aimed to establish whether selective blocking of Ang II improves LVH beyond reducing BP and, consequently, reduces cardiovascular morbidity and death.

INTERPRETATION. Losartan prevents more cardiovascular morbidity and death than atenolol for a similar reduction in BP and is better tolerated. Losartan seems to confer benefits beyond reduction in BP.

Comment

The amount of effort put into making the LIFE study has been proven by its continuing productivity of numerous high standard original papers in this high-risk hypertensive patient group with LVH. These studies have not only provided us a deeper understanding of the pathophysiology of hypertension-related LV remodelling and its diversity of associations with other disease states, such as insulin resistance, but has also provided us with a better insight into the many research methodologies used in the study. Most importantly, it will continue to provide us with a rationale of treating these high-risk patients.

Indeed, LIFE suggests that losartan reduces cardiovascular morbidity and mortality compared with atenolol, beyond that which could be achieved by its BP lowering effect. The underlying mechanism(s) through which this beneficial effect came about with ARB losartan is yet to be elucidated, but it is likely related to modulating the angiotensin system systemically and/or locally at the myocardial level. It is well known that Ang II is associated with the development of LVH; selective blockade of Ang II may reverse the hypertrophy and lead to decreased cardiovascular morbidity beyond just lowering BP. The results of this trial are both interesting and relevant to what is an expanding use of angiotensin-receptor blockers in the hypertensive population.

Table 16.1 Major clinical end-points: Losartan-based therapy versus Atenolol-based therapy in essential hypertension with signs of LVH

End-point	Losartan n (%)	Rate	Atenolol n (%)	Rate	Adjusted hazard ratio (95% CI)	P value
Primary composite end-point (cardiovascular mortality, stroke and MI)	508 (11%)	23.8	588 (13%)	27.9	0.87 (0.77–0.98)	0.021
Cardiovascular mortality	204 (4%)	9.2	234 (5%)	10.6	0.89 (0.73–1.07)	0.206
Stroke	232 (5%)	10.8	309 (7%)	14.5	0.75 (0.63–0.89)	0.001
MI	198 (4%)	9.2	188 (4%)	8.7	1.07 (0.88–1.31)	0.491
Total mortality	383 (8%)	17.3	431 (9%)	19.6	0.90 (0.78–1.03)	0.128
Angina admission	160 (3%)	7.4	141 (3%)	6.6	1.16 (0.92–1.45)	0.212
HF admission	153 (3%)	7.1	161 (4%)	7.5	0.97 (0.78–1.21)	0.765
Revascularization	261 (6%)	12.2	284 (6%)	13.3	0.94 (0.79–1.11)	0.441

Source: The LIFE Study Group (2002).

LIFE was a double-blind trial that involved a total of 9193 patients (aged 55–80 years; 54% female and 92% white, 13% diabetic, with 16% having a history of coronary artery disease and 8% a history of cerebrovascular disease), with hypertension (previously treated 72% or untreated 28%) and electrocardiographic (ECG) evidence of LVH randomized to receive the ARB losartan ($n = 4605$) or the beta-blocker atenolol ($n = 4588$) (mean daily doses, 82 mg and 79 mg, respectively). More than half of both groups received concomitant hydrochlorothiazides and other anti-hypertensive medications as needed to obtain a BP goal of less than 140/90 mmHg, but no patients were allowed to take ACEI, other ARBs, or other beta-blockers. Exclusion criteria included secondary hypertension; MI or stroke within the last 6 months; angina pectoris requiring treatment with beta-blockers or calcium channel blockers (CCB); and HF or LV ejection fraction 40% or less. Follow-up was 99%.

During follow-up (mean, 4.8 years), after adjusting for differences in achieved BP levels incidence of the primary composite end-point (cardiovascular death, MI or stroke) was lower with losartan than with atenolol (11% vs 13%, [relative risk (RR) 0.87, 95% confidence interval (CI) 0.77–0.98, $P = 0.02$], numbers needed to treat [NNT] = 244 patients per year). Most of the benefit was driven by a 25% reduction in the risk of fatal and non-fatal stroke (RR 0.75, 95% CI 0.63–0.89, $P = 0.001$), with no benefit seen for fatal and non-fatal MI (RR 1.07, 95% CI 0.88–1.31, $P = 0.5$) or cardiovascular death (RR = 0.89; 95% CI, 0.73–0.07) and all-cause mortality (RR = 0.90; 95% CI, 0.78–1.03). BP fell by 30.2/16.6 (SD 18.5/10.1) and 29.1/16.8 mmHg (19.2/10.1) in the losartan and atenolol groups, respectively.

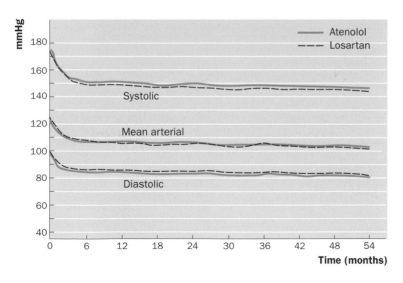

Fig. 16.1 BP during follow-up. Source: The LIFE Study Group (2002).

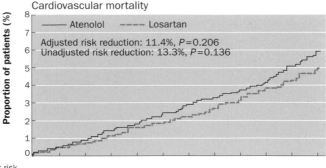

Number at risk

Losartan	4605	4563	4532	4496	4448	4410	4373	4327	4284	4152	2005	976
Atenolol	4588	4553	4513	4474	4442	4388	4341	4299	4252	4107	2006	965

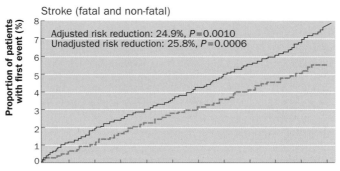

Number at risk

Losartan	4605	4528	4469	4408	4332	4273	4224	4166	4117	3974	1928	925
Atenolol	4588	4490	4424	4372	4317	4245	4180	4119	4055	3894	1901	897

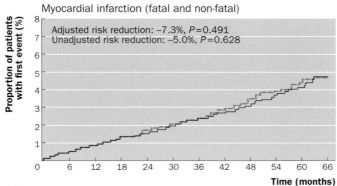

Number at risk

Losartan	4605	4525	4478	4430	4367	4307	4258	4196	4139	3999	1953	936
Atenolol	4588	4517	4466	4415	4364	4302	4243	4192	4134	3975	1953	937

Fig. 16.2 Kaplan–Meier curves for individual end-points. Source: The LIFE Study Group (2002).

Despite comparable BP lowering with the two drugs, LVH regressed more with losartan than with atenolol. However, only 30% of the benefit on study outcome was explained by the degree of ECG LVH regression.

In a pre-specified subgroup of 1195 diabetics (see below, Lindholm *et al.* 2002), losartan fared significantly better than atenolol regarding the primary composite end-point and regarding all-cause mortality, cardiovascular mortality, and admission for HF. MI and stroke rates were not different between the two treatment arms in diabetics.

Moreover, new-onset diabetes was less common (25% reduction) with losartan (see below). Even among 'low-risk' patients, that is, those without vascular disease or diabetes, there was an 18% reduction in the primary end-points in those taking losartan. Losartan was also better tolerated and caused fewer study dropouts.

The authors conclude that in patients with essential hypertension and ECG LVH, treatment based on losartan, as compared with a treatment regimen based on atenolol, was associated with less overall cardiovascular morbidity and mortality, stroke and new onset of diabetes; however, no difference was noted between groups in the occurrence of MI or cardiovascular death. In addition, losartan was better tolerated and caused greater regression of ECG LVH for a similar amount of BP reduction. Losartan appears to confer benefits beyond BP reduction in older patients with hypertension and ECG LVH |**22,23**|.

It is clear that in patients with essential hypertension and signs of LVH, losartan reduced strokes and new-onset diabetes more than atenolol. In addition, losartan also provided at least as much cardioprotection as atenolol, whether or not either drug was used with a low-dose hydrochlorothiazide. Certainly, it is known from previous hypertensive trials that atenolol effectively reduce both the risk of MI and stroke. The Joint National Committee (JNC) VI report |**24**| also recommends diuretics and beta-blockers to prevent the occurrence of initial stroke in those with uncomplicated hypertension. It is interesting that losartan-based treatment appears statistically no different from atenolol in preventing MI in high-risk hypertensive with LVH. A 25% further reduction in stroke with losartan in this high-risk group is therefore impressive as stroke is a major cause of death and disability and was more frequent than MI in this study and others during the past decade. The possibility arises that ARBs seem to provide cardioprotection beyond BP lowering and ought to underlie any antihypertensive treatment strategy.

It is possible that losartan achieved the overall cardiovascular benefits beyond its effect on lowering BP alone. However, the data and the study conclusions should be interpreted with caution, especially when stroke was the only significant primary composite end-point. It is of note that the observed benefit was small in a select group of patients and there was no additional reduction demonstrated in all-cause mortality compared with less expensive atenolol. In addition, cardiovascular mortality was not significantly affected, and the risk of MI, although not significantly different, was 7% more likely to have occurred in the losartan group, a trend that remains unexplained. Furthermore, most patients required more than one agent to reach target-level BP. Use of multiple agents could therefore confound the comparison between the two agents in reducing risk. Thus, in this study it was the regimen *per se* and not losartan alone that probably provided the benefit. Furthermore, the benefit of losartan over atenolol was more pronounced in a separate trial of hypertensive diabetic patients with LVH (NNT = 122 patients per year) (as discussed in Lindholm *et al.* 2002).

Rather surprisingly, in this study of high-risk hypertensive patients the target BP of lower than 140/90 mmHg was only achieved in fewer than 50% of patients in both groups. Mean BP was not lowered as much in the atenolol group as in the losartan group, which suggests that a higher dose of atenolol might have been necessary to compare genuinely the efficacy of the two drugs. In fact, only about 10% of patients in each study group reached goal BP with monotherapy—the remainder did so with the addition of hydrochlorthiazide or other agents. As the distribution of additional drugs is said not to differ between the two groups, almost all patients required additional therapy with a thiazide diuretic. As 'other drugs', a CCB (not specifically mentioned in the paper), was probably also required in about one-half of the patients.

The cardiovascular benefits of ARBs probably resulted from interference with the deleterious effects of Ang II. The results should be applicable to other ARBs, i.e. a class effect. However, it is of note that recently, the US FDA has approved labelling changes that candesartan is better than losartan in lowering BP. The data from three randomized trials, including two forced-titration trials, have shown that at the maximum recommended daily dose, 32 mg of candesartan reduced blood SBP and DBP by about 3/2 mmHg more at trough than did 100 mg of losartan. However, there is no evidence to support that the 3/2 mmHg more reduction in BP with candesartan will translate to better outcome measures. The Valsartan Antihypertensive Long-term Use Evaluation (VALUE) trial, comparing another ARB valsartan with the CCB amlodipine in high-risk hypertensive patients will become available in 2004. This

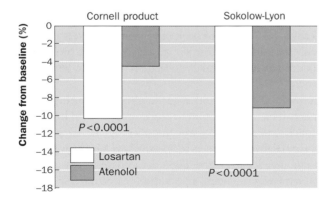

Fig. 16.3 Change in Cornell voltage-duration product and Sokolow–Lyon from baseline. *P* is for between-group differences. Source: The LIFE Study Group (2002).

trial will provide evidence whether drugs within this class would provide similar benefit in high-risk patients. And, more specifically, to clarify further the question of whether or not specific stroke protection benefits exist for the ARB class beyond BP reduction.

It is also possible that ARB interact with thiazide diuretic differently (from interaction between beta-blocker and diuretic), and thus in favour of the losartan-based treated patients. How compounds that interact with the renin–angiotensin axis protect against stroke is unclear at this time. It is known that LVH (both on ECG and echocardiography) is a BP-independent predictor of cerebrovascular events, and LV mass regressed more so with losartan in the LIFE trial. This was sufficient to explain about one-third of the difference in stroke rate.

In the HOPE, involving 4600 people aged 55 or older who are at high risk for coronary heart disease (CHD) and stroke, have reported that patients on ramipril had a lower risk of stroke, MI, cardiovascular death and developing diabetes, despite only a modest reduction in 'clinic' BP readings. However, substudy with 24-hour BP monitoring suggested that more of the benefits of ramipril in HOPE may actually be related to BP reduction (especially during night-time) to a larger extent than previously ascribed |12|.

Although ACEIs have not yet been compared directly (probably never will be) with ARBs in these high-risk patients, there is no reason to believe that the benefit of losartan shown in this study is superior to (and may actually be less than) that of less expensive ACEI, given the fact that captopril (an ACEI) was superior than losartan in the treatment of HF in the Losartan Heart Failure Survival Study (ELITE II) study (Pitt *et al.*) |25|. Furthermore, losartan also failed to show benefits over the ACEI captopril in the Optimal Trial in Myocardial Infarction with the Angiotensin II Antagonist Losartan (OPTIMAAL) in post-MI patients (see page 341) |26|. In fact, captopril showed a trend toward superiority. Nevertheless, losartan was better tolerated. It remains unknown whether combining ARB and ACEI is more beneficial in these high-risk groups. Of note, patients in the HOPE trial, who had previously been treated with aspirin, tended toward a reduced stroke benefit from ramipril compared with patients who had not been treated with aspirin. As of yet, the LIFE study has not reported whether there was an aspirin and losartan interaction. As only 6% of the participants were black, it is unclear if the results can be generalized to all ethnic populations.

It is also unknown whether ARBs are superior to diuretics such as chlorthalidone. ALLHAT (see below) has reported that thiazide diuretic is superior to ACEI lisinopril and dihydropyridine CCB amlodipine in all secondary outcomes. As the achieved BP reduction was similar with chlorthalidone and amlodipine in ALLHAT, the superiority of the diuretic in that comparison is clear. This supports the notion that: 'it does matter how we lower BP, not just lower it'. Thiazide would always be the first choice (if no contraindication) to which other agents added upon when BP goal still not yet achieved.

However, the use of beta-blocker atenolol as a comparator to losartan in this study does not seem appropriate. It would be more informative if losartan was compared with a thiazide diuretic. The average of patients in LIFE is 67 years (55–80 years). Indeed, a meta-analysis by Messerli *et al.* |27| has found that studies generally unfavourable to beta-blockers involve elderly hypertensive patients with mean age about 70 years, and non-compliant stiff vascular systems. Beta-blockers are also generally suspect in their ability to prevent stroke.

One important practical advantage of losartan over atenolol is that losartan has fewer side-effects reported in the study. Indeed, the reduction in side-effects with ARBs was a positive step toward increasing patient satisfaction and compliance. With all the above considerations, it is fair to say that in hypertensive patients with ECG LVH, the selection of the ARB losartan may be a better choice than the beta-blocker atenolol as part of a treatment regimen.

Whether the benefits of losartan in LIFE are related entirely to protection against the adverse effects of Ang II, including its growth promoting properties in the heart and vasculature, or to other actions unique to the losartan molecule is unclear and will require further study.

In the next few years, many more important clinical trials will be completed, including VALUE, (Kjeldsen *et al.*) |28| Valsartan in Acute Myocardial Infarction (VALIANT) (Pfeffer *et al.*) |29|, and Candesartan in Heart Failure Assessment of Reduction in Mortality and Morbidity (CHARM) (Swedberg *et al.*) |30|. These studies will provide important opportunities for learning more about the utility of the ARB in the prevention of cardiovascular events in patients with risk factors for coronary disease or in patients who have already experienced an MI. In addition, a large-scale clinical trial, Ongoing Telmisartan Alone and in Combination with Ramipril Global Endpoint Trial (ONTARGET) (Yusuf *et al.*) |31|, is going to evaluate carefully the utility of the combination of an ACEI and an ARB on cardiovascular outcome.

Cardiovascular morbidity and mortality in patients with diabetes in the Losartan Intervention For Endpoint reduction in hypertension study (LIFE): a randomized trial against atenolol.

Lindholm LH, Ibsen H, Dahlof B, *et al.* and the LIFE study group. *Lancet* 2002; **359**(9311): 1004–10.

B A C K G R O U N D . **The most suitable antihypertensive drug to reduce the risk of CVD in patients with hypertension and diabetes is unclear. In pre-specified analyses, we compared the effects of losartan and atenolol on cardiovascular morbidity and mortality in diabetic patients.**

I N T E R P R E T A T I O N . Losartan was more effective than atenolol in reducing cardiovascular morbidity and mortality as well as mortality from all causes in patients with hypertension, diabetes and LVH. Losartan seems to have benefits beyond BP reduction.

Comment

There were 1195 diabetics (mean age 67 years, 586 treated with losartan) in this subgroup analysis. The baseline Framingham risk score and ECG LVH were used as covariates to compare the effects of the drugs on the primary composite end-point of cardiovascular morbidity and mortality (cardiovascular death, stroke or MI). After a mean follow-up of 4.8 years, the reduction of mean BP was also not different between the two groups. There was a 24% reduction (more favourable than the 13% reduction seen in the overall trial) in risk of the primary end-point in the losartan group ($P = 0.031$), 37% reduction in the risk of cardiovascular death (although there was no benefit on the specific end-point of cardiovascular mortality in the entire study), and a notable 39% reduction in all-cause mortality (see Table 16.2). Admission for HF was also reduced by 40% in the losartan group. As in the overall trial, there was no difference in the risk of MI between the two groups. Interestingly, at the conclusion of the trial, although SBP was reduced 2 mmHg more in the losartan-based (146/79 mmHg) than in the atenolol-based group (148/79 mmHg), there was no difference in the risk of stroke, which accounted for the majority of benefit in the overall analysis.

The losartan-based regimen was also more effective than atenolol-based regimen in reversing LVH. Interestingly, serum glucose did not differ between the two groups throughout the study. Although the percentage of patients with clinical nephropathy (at least 300 mg of protein/g creatinine per day) was similar in the two groups at study entry, fewer patients in the losartan group still had evidence of nephropathy at the study's conclusion.

The benefit of losartan over atenolol was especially marked in the small group (20%) of diabetic patients who had not been treated for hypertension before the

Table 16.2 Losartan-based therapy vs atenolol-based therapy in diabetes with essential hypertension and signs of LVH

End-point	Losartan-treated diabetics (%) (n = 586)	Atenolol-treated diabetics (%) (n = 609)	Adjusted relative risk (95% CI)	P value	NNT (CI)
Primary end-point (cardiovascular death, stroke or MI)	103 (18%)	139 (23%)	0.76 (0.58–0.98)	0.031	21 (12–250)
Cardiovascular deaths	38 (6%)	61 (10%)	0.63 (0.42–0.95)	0.028	28 (18–211)
All-cause mortality	63 (11%)	104 (17%)	0.61 (0.45–0.84)	0.002	16 (12–40)
Admission for HF	32 (5%)	55 (9%)	0.59 (0.38–0.92)	0.019	28 (19–145)

NNT, number needed to treat to prevent one event.
Source: Lindholm et al. (2002).

study. Hypertensive diabetic patients with LVH seem to benefit more from a losartan-based regimen (together with a thiazide diuretic) than atenolol-based regimen. The more benefits gained with losartan than with atenolol in the even higher-risk patients with diabetes (i.e. LVH + diabetes + hypertension) than those without diabetes is in fact consistent with current treatment guideline recommendations which recommend the use of a specific class of agents as initial therapy in the presence of compelling indications (in this case diabetes mellitus). The current treatment guideline recommendations support the use of agents that block the angiotensin system as first line treatment in hypertensives with diabetes mellitus. This does seem to support the notion that 'it does matter which class of agent we lower BP, not just we lower it by any agent', particularly when one is dealing with a special group of patients with high cardiovascular risk. In fact, the data showed no better beneficial effects of losartan-based over atenolol-based therapy for patients without diabetes.

In the losartan-treated group, proteinuria was present in 11% of patients at study entry and was reduced to 8%, whereas the atenolol-treated group was associated with an 11–12% reduction at the study's conclusion suggesting that an ARB may be more effective in reducing clinical nephropathy than a beta-blocker. These results seem comparable with trials that have shown renoprotective and/or cardioprotective beneficial effects with the use of ARB, the 'sartans' in type 2 diabetic patients with hypertension, and microalbuminuria or proteinuria (a marker of target organ damage, in this case renal damage, perhaps equivalent to LVH as in the LIFE study). These trials include the RENAAL (Reduction of Endpoints in NIDDM with the Angiotensin II Antagonist Losartan) |32|, the IDNT (Irbesartan Diabetic Nephropathy Trial) |33|, and the IRMA II (IRbesartan MicroAlbuminuria) |34|. Taken together with the LIFE study, these trials have shown very similar results point to a cardiovascular protective effect afforded by ARB that cannot be accounted for exclusively by the BP reduction *per se*. Thus, ARBs are beneficial for high-risk diabetic patients with target organ damage (LVH or proteinuria), and that the benefit may supersede the BP effect. However, it is of interest to note that the UKPDS (UK Prospective Diabetes Study) study in more than 1100 type 2 diabetic patients over an 8+ year period failed to demonstrate a difference in cardiovascular outcome where an ACEI group of subjects was compared with a group of patients on a beta-blocker-based regimen |35|.

Stroke was the most likely primary end-point to occur among the three composite end-points and continues to be the most devastating consequence of hypertension. Certainly, LVH remains a BP-independent predictor for stroke. Finally, there appears to be few caveats in this study. Of note, the main benefit with losartan-based therapy was seen in patients with diabetes as the primary outcome does not seem to differ when these are subtracted from the total cohort. Few patients remained only on the blinded medicine (9%) as almost all participants ended up on two or more medicines and still fell short of the BP goal recommended for those with diabetes (<130/80 mmHg). Although the authors adjusted for the 2 mmHg greater reduction in SBP seen in those on losartan, this should have accounted for a further reduction in stroke as seen in the overall trial but not in the diabetic cohort. It is also interesting to note that in the non-diabetic patients, the almost 15% reduction of the primary outcome was driven by the 25% reduction in stroke, whereas in the diabetic patients, the 24% reduction in the primary end-point was driven mostly by a reduction in cardiovascular and total mortality. However, the number of stroke events occurred was at least 1.5–1.8 times higher in the diabetic patients compared with the non-diabetic patients, i.e. higher stroke risk in diabetics. Furthermore, the reduction in stroke and MI events was not different between the two treatment arms in the diabetic substudy. Finally, there were no other benefits with losartan-based therapy other than for stroke reduction in the total cohort.

Such discrepancies are difficult to dissect. It is of interest to speculate on possible differences in the groups at baseline in the presence of atrial fibrillation. Did those patients on atenolol have more CVD before the study started? The LIFE trial suggests that LVH reversal leads to an improvement in outcome in the diabetic. In addition, the selection of atenolol, and for that matter a beta-blocker, as the control therapy could explain some of the difference between the treatment groups.

As the diabetic cohort usually accounts for the greatest clinical benefit seen within a trial, the discordant findings between the overall cohort and the diabetic cohort on the primary end-points seem rather worrying as the paper seem to give an impression that losartan is superior to atenolol in preventing cardiovascular death in diabetics, but in actual fact the number of MI and stroke events occurred were not different between the two regimens. It seems that losartan-based therapy in LIFE saves lives but does not prevent heart attacks and stroke. Nevertheless, the initial use of the ARB as a component of therapy (with a thiazide) appears to be more beneficial than the initial use of the beta-blocker in patients with hypertension, diabetes and ECG LVH.

Risk of new-onset diabetes in the Losartan Intervention For Endpoint reduction in hypertension study.

Lindholm LH, Ibsen H, Borch-Johnsen K, et al.; For the LIFE study group.
J Hypertens 2002; **20**(9): 1879–86.

BACKGROUND. There has been uncertainty about the risk of new-onset diabetes in hypertensive individuals treated with different BP-decreasing drugs. The objective of this study was to study this risk in hypertensive individuals who were at risk of developing diabetes mellitus in the LIFE study.

INTERPRETATION. New-onset diabetes could be strongly predicted by a newly developed risk score using baseline serum glucose concentration (non-fasting), body mass index, serum high-density lipoprotein (HDL) cholesterol concentration, SBP and history of prior use of antihypertensive drugs. Independently of these risk factors, fewer hypertensive patients with LVH developed diabetes mellitus if they were treated with losartan than if they were treated with atenolol.

Comment

In this subgroup analysis, there was less new-onset diabetes developed in patients taking losartan compared with those receiving atenolol during the course of the trial, regardless of other risk factors for diabetes. Of 7998 patients at baseline who did not have diabetes, 562 developed the disease over the course of the study. Those taking losartan in addition to other antihypertensive therapy had a 25% lower risk of developing diabetes than those assigned to the beta-blocker; of 4019 patients taking losartan, 242 (6%) developed diabetes, compared with 320 (8%) of the 3979 on atenolol. The strongest predictor of new-onset diabetes was serum glucose, followed by BMI and low HDL.

The lower rate of new-onset diabetes (difference of 25%) with losartan confirms findings from prior studies with the ACEI ramipril and captopril. This finding could have related to a differential effect on insulin resistance—the precursor condition for overt diabetes—favouring losartan. However, it appears that such observation is not due to a benefit of losartan but rather due to a potentially negative effect of atenolol as beta-blocker was associated with worsening insulin sensitivity over time. Indeed, in those receiving atenolol, insulin sensitivity fell throughout the study. Of interest is the observation that body weight decreased similarly in both treatment groups (84.3–82.5 kg and 84.3–82.6 kg for losartan and atenolol, respectively). Typically, body weight increases with long-term beta-blocker therapy.

Effects of losartan on cardiovascular morbidity and mortality in patients with isolated systolic hypertension and left ventricular hypertrophy.

Kjeldsen SE, Dahlof B, Devereux RB, *et al.*; LIFE (Losartan Intervention for Endpoint Reduction) Study Group. *JAMA* 2002; **288**: 1491–8.

BACKGROUND. Drug intervention in placebo-controlled trials has been beneficial in isolated systolic hypertension (ISH). The objective is to test the hypothesis that losartan improves outcome better than atenolol in patients with ISH and ECG LVH.

INTERPRETATION. These data suggest that losartan is superior to atenolol in treatment of patients with ISH and ECG LVH.

Comment

This substudy involved 1326 patients with SBPs of 160–200 mmHg and DBPs of less than 90 mmHg (mean, 174/83 mmHg) and ECG LVH.

BP was reduced by an identical amount 28/9 mmHg in both groups. The primary end-point a composite of cardiovascular death, stroke, and MI was reduced by 25% in the losartan group, which was not quite statistically significant (RR 0.75; 95% CI 0.56–1.01; $P = 0.06$, adjusted for risk and degree of ECG LVH; unadjusted RR 0.71; 95% CI 0.53–0.95; $P = 0.02$). When individual components of the composite end-point are looked at, both cardiovascular death (RR 0.54; 95% CI 0.34–0.87; $P = 0.01$)

and stroke (RR 0.60; 95% CI 0.38–0.92; $P = 0.02$) were reduced significantly in the losartan group. However, there was no difference in the incidence of MI. New-onset diabetes (RR 0.62; 95% CI 0.40–0.97; P = 0.04) and total mortality (RR 0.72; 95% CI 0.53–1.00; $P = 0.046$) also occurred less frequently with losartan. In addition, losartan decreased ECG LVH more than atenolol ($P <0.001$) and was better tolerated.

As discussed already above, the LIFE study should be generalized with care to a younger patient population. Beta-blocker probably is a better antihypertensive agent in younger and middle-aged patients as there is evidence to suggest that beta-blockers are less beneficial in older hypertensives patients, whereas dihydropyridine CCB and diuretics have been shown to be more effective in elderly patients in whom ISH is more prevalent. The results of this substudy may therefore be viewed as beta-blockers having different effects in younger vs older patients, and that the early benefits observed may not be ascribed to losartan-treated effects, but rather it is likely to be due to the unfavourable effects of atenolol-based treatment in this particular group of patients. Of note, there are so far no placebo-controlled outcome trials with beta-blockers in patients with ISH. This study also does not give information on whether losartan is superior to diuretics or calcium blockers as a first-line treatment for ISH.

Table 16.3 LIFE: Major clinical end-points in patients with ISH

End-point	Losartan (n = 660)	Atenolol (n = 666)	Adjusted RR (95% CI)	P
CV death/stroke/MI	11.4%	15.6%	0.75 (0.56–1.01)	0.06
CV death	4.1%	7.8%	0.54 (0.34–0.87)	0.01
Stroke	4.8%	8.4%	0.60 (0.38–0.92)	0.02
MI	4.7%	5.4%	0.89 (0.55–1.44)	0.64
Total mortality	10.0%	14.0%	0.72 (0.53–1.00)	0.046
New-onset diabetes	5.8%	9.0%	0.62 (0.40–0.97)	0.04

Source: Kjeldsen *et al.* (2002).

Table 16.4 LIFE: Major clinical end-points in patients without ISH

End-point	Losartan (n = 3945)	Atenolol (n = 3922)	Adjusted RR (95% CI)	P
CV death/stroke/MI	11.0%	12.3%	0.90 (0.79–1.02)	0.11
CV death	4.5%	4.6%	0.99 (0.80–1.22)	0.90
Stroke	5.1%	6.5%	0.79 (0.66–0.95)	0.01
MI	4.2%	3.9%	1.12 (0.90–1.40)	0.30
Total mortality	8.0%	8.6%	0.95 (0.82–1.11)	0.51
New-onset diabetes	6.1%	7.9%	0.77 (0.64–0.92)	0.005

Source: Kjeldsen *et al.* (2002).

Table 16.5 Outcomes in LIFE compared with SHEP and SYST-EUR

Outcome	SHEP (%)	SYST-EUR (%)	LIFE losartan group (%)	LIFE atenolol group (%)
All-cause mortality	19.3	20.5	21.2	30.2
Cardiovascular mortality	8.2	9.8	8.7	16.9
Stroke	10.4	7.9	10.6	18.9
All cardiovascular events	17.8	23.3	25.1	35.8

Source: Kjeldsen *et al.* (2002).

Table 16.5 shows the differences in all-cause mortality, cardiovascular mortality, stroke and total mortality between LIFE and 2 placebo-controlled trials in patients with ISH-SHEP (Systolic Hypertension in the Elderly Program), which used chlor-thalidone and atenolol, and SYST-EUR (Systolic Hypertension in Europe), which used the CCB nitrendipine together with enalapril and hydrochlorothiazide. However, it should be noted that the latter two trials did not specifically recruit patients with ECG LVH, that is, at different cardiovascular risk.

It is also possible that ARBs interact with thiazide diuretics differently (compared with the interaction between beta-blocker and diuretic), and thus in favour of the losartan-based-treated patients. How compounds that interact with the renin–angiotensin axis protect against stroke is unclear at this time.

What about patients without clinically evident vascular disease?

Concerns have been raised that many patients in the LIFE study had no overt vascular disease and were therefore at lower risk. A subsequent analysis of the LIFE data (presented at the 2002 Scientific Sessions of the American Heart Association) in these patients, has shown even greater reductions in both the composite end-point and the components of the primary end-point for losartan compared with atenolol |**36**|.

The subgroup of patients without vascular disease comprised a total of 6886 patients (3402 assigned to losartan and 3484 to atenolol). The Framingham 5-year predictive risk score (predicted incidence of coronary events over 5 years) for these patients was 21.5%. Baseline clinical characteristics were similar in each treatment group. Cox regression analysis with baseline Framingham risk score and ECG LVH as covariates was used to compare the effects of the two regimens on the occurrence of a first primary event (cardiovascular death, MI or stroke).

The results showed that the combined risk of cardiovascular death, MI and stroke was still significantly reduced by 19% with losartan compared with atenolol ($P = 0.008$) in this population (see Table 16.6). Stroke was reduced by 34% in the losartan-treated patients compared with the atenolol-treated group ($P = 0.0003$). A slight trend in favour of atenolol was seen for risk of MI and in favour of losartan for

Table 16.6 Primary and secondary outcomes in LIFE patients without clinically evident vascular disease

	Losartan (n = 3402)	Atenolol (n = 3484)	Adjusted RR (%)	P	Unadjusted RR (%)	P
Primary composite end-point	282	355	−19	0.008	−20	0.006
Cardiovascular mortality	103	132	−20	0.092	−20	0.091
Stroke	125	125	−34	<0.001	−34	<0.001
MI	110	100	+14	0.36	+13	0.39
Total mortality	225	268	−15	0.06	−15	0.08
New-onset diabetes mellitus	173	254	−31	<0.001	−31	<0.001

Source: Devereaux RB et al. (2002).

total mortality. A significantly lower rate of new onset of diabetes was also seen with losartan ($P < 0.001$). However, in these patients without clinical evidence of vascular disease, losartan-based treatment failed to prevent MI when compared with atenolol-based treatment. The relative risk of MI was 14% higher in losartan-treated than atenolol-treated patients.

LIFE and atrial fibrillation

Data on the subgroup of patients in LIFE who had atrial fibrillation were presented at the European Society of Cardiology meeting in 2002 |37|. In LIFE, 324 patients had atrial fibrillation and as with the main trial, all had hypertension (160–200 mmHg SBP and 95–115 mmHg DBP) and ECG LVH (Cornell). At the end of the trial, strokes occurred in 12% ($n = 8$) of the losartan-treated group, compared with 21.3% ($n = 37$) of the atenolol-treated group. This translated to a 49% risk reduction (adjusted hazard ratio 0.50; 95% CI 0.29–0.89) in the risk of stroke ($P = 0.018$). Expressed another way, 11 patients treated with losartan instead of atenolol for 4.8 years will prevent one stroke.

The efficacy and tolerability of losartan vs atenolol in patients with isolated systolic hypertension. Losartan ISH Investigators Group.
Farsang C, Garcia-Puig J, Niegowska J, Baiz AQ, Vrijens F, Bortman G.
J Hypertens 2000; **18**(6): 795–801.

BACKGROUND. To compare the efficacy and tolerability of Ang II antagonist losartan and the beta-blocker atenolol in the treatment of patients with ISH after 16 weeks of treatment.

INTERPRETATION. It is concluded that 50 mg losartan and 50 mg atenolol produced comparable reductions in sitting SBP in patients with ISH but losartan was better tolerated. This is the first demonstration of the therapeutic value of selective Ang II receptor blockade with losartan in the treatment of ISH.

Comment

This was a double-blind, randomized, multi-country study in 273 patients with ISH (sitting SBP of 160–205 mmHg, and a sitting DBP <90 mmHg) randomized to receive 50 mg losartan or 50 mg atenolol once daily for 16 weeks. Additional hydrochlorothiazide was given at 8 and 12 weeks when the BP was still ≥160 mmHg.

The effect of a losartan-based treatment regimen on isolated systolic hypertension.

Cushman WC, Brady WE, Gazdick LP, Zeldin RK. *J Clin Hypertens* 2002; **4**(2): 101–7.

BACKGROUND. This study was conducted to compare the antihypertensive efficacy and tolerability, over 12 weeks, of a losartan-based treatment regimen and placebo in patients with ISH.

INTERPRETATION. In patients with ISH, a once-daily losartan-based treatment regimen significantly lowered SBP. The losartan-based regimen exhibited antihypertensive efficacy that was superior to that of placebo, with a similar tolerability profile.

Comment

This is a small placebo-controlled trial with 308 patients, age ≥35 years with ISH (defined as trough sitting SBP 140–200 mmHg and DBP 70–89 mmHg) randomized to losartan 50 mg ($n = 157$) or placebo ($n = 151$) once daily, with titration as necessary to achieve a goal trough sitting SBP <140 mmHg. Baseline SBP was similar between the two groups (losartan, 165.3 mmHg; placebo, 166.1 mmHg). At 12 weeks, mean trough sitting SBP decreased significantly (P <0.001) in both the losartan-based treatment group (by 19.2 mmHg) and in the placebo group (by 7.6 mmHg). The reduction in sitting SBP was significantly greater for losartan than placebo (−11.6 mmHg; 95% CI −14.8 to −8.4).

ISH is thought to arise primarily from stiffening of the large arteries, with a result-ant reduction in distensibility and elasticity. ARBs can reduce arterial stiffness via several mechanisms by modulating the renin–angiotensin system. In addition, losartan has been shown to inhibit Ang II-mediated adverse vascular remodelling of the arterial wall and to normalize endothelial function of small arteries in patients with essential hypertension, effects that may render them useful in the treatment of ISH; these are the rationale behind this study. Indeed, as compared with placebo, losartan reduced SBP to a greater degree in patients with ISH. This study was not designed to determine the impact of treatment of ISH with a losartan-based regimen on cardiovascular morbidity and mortality.

The data from this study extend those of the study by Farsang *et al.* (2000, see above), a randomized, double-blind comparison of losartan and atenolol in the treatment of ISH. In that study, patients received losartan 50 mg or atenolol 50 mg once daily over a 16-week treatment period with hydrochlorthiazide added at weeks 8 and 12 if necessary. Both the losartan- and atenolol-based regimens effectively reduced baseline sitting SBP in patients with ISH (173.7 mmHg reduced to 149.0 mmHg with losartan and 173.5 mmHg reduced to 148.2 mmHg with atenolol).

Is cardiovascular remodeling in patients with essential hypertension related to more than high blood pressure? A LIFE substudy.

Olsen MH, Wachtell K, Hermann KL, *et al. Am Heart J* 2002; **144**(3): 530–7.

BACKGROUND. Blocking the renin–aldosterone–Ang II system has been hypothesized to induce BP-dependent as well as BP-independent regression of cardiovascular hypertrophy. However, the relative influence of elevated BP and various neurohormonal factors on cardiovascular remodelling in hypertension is unclear.

INTERPRETATION. Apart from being associated with a high BP burden, cardiovascular remodelling was associated with high levels of circulating adrenalin, aldosterone, as well as Ang II, suggesting a beneficial effect above and beyond the effect of BP reduction when using antihypertensive agents blocking the receptors of these neurohormonal factors.

Comment

LVH is a major cardiovascular risk factor for morbidity and mortality. It is caused by arterial hypertension, although various haemodynamic and non-haemodynamic factors contribute to its development. Especially, the RAAS is involved in the pathophysiology of LVH. Ang II has been shown to have several direct and indirect actions on cardiac cells that might influence cardiac hypertrophy. These include actions on cardiomyocytes, fibroblasts, sympathetic nerves, coronary vascular smooth muscle and coronary endothelial cells. All these effects could thus be blocked by losartan and are, by convention, designated Ang II receptor type 1 (or AT1 receptor) mediated.

The relative importance of haemodynamic burden (24-hour SBP) vs neurohormonal factors (serum insulin, and plasma levels of adrenalin, noradrenalin, renin, Ang II, aldosterone and endothelin) on cardiovascular hypertrophy and remodelling is unclear. To investigate this and the relationship between LVH and vascular hypertrophy, remodelling, and stiffness, the authors measured LV mass by echocardiography, as well as by magnetic resonance imaging (i.e. combining the most clinically used method with the more accurate method) in 43 untreated hypertensive patients with ECG LVH. They found that the relative association of BP and neurohormonal factors to remodelling of the myocardium, the conduit and the resistance arteries, respectively, differed from one part of the cardiovascular system to the other. Higher LV mass index was associated with higher median 24-hour SBP, whereas higher relative wall thickness (measured by echocardiography), indicating concentric LV geometry, was associated with higher levels of circulating adrenalin and aldosterone. Higher intima-media thickness of the common carotid arteries was also associated with higher median 24-hour SBP as well as higher levels of circulating adrenalin, whereas lower distensibility was associated with higher median 24-hour SBP as well as higher levels of circulating Ang II. Remodelling of the subcutaneous resistance arteries (by measuring media/lumen ratio of isolated subcutaneous resistance arteries), examined *in vitro*, was associated with higher levels of circulating adrenalin. In addition, the degree of cardiac and vascular hypertrophy was interrelated. LVH was related to hypertrophy of the common carotid arteries, vascular remodelling in the forearm, and low distensibility of the subcutaneous resistance arteries partly independently of the BP.

The results of this study supports earlier findings that cardiac myocyte growth is primarily related to load (SBP), whereas smooth muscle cell growth is related to neurohormonal stimuli, but indicate also an influence of circulating neurohormonal factors on LV geometry through LV remodelling. In addition, cardiac load is dependent on brachial BP as well as vascular structure, supporting the present finding of a relationship between cardiac mass and vascular structure and stiffness not explained by their common relationship to the BP. These findings suggested that a beneficial effect above and beyond the effect of BP reduction may be gained by using antihypertensive agents blocking the receptors of these neurohormonal factors such as ARBs, aldosterone inhibitors or ACEIs as well as beta-blockade. However, in the REGAAL Study (as we will discuss below), subpopulation of patients in whom neurohormones were measured losartan, but not atenolol, significantly decreased the concentrations of atrial natriuretic peptide, brain natriuretic peptide (brain natriuretic peptide) and immunoreactive amino-terminal pro-brain natriuretic peptide. *In vitro* data have shown that Ang II may play a part in mediating upregulation of atrial natriuretic peptide and brain natriuretic peptide genes, thus suggest a direct role of Ang II receptor blockade in the cardiac effects of losartan.

Indeed, the selection of atenolol, a beta-blocker, as the control therapy may explain some of the difference between the treatment groups in the LIFE study. In this regard, central pressure determinants are increasingly viewed as a truer reflection of cardiovascular risk than is the case with peripheral BP readings. It is plausible that the findings in the LIFE trial are the differing effects of beta-blockers and ARBs on central pulse pressure and blood vessel stiffness despite similar peripheral BPs. Although these parameters were not determined in the LIFE trial it might be expected that ARBs more favourably impacted these measures than did beta-blockade, and therein reduced central pressures to a greater degree. Indeed, Schiffrin *et al.* |38| have also previously shown that treatment with losartan provided a greater reduction in small arterial wall thickness than did atenolol for equal peripheral BP control.

Effects of losartan and atenolol on left ventricular mass and neurohormonal profile in patients with essential hypertension and left ventricular hypertrophy.

Dahlof B, Zanchetti A, Diez J, *et al.* for the REGAAL Study Investigators.
Journal of Hypertension 2002; **20**(9): 1855–64.

BACKGROUND. To compare the effects of the Ang II antagonist, losartan, with those of atenolol on LVH, BP and neurohormone concentrations in hypertensive patients with LVH.

INTERPRETATION. Both losartan- and atenolol-based regimens effectively decreased BP. Losartan was non-inferior and numerically superior to atenolol in regression of LVH. The reduction in hypertrophy with losartan treatment was accompanied by reductions in circulating concentrations of cardiac natriuretic peptides. Losartan, by specifically blocking Ang II, may therefore have effects on the heart beyond those expected from the decrease in BP alone. Losartan was better tolerated than atenolol.

Comment

The REGAAL study is a 36-week, randomized, multi-centre, double-blind, parallel-group study comparing the effects of losartan with those of atenolol on LV mass index in 225 patients (aged 21–80 years) with mild-to-moderate essential hypertension and echocardiographically documented LVH assessed up to 30 days before enrolment. Hydrochlorothiazide is added to patients not achieving the goal BP (<140/90 mmHg) by the sixth week or 12th week after randomization. The primary efficacy analysis was based on the week 36 change from baseline in LV mass index.

Despite generally comparable reductions in sitting DBP and SBP, the losartan-based regimen significantly reduced LV mass index compared with baseline after 36 weeks (primarily because of a decrease in LV wall thickness), whereas the atenolol-based regimen had no significant effect. The numerically greater reduction in LVH in the losartan regimen is consistent with the findings of previous clinical trials comparing atenolol with blockers of the renin–angiotensin system, including valsartan, irbesartan and ramipril, in hypertensive patients. At first glance, this study appears as a smaller-scale replicate of the LIFE substudy. Based on their findings that changes in neurohormones in losartan-treated patients, but not in atenolol-treated patients, they support the concept that the effects of the two agents on LVH may be substantially different. Accordingly, the use of specific agents such as Ang II type 1 receptor blocker that not only lower BP load but also attenuate the adverse neurohormonal drive of Ang II may be more beneficial.

Ethnic differences in electrocardiographic criteria for left ventricular hypertrophy: the LIFE study. Losartan Intervention For Endpoint.

Okin PM, Wright JT, Nieminen MS, *et al. Am J Hypertens* 2002; **15**(8): 663–71.

BACKGROUND. African-Americans have greater precordial QRS voltages than white people, with concomitant higher prevalences of ECG LVH and lower specificity of ECG LVH criteria for the identification of anatomic hypertrophy. However, the high mortality associated with LVH in African-American patients makes more accurate ECG detection of LVH in these patients a clinical priority.

INTERPRETATION. When standard, non-ethnicity-specific thresholds for the identification of LVH are used, Sokolow–Lyon and 12-lead voltage overestimate and Cornell voltage underestimates the presence and severity of LVH in African-Americans relative to white individuals. However, these apparent ethnic differences in test performance disappear when ethnic differences in the distribution of ECG LVH criteria are taken into account. These findings demonstrate that ethnicity-specific ECG criteria can equalize detection of anatomical LVH in African-American and white patients.

Comment

Accurate ECG detection of LVH is a clinical challenge in African-American hypertensive individuals that is accentuated by the increased morbidity and mortality associated with anatomical LVH. Although African-American patients have a higher prevalence of ECG LVH than white patients, the traditional ECG criteria for the identification of LVH in African-Americans has been significantly less accurate than in other populations due to the apparent lower specificity of voltage criteria in African-American individuals.

The higher prevalence of ECG LVH in African-Americans is out of proportion to ethnic differences in BP, and occurs despite similar rates of echocardiographic LVH in African-American and white patients, and greatly exceeds the minor ethnic differences in LV dimensions and mass observed using echocardiography. Thus, the increased QRS amplitudes in African-American patients are in part independent of increases in LV mass. Although ECG LVH has been associated with increased morbidity and mortality in predominantly white populations, some uncertainty remains regarding the risk of ECG determined LVH in African-American populations.

The aims of the present study were as follows: (i) to examine ethnic differences in ECG criteria for LVH; (ii) to determine whether these differences in ECG LVH persist after controlling for possible ethnic differences in LV mass and body habitus; and (iii) to establish whether there are true ethnic differences in performance of ECG criteria for the detection of echocardiographic LVH, or whether apparent ethnic differences reflect the use of identical test partitions that have different performance characteristics in African-American and white individuals.

After adjusting for ethnic differences in LV mass, body mass index, sex and prevalence of diabetes, mean Sokolow–Lyon and 12-lead sum of voltage were significantly

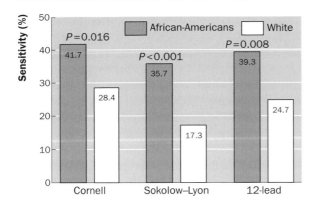

Fig. 16.4 Comparison of sensitivity of electrocardiographic voltage criteria for left ventricular hypertrophy in African-American (**dark-filled bars**) and white (**light-filled bars**) hypertensive patients, using sex- and ethnicity-specific partitions with matched specificity of 83% in this population, but with specificities of 97% in a population of working adults. Threshold partitions used were as follows: Cornell voltage: African-American women >33.0 mm, white women >26.6 mm; African-American men >25.5 mm, white men >31.7 mm; Sokolow–Lyon voltage: African-American women >33.0 mm, white women >38.1 mm; African-American men >48.2 mm, white men >43.5 mm; 12-lead voltage: African-American women >191.5 mm, white women >199.3 mm; and African-American men >225.1 mm, white men >224.6 mm. Source: The ALLHAT Officers and Coordinators for the ALLHAT Collaborative Research Group (2002a).

higher, but Cornell voltage was lower, in African-Americans than in whites. As a consequence of these differences, when identical partition values were used in both ethnic groups, Sokolow–Lyon and 12-lead voltage criteria had lower specificity in African-Americans than white people (44% vs 69%, $P = 0.007$ and 44% vs 59%, $P = 0.10$) but had greater sensitivity in African-Americans (51% vs 27%, $P < 0.001$ and 62% vs 45%, $P = 0.003$). In contrast, Cornell voltage specificity was higher (78% vs 62%, $P = 0.09$) but sensitivity was slightly lower (49% vs 57%, $P = 0.16$) in African-Americans. However, when overall test performance was compared using receiver operating curve analyses that were independent of partition value selection, ethnic differences in test performance disappeared, with no differences in accuracy of any of the ECG voltage criteria for the identification of LVH between African-American and white hypertensive individuals.

These findings demonstrate that mean values of both voltage and voltage-duration product criteria for LVH are strongly related to ethnicity, producing apparent ethnic differences in test performance of these ECG criteria for the detection of echocardiographic LVH when identical test criteria were used in African-American and white patients. However, when ethnic differences in QRS voltages and voltage duration products were taken into account by comparing overall test performance of these criteria using receiver operating curve area analyses that were independent of

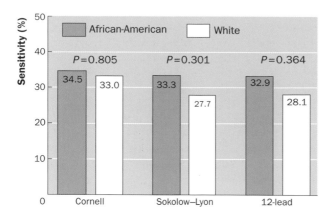

Fig. 16.5 Comparison of sensitivity of electrocardiographic voltage-duration criteria for left ventricular hypertrophy in African-American (**dark-filled bars**) and white (**light-filled bars**) hypertensive patients, using sex- and ethnicity-specific partitions with matched specificity of 83% in this population, but with specificities of 97% to 100% in a population of working adults. Threshold partitions used were as follows: Cornell voltage: African-American women >2972 mm x msec, white women >2731 mm x msec; African-American men >2797 mm x msec, white men >3346 mm x msec; Sokolow–Lyon voltage: African-American women >3597 mm x msec, white women >3708 mm x msec; African-American men >5267 mm x msec, white men >4611 mm x msec; 12-lead voltage: African-American women >22 980 mm x msec, white women >20 527 mm x msec; and African-American men 24 035 mm x msec, white men >25 004 mm x msec. Source: The ALLHAT Officers and Coordinators for the ALLHAT Collaborative Research Group (2002a).

partition value selection, there were no ethnic differences in the accuracy of these ECG voltage and voltage-duration product criteria for the detection of echocardiographic LVH. These findings demonstrate the need for ethnicity-specific ECG LVH criteria to optimize detection of anatomical LVH in both African-American and white individuals.

Correlates of pulse pressure reduction during antihypertensive treatment (losartan or atenolol) in hypertensive patients with electrocardiographic left ventricular hypertrophy (the LIFE study).

Gerdts E, Papademetriou V, Palmieri V, *et al. Am J Cardiol* 2002; **89**(4): 399–402.

BACKGROUND. In hypertensive patients, pulse pressure has been related to hypertension-induced target organ damage and risk of cardiovascular events. However,

correlates of pulse pressure reduction during antihypertensive treatment have been less extensively investigated.

INTERPRETATION. In hypertensive patients with ECG LVH, older age, less reduction in mean BP, concomitant diabetes mellitus and shorter stature are associated with attenuated pulse pressure reduction during antihypertensive treatment.

Comment

Previous outcome studies in hypertensive patients have demonstrated pulse pressure to be a predictor of cardiovascular morbidity and mortality, but less is known about factors associated with pulse pressure reduction during antihypertensive treatment. Of note, the reduction in pulse pressure during antihypertensive treatment does not necessarily parallel that of SBP and DBP. Thus, to describe further factors associated with pulse pressure reduction during antihypertensive treatment, 767 patients aged 55–80 years in the LIFE study were evaluated. The study found that over 2 years of treatment, BP and pulse pressure were reduced from 173/98 to 147/84 mmHg and from 75 to 63 mmHg, respectively, both P <0.001. When dividing the study population into two groups using a prognostically validated partition for pulse pressure, patients with pulse pressure ≥63 mmHg after 2 years of antihypertensive treatment ($n = 349$), they identified four clinical variables, besides initial pulse pressure, as independent correlates of an attenuated pulse pressure reduction: older age, shorter stature, concomitant diabetes mellitus and less reduction in mean BP. It would be interesting to see further analyses on unblinded study treatment (atenolol vs losartan) on pulse pressure in relation to outcomes.

The Antihypertensive and Lipid-Lowering Treatment to Prevent Heart Attack Trial (ALLHAT-LLT) ... the world's largest drug trial

Major outcomes in moderately hypercholesterolemic, hypertensive patients randomized to pravastatin vs usual care. The Antihypertensive and Lipid-Lowering Treatment to Prevent Heart Attack Trial (ALLHAT-LLT).
The ALLHAT Officers and Coordinators for the ALLHAT Collaborative Research Group. *JAMA* 2002a; **288**: 2998–3007.

BACKGROUND. Studies have demonstrated that statins administered to individuals with risk factors for CHD reduce CHD events. However, many of these studies were too small to assess all-cause mortality or outcomes in important subgroups. The objective of this study was to determine whether pravastatin compared with usual care reduces all-cause mortality in older, moderately hypercholesterolaemic, hypertensive participants with at least one additional CHD risk factor.

INTERPRETATION. Pravastatin did not reduce either all-cause mortality or CHD significantly when compared with usual care in older participants with well-controlled hypertension and moderately elevated low-density lipoprotein (LDL) cholesterol. The results may be due to the modest differential in total cholesterol (9.6%) and LDL cholesterol (16.7%) between pravastatin and usual care compared with prior statin trials supporting CVD prevention.

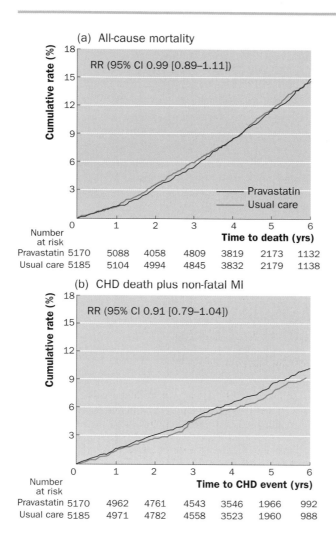

Fig. 16.6 Kaplan–Meier curves for all-cause mortality and cumulative CHD death plus non-fatal MI. Source: The ALLHAT Officers and Coordinators for the ALLHAT Collaborative Research Group (2002a).

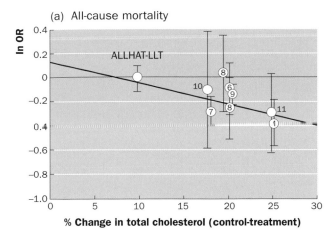

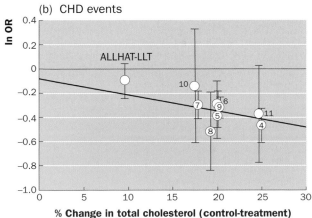

Fig. 16.7 Reductions in mortality and CHD event rates vs total cholesterol differential. Log odds ratios (ln OR) and 95% CIs for active treatment vs control for nine large statin trials (Table 16.7) are compared with regression lines (solid) from meta-analyses of 45 long-term trials using statins and other cholesterol-lowering interventions published before 31 December 2000.[25] Numbers inside data markers are references (See Table 16.7). Source: The ALLHAT Officers and Coordinators for the ALLHAT Collaborative Research Group (2002a).

[25] Gordon DJ, Proschan MA, Rossouw JE. Cholesterol lowering and cardiovascular disease. Presented at the Sixth International Symposium on Global Risk of Coronary Heart Disease and Stroke: Assessment, Prevention and Treatment. Florence, Italy. 2002 June 12–15.

Table 16.7 Comparison of the ALLHAT-LLT to other large, long-term statin trials*

| | | | Odds ratio (95% CI)† | |
Trial	Sample size	% Change in total cholesterol†	All-cause mortality	CHD events
Prior trials†	54 381	20.2	0.83 (0.78–0.88)	0.70 (0.67–0.74)
4S[4]	4444	25.0	0.69 (0.56–0.84)	0.62 (0.54–0.72)
LIPS[11]	1677	24.7	0.72 (0.46–1.11)	0.68 (0.45–1.01)
HPS[9]	20 536	20.3	0.86 (0.80–0.94)	0.72 (0.66–0.78)
WOSCOPS[5]	6595	20.0	0.78 (0.60–1.01)	0.69 (0.56–0.84)
CARE[6]	4159	20.0	0.91 (0.74–1.12)	0.75 (0.62–0.90)
AFCAPS[8]	6605	19.3	1.04 (0.76–1.43)	0.60 (0.43–0.83)
LIPID[7]	9014	17.9	0.76 (0.67–0.86)	0.75 (0.66–0.84)
PostCABG[10]	1351	17.6	0.91 (0.57–1.48)	0.87 (0.54–1.38)
ALLHAT-LLT	10 355	9.6	0.99 (0.89–1.11)	0.91 (0.79–1.04)
All Trials†	64 736	18.5	0.86 (0.82–0.90)	0.73 (0.69–0.77)

* ALLHAT indicates Antihypertensive and Lipid-Lowering Treatment to Prevent Heart Attack Trial; LLT, Lipid-Lowering Trial; and CHD, coronary heart disease. Other trial names are listed in their corresponding references (superscript numbers). Statin trials of at least 2 years' duration and with at least 1000 participants were eligible for inclusion.
† The percentage change in total cholesterol is the approximate differential in total cholesterol during the trial in the statin group relative to the control group. The odds ratios (statin/control) and corresponding 95% confidence intervals (CIs) summarize the relative differences in all-cause mortality and CHD events across trials, which had varying lengths of follow-up.
‡ Meta-analysis was performed using the method of Peto R et al. (Br J Cancer, 1977; **35**: 1–39), which sums the difference between observed and expected events in the active treatment groups and variances for the component trials and computes the overall odds ratio as the ratio of the sum of observed minus expected events to the sum of variances. Note that odds ratios are based on simple proportions of events and often differ slightly from published hazard ratios for these trials.
 [4] The Scandinavian Simvastatin Survival Study (4S)
 [5] The West of Scotland Coronary Prevention Study (WOSCOP)
 [6] The Cholesterol and Recurrent Events Trial (CARE)
 [7] The Long-Term Intervention with Pravastatin in Ischaemic Disease (LIPID) Study
 [8] The AFCAPS/TexCAPS
 [9] The Heart Foundation Study (HPS)
 [10] The Post Coronary Bypass Graft Trial (PostCABG)
 [11] The Lescol Intervention Prevention Study (LIPS)
Source: The ALLHAT Officers and Coordinators for the ALLHAT Collaborative Research Group (2002a).

Major outcomes in high-risk hypertensive patients randomized to angiotensin-converting enzyme inhibitor or calcium channel blocker vs diuretic: The Antihypertensive and Lipid Lowering Treatment to Prevent Heart Attack Trial (ALLHAT).

The ALLHAT Officers and Coordinators for the ALLHAT Cooperative Research Group. *JAMA* 2002b; **288**: 2981–97.

B A C K G R O U N D . **Antihypertensive therapy is well established to reduce hypertension-related morbidity and mortality, but the optimal first-step therapy is** unknown. **The objective of the study is to determine whether treatment with a CCB or an ACEI lowers the incidence of CHD or other CVD events vs treatment with a diuretic.**

INTERPRETATION. Thiazide-type diuretics are superior in preventing 1 or more major forms of CVD and are less expensive. They should be preferred for first-step antihypertensive therapy.

Comment

'All too few clinicians are aware that possibly the most successful antihypertensive drugs are the thiazide diuretics. They have been shown in many studies, particularly in older patients, to be the best option for lowering BP as well as preventing heart attacks and strokes. They are also much more cost-effective than other first-line agents' |39|.

One could now argue that die-hard diuretic enthusiasts have (probably) been vindicated with the publication of the results of the largest hypertension clinical trial ever conducted—the Antihypertensive and Lipid-Lowering Treatment to Prevent Heart Attack Trial (ALLHAT) (2002a). ALLHAT was a randomized, double-blind, active-controlled trial designed to compare the rate of CHD events in 'high-risk' hypertensive patients initially randomized to a diuretic (chlorthalidone) vs each of three 'alternative' antihypertensive drugs: an a-adrenergic blocker (doxazosin), an ACEI (lisinopril), and a CCB (amlodipine), as well as the effects of lipid lowering therapy in these 'high-risk' hypertensives—The ALLHAT Officers and Coordinators for the ALLHAT Cooperative Research Group (2002a,b). This study reported that the incidence primary end-points of fatal CHD and non-fatal MI was identical with a thiazide diuretic, an ACEI, and a dihydropyridine CCB.

Eligible patients were aged $\geq$55 years with stage 1 or 2 hypertension or who were already taking antihypertensive medication, and with at least one other CHD risk factor. These risk factors included previous MI or stroke, LVH by ECG or echocardiogram, a history of type 2 diabetes mellitus, current cigarette smoking, and low HDL cholesterol levels. The original trial population comprised of 42 418 patients, but the doxazosin arm of the trial was stopped prematurely in January 2000 because of a 25% higher rate of combined cardiovascular events and a twofold higher rate of admission for HF compared with chlorthalidone |40|. The remaining 33 357 patients

Table 16.8 ALLHAT: primary end-point

Drug	6-year rate of events (%)	RR (95% CI)	P vs chlorthalidone
Chlorthalidone	11.5	–	–
Lisinopril	11.4	0.99 (0.91–1.08)	0.81
Amlodipine	11.3	0.98 (0.90–1.07)	0.65

Source: The ALLHAT Officers and Coordinators for the ALLHAT Cooperative Research Group (2002b).

stayed on their study drugs until the end of the study. Of these, 15 255 were randomized to chlorthalidone (12.5–25.0 mg/day), 9048 to amlodipine (2.5–10.0 mg/day),
and 9054 to lisinopril (10–40 mg/day). If BP was not controlled to below
140/90 mmHg with the step 1 drug (after dose optimization), open-label treatment
drugs from other classes (atenolol, clonidine or reserpine as step 2 drugs, and
hydralazine as step 3) could be added at the physician's discretion. The mean age of
participants was 67 years; 47% were women, 35% were black, 19% Hispanic and 36%
were diabetic.

After a mean follow-up of 4.9 years, primary outcome events occurred in 2956
patients, with virtually identical frequencies in each of the three treatment groups.
Compared with chlorthalidone (6-year rate, 11.5%), the relative risks were 0.98 (95%
CI 0.90–1.07) for amlodipine (6-year rate, 11.3%) and 0.99 (95% CI 0.91–1.08) for
lisinopril (6-year rate, 11.4%). Likewise, all-cause mortality was not different
between the three groups. There were significant differences in the secondary outcomes for both of the newer drugs compared with the diuretic. Compared with those
taking chlorthalidone, patients on amlodipine had, on average, 0.8 mmHg higher
SBP, 38% higher risk of developing HF (P <0.001) (6-year absolute risk, 2.5%), and
35% higher risk of hospitalization or fatal HF (P <0.001). Interestingly, the ACEI
lisinopril appeared to be worse than chlorthalidone—those taking lisinopril had, on
average, about a 2 mmHg higher follow-up SBP (4 mmHg higher in black people),
15% higher risk of stroke (P <0.02, but 40% higher risk in black people, P = 0.01),
and 10% higher risk of combined CVD (P <0.001) (6-year absolute risk, 2.4%, but
19% higher risk in black people, P = 0.04) with 11% higher risk of hospitalization or
treated angina (P = 0.01) as well as 10% higher risk of coronary revascularization

Table 16.9 Secondary outcomes: amlodipine vs chlorthalidone

End-point	Amlodipine (%)	Chlorthalidone (%)	RR (95% CI)	P
6-year rate of HF	10.2	7.7	1.38 (1.25–1.52)	<0.001

Source: The ALLHAT Officers and Coordinators for the ALLHAT Cooperative Research Group (2002b).

Table 16.10 Secondary outcomes: lisinopril vs chlorthalidone

End-point	Lisinopril (%)	Chlorthalidone (%)	RR (95% CI)	P
6-year rate of combined CVD	33.3	30.9	1.10 (1.05–1.16)	<0.001
6-year rate of stroke	6.3	5.6	1.15 (1.02–1.30)	0.02
6-year rate of HF	8.7	7.7	1.19 (1.07–1.31)	<0.001

Source: The ALLHAT Officers and Coordinators for the ALLHAT Cooperative Research Group (2002b).

(a) Mean systolic blood pressure

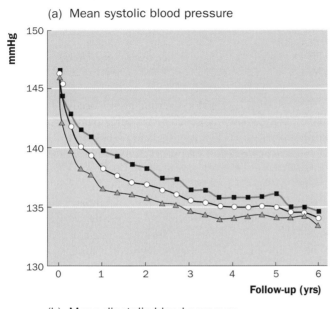

(b) Mean diastolic blood pressure

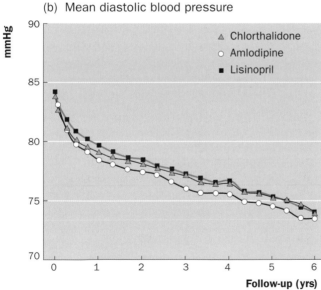

Fig. 16.8 Mean systolic and DBP by year during follow-up. The end of the CCB saga after ALLHAT? Source: The ALLHAT Officers and Coordinators for the ALLHAT Cooperative Research Group (2002b).

(P = 0.05). Rather surprisingly, patients on lisonopril also had 19% higher risk of developing HF (P <0.001) and 10% higher risk of being hospitalized or fatal HF (P = 0.11).

The international consensus for thiazide diuretics as the first-line antihypertensive agent is unchanged over the years, although guidelines for treatment of hypertension have changed significantly in the last decade, especially regarding the role of ACEI and CCBs as first-line agents.

Current guidelines, including the JNC VI |24| have renewed emphasis on the use of CCBs as first-line antihypertensive agents for treating ISH in older patients or those with angina or diabetes. However, the use of CCBs as first-line agents have again been subjected to heavy debate as another meta-analysis by Psaty *et al.* |3| found CCBs to be less effective in preventing cardiovascular events (with the exception of stroke) compared with other first-line antihypertensives.

It should be noted that CCBs are a very heterogeneous group of drugs with properties differing significantly from one drug to another. Even different formulations of the same molecule have significantly different effects on cardiovascular pathophysiology, besides lowering BP. The data from the various meta-analyses of the use of CCBs in preventing hard end-points were largely fragmented because of many possible subgroupings across the class (e.g. dihydropyridine vs non-dihydropyridine CCBs), patients (diabetics vs non-diabetics) and end-points (cardiovascular vs renal). Such meta-analyses have limited statistical power to determine really whether the small, but often significant, differences detected can be generalized to all CCBs. The clinical effectiveness of every formulation must be evaluated separately in well-designed clinical studies.

However, CCBs do fail to prevent HF, an observation that has been consistently reported in many studies. For example, in the INSIGHT (Intervention as a Goal in Hypertension Treatment) trial |41|, HF was approximately twice as frequent in the CCB, compared with the diuretic arm. Not unexpectedly, chlorthalidone was superior to amlodipine in preventing HF in ALLHAT. The BP differences between amlodipine and chlorthalidone were small (<1 mmHg) and balanced (lower SBP in chlorthalidone but lower DBP for amlodipine), and cannot account for the observed difference in HF incidence. None the less, it is of note that amlodipine has a 'neutral effect' on HF, it neither prevents nor precipitates HF, whereas diuretics are very useful for symptom control. Indeed, it is impossible to prove or disprove whether thiazide merely delayed the onset and thus the diagnosis of HF rather than altering the end course of the disease, i.e. death, which was not significantly different between the amlodipine and chlorthalidone group.

In addition, it is some relief that there were no significant differences in both CHD and stroke rates found between amlodipine and chlorthalidone-base therapy in ALLHAT. As a matter of fact, 6-year stroke and CHD rates were actually lower in patients on amlodipine compared with patients on lisinopril. Importantly, there was no increased risk of cancer, gastrointestinal bleeding or non-cardiovascular deaths in patients on amlodipine. In fact, the bleeding rates were significantly lower relative to the ACEI (6-year event rates per 100 persons: 8.0 vs 9.6, respectively).

Stroke prevention with angiotensin-converting enzyme inhibitors

Use of ramipril in preventing stroke: double blind randomized trial.
Bosch J, Yusuf S, Pogue J, *et al.*, on behalf of the HOPE investigators.
Br Med J 2002; **324**: 699–702.

BACKGROUND. Strokes can be prevented by lowering BP in people with hypertension and by the use of antiplatelet agents in people with vascular disease. Although a person's risk of stroke increases with BP, the population attributable risk of stroke is greatest at pressures that would not currently be treated with drugs. We therefore need additional strategies that lower the risk of stroke across a broad range of patients at high risk. This study was to determine the effect of the ACEI ramipril on the secondary prevention of stroke.

INTERPRETATION. Ramipril reduces the incidence of stroke in patients at high risk, despite a modest reduction in BP.

Comment

Preclinical and clinical data suggest that ACEIs or ARBs may reduce the risk for ischaemic events independent of the drugs' BP-lowering effects. As previously shown in the HOPE study, patients 55 years of age and over had a reduction in the risk of MI, stroke, cardiovascular death, as well as total mortality, when the ACEI ramipril was added to the patients' established therapy compared with a group of subjects on other agents that did not include an ACEI. New data from this subanalysis of the 9297 patients who participated in the original HOPE trial on the secondary prevention of stroke, transient ischaemic attack (TIA), and cognitive function were evaluated. Stroke was confirmed by computed tomography, magnetic resonance imaging or autopsy in 84% of the cases. Strokes not documented by computed tomography, magnetic resonance imaging (within 14 days of onset) or autopsy evidence were classified as 'uncertain'. Haemorrhagic strokes and strokes of uncertain type are combined as 'non-ischaemic' strokes in Table 16.11.

By 4.5 years, in those who received an ACEI plus other drugs, compared with a regimen that did not include an ACEI, the risk of overall stroke was decreased by 32% (absolute risk 3.4 vs 4.9%), and by 31% among diabetics while the risk of fatal stroke was reduced by 61%, and non-fatal stroke was reduced by 24%. In addition, recurrent strokes were also reduced by about 33%. Ischaemic and haemorrhagic strokes were both reduced, by 36% and 26% respectively.

Ramipril lowered mean baseline BP (139/79 mmHg) modestly: by 3.8/2.8 mmHg. After adjusting for differences in baseline BP as well as changes in BP in those who received ramipril, there was still a 28% reduction in the risk of stroke in this group.

The BP benefit was seen across BP levels, medication use (e.g. among the 76% of patients taking aspirin) and condition (previous stroke/TIA, diabetes, hypertension, etc.).

The results demonstrated a benefit of treatment with the ACEI ramipril over placebo in preventing strokes, both total stroke and all stroke subtypes. The data seem to be more widely applicable than that published in the diabetic group as data now have shown similar benefit in stroke prevention regardless of their diabetic status—the benefits were seen across all subgroups—in patients with (11%) and without previous stroke, patients with underlying coronary artery disease (80%), peripheral arterial disease (43%) or diabetes (38%). In addition, the benefit was seen at all levels of BP, including those hypertensive and those with an initial BP <120/70 mmHg. Moreover, patients who had a stroke while on ramipril also tended to have less severe motor and cognitive deficits compared with those on placebo. Characterization of cognitive and motor changes after a stroke while on assigned therapy showed that patients taking ramipril had less severe deficits than those on placebo. Changes such as those in cognition or consciousness, ocular or visual symptoms, face or limb weakness, dysarthria or dysphasia, or frank dysphagia, were significantly less frequent among those on treatment.

The authors concluded that patients at high risk for stroke should continue to receive aspirin and, in addition to other BP lowering agents required to achieve BP control, an ACEI. They believe the widespread use of an ACEI, such as ramipril, in those at high risk for stroke, may have a major impact on public health.

The HOPE study, in which 11% of the patients enrolled had a history of a stroke or TIA, found that treatment with an ACEI (plus other medications) reduced the risk of fatal and non-fatal stroke and TIA at all levels of entry BP. Again as in the overall study, the estimates of treatment benefit were consistent across all subgroups examined: those with and without hypertension, with and without prior CHD, with and without prior peripheral vascular disease, with and without diabetes. The benefit was seen in all subtypes of stroke and, according to the authors, was independent of the modest reduction in BP that occurred with ramipril (3/2 mmHg), compared with other agents. In the HOPE study, BP was only measured several times throughout the study.

In the PROGRESS study [13], in which 100% of the 6105 patients had a previous stroke or TIA, randomized to placebo or 4 mg of perindopril, with the addition of 2.5 mg of indapamide if needed have also provided similar results. Overall, the risk of recurrent stroke was reduced by 28% with an average BP reduction of 9/4 mmHg. In

Table 16.11 Results on stroke reduction in HOPE

Stroke type	Ramipril	Placebo	RR (95% CI)
Total stroke	3.4%	4.9%	0.68 (0.56–0.84)
Ischaemic stroke	2.2%	3.4%	0.64 (0.50–0.82)
Non-ischaemic stroke	1.4%	1.7%	0.80 (0.57–1.12)

Source: Bosch et al. (2002).

the 58% of patients on combination therapy who experienced a BP reduction of 12/5 mmHg, the reduction in stroke risk was 43%, whereas in the 42% of patients treated only with perindopril, in whom BP was reduced by only 5/3 mmHg, there was no reduction in stroke. The benefit of combination therapy over single-drug therapy occurred in those both with and without hypertension. Most patients were on antiplatelet therapy and almost one-half of the patients were also on concomitant antihypertensive therapy. In this trial, BP was measured five times during the first year and twice a year during the second and subsequent 4 years of the trial. In HOPE, BP was recorded at study entry, after 2 years, and at the study's 4-year conclusion with the lower of the two values at each visit recorded.

One must interpret the data cautiously, however. The numbers needed to treat to prevent one stroke are relatively high. Furthermore, certain subgroups may experience less benefit (e.g. those with prior stroke or TIA; aspirin or CCB users). As the accompanying editorial points out, this limitation for aspirin users raises the nagging question of whether ACEI interact negatively with aspirin.

As opposed to the HOPE study, the PROGRESS trial emphasizes that the degree of BP reduction achieved with an ACEI/diuretic based combination appears more important than less effective BP reduction with ACEI monotherapy. It should be noted that most of the patients included in the HOPE study were on diuretic therapy at entry. Therefore, BP reduction with treatment with an ACEI/diuretic combination appears beneficial in reducing the risk of first and recurrent stroke in high-risk patients with and without hypertension.

Furthermore, in an ambulatory BP-monitoring substudy of the HOPE trial |12|, there were more profound BP-lowering effects at night than those measured in the daytime ambulatory clinic (ramipril was given in the evening). Thus, there may be more to the story of 'modest' BP lowering in the HOPE trial.

If one considers both the HOPE and PROGRESS study, there is consistent and mounting evidence that ACEIs are important treatments in preventing first and recurrent stroke. However, the results from ALLHAT have confirmed the superiority of thiazide diuretic over either ACEI or CCB in preventing stroke. Thus, a thiazide should be the initial agent to use with other agent added if necessary. This HOPE subanalysis supports the use of these agents in patients with a history of stroke or TIA, regardless of their initial hypertension status; however, benefit is greater in patients with hypertension.

Effect of losartan and captopril on mortality and morbidity in high-risk patients after acute myocardial infarction: the OPTIMAAL randomized trial.

Dickstein K, Kjekshus J and the OPTIMAAL Steering Committee. *Lancet* 2002 Sep 7; **360**(9335): 752–60.

BACKGROUND. ACEI attenuate the detrimental effects of Ang II, and improve survival and reduce morbidity in patients with acute MI and evidence of HF or LV dysfunction.

Selective antagonism of the angiotensin type 1 receptor represents an alternative approach to inhibition of the renin–angiotensin system. The purpose of this multi-centre, randomized trial is to test the hypothesis that the Ang II antagonist losartan would be superior or non-inferior to the ACEI captopril in decreasing all-cause mortality in high-risk patients after acute MI.

INTERPRETATION. As we saw a non-significant difference in total mortality in favour of captopril, ACEI should remain first-choice treatment in patients after complicated acute MI. Losartan cannot be generally recommended in this population. However, it was better tolerated than captopril, and was associated with significantly fewer discontinuations. Although the role of losartan in patients intolerant of ACE inhibition is not clearly defined, it can be considered in such patients.

Comment

Losartan failed to show benefits over the ACEI captopril in post-MI patients. Indeed, captopril showed a trend toward superiority. As expected, losartan was significantly better tolerated than captopril with fewer discontinuations of treatment.

The study included 5477 patients 50 years of age or older (mean age 67.4 years), with confirmed acute MI and HF during the acute phase or a new Q-wave anterior infarction or reinfarction (i.e. high-risk patients for LV dysfunction), randomized and titrated to a target dose of losartan (50 mg once daily) or captopril (50 mg three times daily) as tolerated, and were followed for a mean of 2.7 years. Patients were recruited from 329 centres in seven European countries.

The primary end-point, all-cause mortality, trended in favour of captopril but was not statistically significant. One predefined end-point, cardiovascular death was significantly improved with the ACEI, with most of the other end-points showing a slight trend in favour of captopril. All the mortality difference occurred in the first 7 months, with the curves running parallel thereafter.

The OPTIMAAL results are very similar to those of ELITE-2 in HF, which also showed a trend toward a better effect with captopril than with losartan. ELITE-2 also used a 50-mg daily dose of losartan, and it remains unclear whether ACEI are

Table 16.12 OPTIMAAL: Major efficacy end-points

End-point	Losartan (%)	Captopril (%)	RR (95% CI)	P
Death	18.2	16.4	1.13 (0.99–1.28)	0.069
Re-MI	14	13.9	1.03 (0.89–1.18)	0.722
Death/MI	27.2	25.2	1.10 (0.99–1.22)	0.085
CV death	15.3	13.3	1.17 (1.01–1.34)	0.032
Stroke	5.1	4.8	1.07 (0.84–1.36)	0.587

Source: Dickstein K, Kjekshus J and the OPTIMAAL Steering Committee (2002).

actually superior to Ang II blockers or whether Ang II blockers may be better if used at higher doses or in combination with ACEI. It is of note that in LIFE and RENAAL, 100 mg doses had shown beneficial results, although in different populations. Ongoing HEAAL (Heart Failure Endpoint Evaluation with the Angiotensin II Antagonist Losartan) comparing 50-mg and 150-mg doses of losartan would help to 'settle the issue'.

Similarly, the VALIANT trial is also ongoing, testing a much higher dose of an angiotensin antagonist (160-mg valsartan twice daily) against the same dose of captopril in similar high-risk population as used in OPTIMAAL should also help to clarify the issue.

Table 16.13 Tolerability—drug discontinuations

Discontinuation reason	Losartan	Captopril	RR	P
Discontinuation for any reason	17%	23%	0.70	<0.0001
Discontinuation due to ADRs (adverse drug reactions)	7%	14%	0.50	<0.0001

Source: Dickstein K, Kjekshus J and the OPTIMAAL Steering Committee (2002).

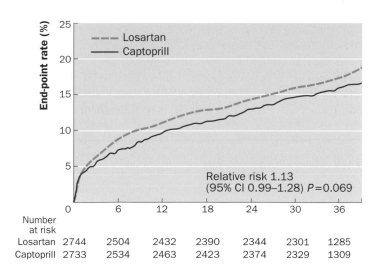

Fig. 16.9 Kaplan–Meier curve for primary end-point (all-cause mortality). Source: Dickstein K, Kjekshus J and the OPTIMAAL Steering Committee (2002).

Angiotensin receptor blockers in heart failure: meta-analysis of randomized controlled trials.

Jong P, Demers C, McKelvie RS, Liu PP. *J Am Coll Cardiol* 2002; **39**(3): 463–70.

BACKGROUND. There is uncertainty regarding the efficacy of ARBs as substitute or adjunctive therapy to ACEIs in the treatment of HF. This meta-analysis sought to determine the effect of ARBs on mortality and hospitalization in patients with HF.

INTERPRETATION. This meta-analysis cannot confirm that ARBs are superior in reducing all-cause mortality or HF hospitalization in patients with symptomatic HF, particularly when compared with ACEIs. However, the use of ARBs as monotherapy in the absence of ACEIs or as combination therapy with ACEIs appears promising.

Comment

This meta-analysis showed that ARBs have no benefit over ACEI in reducing mortality or hospitalizations in patients with HF. However, the authors reported a trend towards improved outcomes in patients taking ARBs alone, compared with patients on placebo, while patients taking both an ARB and an ACEI fared better than people taking only an ACEI in terms of hospitalizations.

The analysis included 17 randomized controlled trials that compared ARBs with either placebo or ACEIs in patients with symptomatic HF (a pooled total of 12 469 patients). The pooled outcomes were all-cause mortality and hospitalization for HF. Only five of the 17 trials studied compared an ARB with placebo without ACE inhibition as background therapy. Interestingly, when against placebo, ARBs showed a trend towards benefit in reducing hospitalizations, although only one trial included in the meta-analysis looked at hospitalizations with ARBs vs placebo: mortality (0.68; 0.38–1.22) and hospitalization (0.67; 0.29–1.51). Such a trend is reassurance to the use of ARBs as monotherapy in patients who are intolerant to ACEI, although trials that directly compared ARBs with ACEIs showed no survival benefit for ARBs: pooled rates of death (odds ratio: 0.96; 95% CI 0.75–1.23) or hospitalization (0.86; 0.69–1.06). In contrast, the virtually identical observed risks of both ARBs and ACEI in the stratified analysis is compatible with, though not proof of, the hypothesis that ARBs and ACEI may be interchangeable when clinically warranted.

More decisive answers to the ARB vs ACEI questions should come with the pending results of several trials. These include the VALIANT trial looking at the ARB valsartan in comparison with, and in combination with, captopril in post-MI patients with HF or LV dysfunction. Another is the CHARM trial, looking at candesartan against placebo in different treatment groups, including one group taking ACEI and another on the ARB alone. Both trial results are expected in late 2003. These ongoing clinical trials should help resolve the definitive role of ARBs in the treatment of HF in particular as monotherapy in the absence of ACEI, or as combination therapy with ACEI.

Genetic marker for which hypertensive patients benefit most from diuretics

Diuretic therapy, the α-adducin gene variant, and the risk of myocardial infarction or stroke in persons with treated hypertension.
Psaty BM, Smith NL, Heckbert SR, *et al. JAMA* 2002; **287**: 1680–9.

BACKGROUND. A genetic variant in α-adducin has been associated with renal sodium reabsorption and salt-sensitive hypertension. Whether this genetic variant modifies the effect of diuretic therapy on the incidence of MI and stroke is unknown. The objectives are to estimate the interaction between α-adducin and diuretic therapy on the risk of MI or stroke. Specifically, we hypothesized that in participants with treated hypertension, the risk of MI or stroke associated with diuretic use would be lower in carriers of the adducin variant than in carriers of the adducin wild-type genotype.

INTERPRETATION. In carriers of the adducin variant, diuretic therapy was associated with a lower risk of combined MI or stroke than other antihypertensive therapies. If these findings are confirmed in other studies, this large subgroup of the hypertensive population may be especially likely to benefit from low-dose diuretic therapy.

Comment

Variants of the α-adducin gene are associated with salt-sensitive hypertension. Given the recent published ALLHAT results that have reaffirmed the superiority of thiazide diuretic, it is of interest to investigate whether α-adducin genetic variation influence how diuretic therapy affects risk for MI and stroke in hypertensive patients.

In this population-based, case–control study, Psaty *et al.* studied 206 MI cases, 117 stroke cases, and 715 age- and sex-matched controls; all subjects were being treated for hypertension. Subjects were identified as having the wild-type genotype or as carriers of one or two copies of the Trp460 allele of the α-adducin gene. Main outcome measure is the risk of the combined outcome of first non-fatal MI or stroke.

It was found that more than one-third of subjects had at least one copy of the suspect allele. Compared with subjects with the wild-type genotype who were not taking diuretics (but were taking other antihypertensives), wild-type subjects taking diuretics had a similar risk for the combined outcome of MI or stroke. Among patients with the suspect allele, diuretic therapy was associated with a lower risk of the combined outcome of MI and stroke than other antihypertensive therapies (OR, 0.49; 95% CI 0.32–0.77). The OR in carriers of the adducin variant was less than half of the OR in carriers of the wild-type genotype ($P = 0.005$). The genetic-variant-related reduction in risk with diuretic therapy persisted after adjustment for confounders, including age, sex, diabetes and coronary artery disease. These data

suggest that the antihypertensive benefits of diuretic therapy may be modulated by
α-adducin genetic variation. Clinicians may one day be able to use genetic profiles to
customize antihypertensive regimens.

Combination treatment of angiotensin II receptor blocker and angiotensin-converting-enzyme inhibitor in non-diabetic renal disease (COOPERATE): a randomized controlled trial.

Nakao N, Yoshimura A, Morita H, *et al. Lancet* 2003 Jan 11; **361**(9352): 117–24.

BACKGROUND. Present ACEI treatment fails to prevent progression of non-diabetic renal disease. This study aimed to assess the efficacy and safety of combined treatment of ACEI and ARB, and monotherapy of each drug at its maximum dose, in patients with non-diabetic renal disease.

INTERPRETATION. Combination treatment safely retards progression of non-diabetic renal disease compared with monotherapy. However, as some patients reached the combined primary end-point on combined treatment, further strategies for complete management of progressive non-diabetic renal disease need to be researched.

Comment

In many studies of patients with diabetes and microalbuminuria, ACEI have been more effective than have other agents in the short-term reduction of microalbuminuria. ARBs have many properties that are similar to ACEI. However, they do not inhibit the breakdown of bradykinin, which causes the cough that is the most common side-effect of ACEI therapy. In the CALM (Candesartan And Lisinopril Microalbuminuria) study, candesartan combined with lisinopril for 24 weeks resulted in greater reductions in BP and in the albumin/creatinine ratio than either drug given alone.

Much experimental and clinical evidence has been published that suggests the RAAS system plays an important part in progression of non-diabetic disease. Results

Table 16.14 Primary end-point among three treatment groups after 3 years follow-up

	Primary end-point reached	Hazard ratio (95% CI)	P value
Combined treatment	11%		
Trandolapril alone	23%	0.38 (0.18–0.63)	0.018
Losartan alone	23%	0.40 (0.17–0.69)	0.016

Source: Nakao *et al.* (2003).

of meta-analyses agree that ACEI are more effective than conventional antihypertensive drugs at delaying of progression of non-diabetic renal disease. However, despite use of maximum-dose ACEI, reduction of proteinuria is highly variable among individuals, which can lead to different outcomes, and even patients initially benefiting from the renoprotective properties of these drugs can deteriorate suddenly after a period of several years, with impairment in renal function.

The authors postulated that complete inhibition of the RAAS would be most beneficial in the management of progressive non-diabetic renal disease, and might be achieved by dual blockage with ARBs and ACEI. To prove this hypothesis, they compare the efficacy of three treatments—monotherapy with an ARB (losartan), monotherapy with an ACEI (trandolapril), and the combination of these drugs—on renal survival—the combined primary end-point of time to doubling of serum creatinine concentration or end-stage renal disease (ESRD). Indeed, losartan and trandolapril have been reported to have renoprotective effects beyond those explained by their antihypertensive effects.

The study is of high quality in methodology, and included 263 Japanese with non-diabetic renal disease, randomized to the losartan (100 mg daily) or the trandolapril (3 mg daily) or a combination of both drugs at equivalent doses. Participants were followed-up for 3 years.

At the end of follow-up, 11% of patients in the combination group reached the primary end-point compared with 23% of patients in each of the monotherapy groups (hazard ratio 0.38). Covariates affecting renal survival were combination

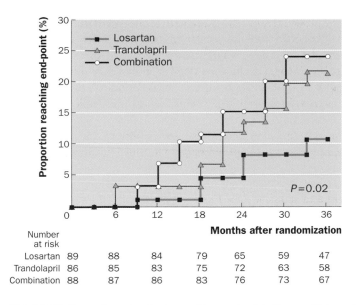

Fig. 16.10 Proportion of patients reaching end-point. Source: Nakao *et al.* (2003).

treatment (hazard ratio 0.38, 95% CI 0.18–0.63, $P = 0.011$), age (1.30, 1.03–2.29, $P = 0.009$), baseline renal function (1.80, 1.02–2.99, $P = 0.021$), change in daily urinary protein excretion rate (0.58, 0.24–0.88, $P = 0.022$), use of diuretics (0.80, 0.30–0.94, $P = 0.043$), and antiproteinuric response to trandolapril (0.81, 0.21–0.91, $P = 0.039$). Importantly, the frequency of side-effects with combination treatment was the same as with trandolapril alone.

The better results in the combination group can be attributed to a 'striking' increase in antiproteinuric effect in this treatment arm. Interestingly, the three treatment groups achieved BP were similar and taken together with the same baseline risk factors, the beneficial effects observed in the combination treatment group seem independent of BP lowering. In addition, the significant antiproteinuric effect of combination treatment was seen irrespective of baseline proteinuria and level of renal function.

Nakao *et al.* noted that, compared with previous studies, few serious adverse reactions were reported, especially cardiovascular events. Whether this occurrence is attributable to the full cardioprotection of each drug at its maximum dose or whether it is because of the cohort's young age, ethnic origin, or both is unknown.

Perhaps the one important practical implication in this study was that the combination regimen was well tolerated, even in patients with advanced renal insufficiency; this suggests that the present practice of avoidance of ACEI or angiotensin blockers to prevent further renal impairment and hyperkalaemia is no longer justified, although gradual increase in dose and careful observation is still recommended.

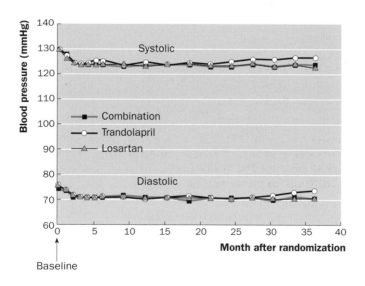

Fig. 16.11 BP by treatment group. Source: Nakao *et al.* (2003)

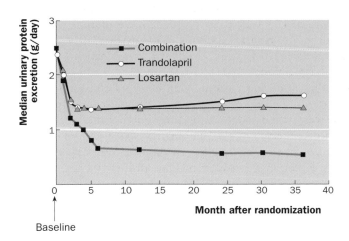

Baseline

Fig. 16.12 Median urinary protein excretion by treatment group. Source: Nakao *et al.* (2003).

But they also caution that as some patients on combination treatment in this study still reached the primary end-point, even with maximum inhibition of the RAAS system, other strategies need to be investigated for complete management of progressive non-diabetic renal disease.

Effect of blood pressure lowering and antihypertensive drug class on progression of hypertensive kidney disease: results from the AASK trial.

Wright JT Jr, Bakris G, Greene T, *et al. JAMA* 2002; **288**(19): 2421–31.

BACKGROUND. Hypertension is a leading ESRD in the USA, with no known treatment to prevent progressive declines leading to ESRD. The objective of this study is to compare the effects of two levels of BP control and three antihypertensive drug classes on glomerular filtration rate (GFR) decline in hypertension.

INTERPRETATION. No additional benefit of slowing progression of hypertensive nephrosclerosis was observed with the lower BP goal. ACEI appear to be more effective than beta-blockers or dihydropyridine CCBs in slowing GFR decline.

Comment

The African American Study of Kidney Disease and Hypertension (AASK) was a 3 × 2 factorial double-blind designed study of 1094 hypertensive African-Americans (non-diabetic) with mild to moderate renal insufficiency, randomized to receive one of three drugs/classes: ramipril, metoprolol or amlodipine with other agents added to achieve one of two BP targets, either an aggressive goal of 125/75 mmHg, or the standard target of 140/90 mmHg. The primary end-point of the trial was the change in GFR slope, including both the total and chronic slopes. The secondary end-point of the study—regarded as potentially more clinically relevant—was a composite of a 50% decrease in the GFR, an absolute decrease in GFR of 25 ml/min per 1.73 m^2, ESRD or death.

This trial is innovative, it is the largest trial focus only on one ethnic group, African-American, designed to evaluate the impact on progression of hypertensive kidney disease. The trial's results are highly contentious and very clinically relevant for a number of facts—the risk of hypertensive ESRD for African-Americans is 20-fold greater than in white people. African-Americans have traditionally been thought to be less responsive to ACEIs. CCBs are currently one of the most commonly prescribed drugs for hypertension in African-Americans. Dihydropyridine CCBs increase proteinuria and may not slow the progression of established renal disease despite substantial reductions in BP.

Indeed, the amlodipine and ramipril arms was prematurely stopped in October 2000 after the trial's data and safety monitoring board (the National Institutes of Health) noted that amlodipine was significantly less effective than ramipril or metoprolol in slowing progression of renal disease especially in patients with baseline evidence of kidney damage (urine protein/creatinine ratio [UP/Cr] >0.22 or proteinuria of approximately 300 mg/day). The ramipril/metoprolol arm was carrying on and this paper reports the full results of the trial.

The primary analysis of GFR slope did not establish a definitive difference among the three drug regimens. However, significant benefits of ramipril vs metoprolol and amlodipine on the main clinical composite outcome and the results of other secondary analyses suggest that ramipril slows hypertensive kidney disease progression compared with the other two regimens. Secondary analyses also suggest that metoprolol may improve renal outcome compared with amlodipine, particularly in participants with higher proteinuria.

Table 16.15 Comparison of antihypertensive agents in reducing GFR, ESRD or death

Drugs compared	RR	P value
Ramipril vs metoprolol	22%	0.042
Ramipril vs amlodipine	38%	0.005
Metoprolol vs amlodipine	19%	0.19
Ramipril vs amlodipine in patients with minimal renal dysfunction*	46%	0.004
Metoprolol vs amlodipine in patients with minimal renal dysfunction*	37%	0.003

* Patients with baseline UP/C of >0.22 or ~300 mg protein/day.
(UP/C, urinary protein to creatinine ratio)
Source: Wright et al. (2002).

In contrast with the comparisons involving amlodipine, the evidence for benefit of ramipril vs metoprolol was noted in the full AASK cohort, irrespective of baseline proteinuria. However, the conclusion of the beneficial effect of ramipril compared with metoprolol is less definitive because the chronic slope was not significant.

In addition, unlike diabetics with hypertension in other trials, non-diabetic patients in AASK showed no difference in benefit from the two BP targets, that is, aiming for BP goals below those recommended in current guidelines does not translate into additional slowing of renal disease progression. This finding is rather surprising given the vast amount of evidence supporting lower BP target especially in patients with target organ damage, in this case renal disease. It should be noted, however, that both the primary and secondary end-points in AASK largely depended on GFR, a surrogate marker of renal disease progression. Furthermore, the trial was not powered to test the differential effect of the two BP targets in preventing harder end-points such as CHD event or stroke, which are the most likely source of morbidity and mortality in the AASK study group with reduced kidney function. Perhaps, the findings extend the paradigm to African-Americans with non-diabetic kidney insufficiency that simply lowering BP is not sufficient to provide optimal protection against adverse kidney outcomes.

Nevertheless, bearing in mind that most patients in AASK also received a thiazide diuretic, the results do support recommendations that ACEI should be considered as first line therapy over beta-blockers and dihydropyridine CCBs in these patients. Moreover, beta-blockers may be more effective than dihydropyridine CCBs in slowing progression among patients with proteinuria.

Furthermore, there is no direct test of the strategy of combined use of ACEI with CCBs or CCBs in combination with an ARB, a common clinical practice. On average, AASK participants in both treatment groups required almost three (an average of 2.75) drugs to attain their target BP and almost assuredly more drugs were required in the group with goal mean arterial pressure less than 92 mmHg. Patients with proteinuria and kidney disease should have their BP brought as close to target (<130/80 mmHg) as possible for cardiovascular and renal protection. Given all these considerations and available evidence as provided by ALLHAT, thiazide diuretic should still be the preferred first antihypertensive choice in black people who are hypertensive with renal disease, with other agents added upon if necessary, preferably ACEI or ARB.

AASK is a landmark study that has shown for the first time the benefit of ACE inhibition in African-Americans in slowing renal disease progression, an under studied group that is at greatly increased risk of serious, costly and fatal disease. The findings effectively trump any lingering concerns over whether ACEI should be used in African-Americans with hypertensive renal disease. However, it is still unclear whether ACEI are equally effective in black hypertensive with LV dysfunction or HF.

Microalbuminuria reduction with valsartan in patients with type 2 diabetes mellitus.

Viberti G, Wheeldon NM for the MARVAL investigators. A blood pressure independent effect. *Circulation* 2002; **106**: 672–8.

BACKGROUND. Elevated urine albumin excretion (UAER) is a modifiable risk factor for renal and CVD in type 2 diabetes. Blockade of the renin–angiotensin system lowers UAER, but whether this effect is independent of BP reduction remains controversial. The MARVAL (MicroAlbuminuria Reduction With VALsartan) study was designed to evaluate the BP-independent effect of valsartan on UAER in type 2 diabetic patients with microalbuminuria.

INTERPRETATION. For the same level of attained BP and the same degree of BP reduction, valsartan lowered UAER more effectively than amlodipine in patients with type 2 diabetes and microalbuminuria, including the subgroup with baseline normotension. This indicates a BP-independent antiproteinuric effect of valsartan.

Comment

In the spectrum of renal disease complicating diabetes, microalbuminuria precedes overt diabetic nephropathy. This stage is readily detectable, is associated with an increased risk for progression to diabetic nephropathy, and is potentially reversible. Once overt nephropathy develops, the goal of therapy is to slow the rate of progression to ESRD.

In this study, 332 type 2 diabetes patients with microalbuminuria (median UAER of three non-consecutive timed overnight urine collections in the range of 20–200 µg/min) with and without hypertension were randomized to 80 mg/day of valsartan, or 5 mg/day of amlodipine, and followed for 24 weeks. A target BP of 135/85 mmHg was attempted for all patients, through dose doubling and the addition of doxazosin or bendrofluazide whenever needed. The primary end-point was the per cent change in UAER from baseline to 24 weeks. From baseline to the end of 24 weeks, the mean (lower and upper quartiles) in UAER was significantly reduced by valsartan (56%, 95% CI 49.6–63.0) compared with amlodipine (92%, 95% CI 81.7–103.7), a highly significant between-group effect ($P < 0.001$). Furthermore, there were more patients reversed to normoalbuminuria with valsartan (29.9% vs 14.5%; $P = 0.001$). Interestingly, valsartan lowered UAER similarly in both the hypertensive and normotensive subgroups, and BP reductions were similar between the two treatments (systolic/diastolic 11.2/6.6 mmHg for valsartan, 11.6/6.5 mmHg for amlodipine) and at no time-point was there a between-group significant difference in BP values in either the hypertensive or the normotensive subgroup.

Other recent studies in similar population have also shown comparable results with MARVAL. In RENAAL (Reduction of Endpoints in Non-insulin-dependent diabetes with the Angiotensin II Antagonist Losartan), 1513 patients (age 31–70 years, 63% men) who had type 2 diabetes and nephropathy randomized to receive losartan,

50–100 mg/day or placebo. Conventional antihypertensive therapy was adjusted to target a SBP and DBP <140 and <90 mmHg, respectively. It was concluded that losartan was renoprotective in patients with type 2 diabetes mellitus and nephropathy beyond that attributable to BP control. Similarly, in the IRbesartan Micro-Albuminuria type 2 diabetes mellitus in hypertensive patients (IRMA II) Parving *et al.* |33| have shown that treating patients who have type 2 diabetes, hypertension and microalbuminuria with irbesartan, 300 mg/day, reduced progression to overt nephropathy at 2 years; though lower doses (e.g. 150 mg/day) were less effective. This beneficial effect of irbesartan was also reported to be independent of BP lowering as well as glycaemic control. In addition, irbesartan was more likely than placebo to cause regression to normoalbuminuria. Furthermore, in the IDNT (Irbesartan Diabetic Nephropathy Trial), Lewis *et al.* |32| also concluded that irbesartan is effective in protecting against the progression of nephropathy due to type 2 diabetes. This protection is independent of the reduction in BP it causes.

Alongside these recent studies of ARBs in diabetic nephropathy, this latest addition from MARVAL helps solidify the belief that ARBs are renoprotective independent of their effects on BP. The authors reported that their findings leave little doubt that AT1 receptor antagonism affects albuminuria also by mechanisms separate from systemic BP changes, i.e. BP independent. They concede, however, that their study was short term and could not establish whether the correction of microalbuminuria by valsartan will be translated into clinical benefit. However, it is of note that the recent LIFE study have reported that diabetic patients with hypertension and ECG LVH (a marker of target organ damage) benefit the most from ARB losartan, also appears to be independent of its BP lowering effect.

The accompanying editorial by Opie and Parving |42| support the fact that ARBs have beneficial renoprotective effects independent of BP lowering, but they question just how much their 'cardioprotective effects' are independent of BP lowering—'there are no human data that prove BP-independent cardioprotection when ARBs are given for renoprotection'. Though the above trials of renal disease progression did have cardiovascular end-points as secondary outcomes there were no significant differences between the ARB and control group except for first hospitalization with HF, where losartan reduced the risk by 32%, but there was a trend, albeit not significant, toward a reduction of MI. However, as none of these were powered or timed to study cardiovascular events, there still remains some concern as to whether or not the ARB would provide cardiovascular risk reduction benefits. In addition, the investigators measured albumin excretion at night but BP during the day. Therefore, without measuring 24-hour BP, it is not possible to be sure that the BPs in the two groups were really identical. BP influences microalbuminuria; therefore, ideally the BP and the microalbuminuria should have been measured over the same period.

Conversely, ACEI have overwhelming data that show substantial risk reduction from cardiovascular events and death in people with type 2 diabetes. It is likely that ACEI provide renoprotection similar to that afforded by ARBs in patients with type 2 diabetes and nephropathy. The MICRO-HOPE (Microvascular Heart Outcomes Prevention Evaluation) study enrolled 3577 patients with diabetes, 32% of whom had microalbuminuria |**43**|. The rate of progression to overt nephropathy was lower in the ramipril group than in the placebo group (relative risk reduction 24%). However, no study exists with clinically important outcomes comparing ARAs with ACEI. A large head-to-head comparative study between ACEI and ARBs with hard end-points in this patient group would seem unlikely given the lack of commercial incentives. However, combination therapy would be attractive and have theoretical advantage. Indeed, the study of Mogensen *et al.* |**44**| provides a preliminary assessment of the role of combination therapy with ARBs and ACEI in the CALM study. They showed that candesartan and lisinopril were effective monotherapies for reducing BP and microalbuminuria; however, their combined use for 24 weeks was well tolerated and more effective for reducing BP in patients with type 2 diabetes, hypertension, and microalbuminuria (albumin/creatinine ratio).

Although further research using clinically important outcomes is required, dual blockade of the renin–angiotensin system with a combined ACEI and ARB seems promising. This combination may offer the best of both treatment strategies and result in lower incidence rates of devastating microvascular and macrovascular complications in persons with type 2 diabetes.

Put in perspective, the new study results support the concept that drugs that block the RAAS offer important cardiovascular and renal advantages as part of multidrug regimens to facilitate better BP control. More studies are needed to answer questions concerning the optimal dosing, best types of combinations to be used, and whether or not there may be some deleterious effects of a combination of these drugs, particularly in patients with congestive HF or renal disease.

Reassessment of National Cholesterol Education Program Adult Treatment Panel-III guidelines: one year later.

Ansell BJ, Waters DD. *Amer J Cardiol* 2002 Sep 1; **90**(5): 524–5.

B ACKGROUND. Since the first Adult Treatment Panel (ATP) guidelines from the National Cholesterol Education Program (NCEP), the goals have evolved from national cholesterol awareness and reduction, to the use of increasingly aggressive lipid-lowering strategies in patients at highest risk for CHD. The most recent NCEP guidelines from the ATP-III |45| appropriately suggest the most aggressive reduction in LDL cholesterol in an expanded group of patients considered to be at highest risk for CHD. Since these guidelines were published approximately 1 year ago, additional clinical trial data suggest that they are already, to a certain extent, out of date.

I NTERPRETATION. It is now clear that cholesterol reduction may not just need to target certain lipid goals, but also be broadly applied to virtually any individual at high risk for atherosclerotic disease.

MRC/BHF Heart Protection Study of antioxidant vitamin supplementation in 20 536 high-risk individuals: a randomized placebo-controlled trial.

Heart Protection Study Collaborative Group. *Lancet* 2002b; **360**: 23–33.

BACKGROUND. It has been suggested that increased intake of various antioxidant vitamins reduces the incidence rates of vascular disease, cancer and other adverse outcomes.

INTERPRETATION. Among the high-risk individuals that were studied, these antioxidant vitamins appeared to be safe. But, although this regimen increased blood vitamin concentrations substantially, it did not produce any significant reductions in the 5-year mortality from, or incidence of, any type of vascular disease, cancer or other major outcome.

MRC/BHF Heart Protection Study of cholesterol lowering with simvastatin in 20 536 high-risk individuals: a randomized placebo-controlled trial.

Heart Protection Study Collaborative Group. *Lancet* 2002c; **360**: 7–22.

BACKGROUND. Throughout the usual LDL cholesterol range in Western populations, lower blood concentrations are associated with lower CVD risk. In such populations, therefore, reducing LDL cholesterol may reduce the development of vascular disease, largely irrespective of initial cholesterol concentrations.

INTERPRETATION. Adding simvastatin to existing treatments safely produces substantial additional benefits for a wide range of high-risk patients, irrespective of their initial cholesterol concentrations. Allocation to 40 mg simvastatin daily reduced the rates of MI, of stroke and of revascularization by about one-quarter. After making an allowance for non-compliance, actual use of this regimen would probably reduce these rates by about one-third. Hence, among the many types of high-risk individual studied, 5 years of simvastatin would prevent about 70–100 people per 1000 from suffering at least one of these major vascular events (and longer treatment should produce further benefit). The size of the 5-year benefit depends chiefly on such individuals' overall risk of major vascular events, rather than on their blood lipid concentrations alone.

Comment

Question: In patients with a high 5-year risk for cardiovascular death, does simvastatin reduce mortality and vascular events? Answer: In patients with a high 5-year risk for cardiovascular death, simvastatin safely reduced all-cause mortality, cardiovascular mortality and cardiovascular events, irrespective of the person's initial blood cholesterol concentrations—the question has been conclusively answered by the world's largest-ever cholesterol-lowering study.

This landmark study included 20 536 UK adults, aged 40–80 years (28% were ≥70 years of age, 75% men) with coronary disease, other occlusive arterial disease, or diabetes or a history of treated hypertension (in men ≥65 years of age), who has non-fasting total cholesterol levels ≥3.5 mmol/l. Patients were randomly allocated to receive 40 mg simvastatin daily (average compliance: 85%) or matching placebo (average non-study statin use: 17%) for an average of 5.5 years. Patients were also randomized in a 2 × 2 factorial design to antioxidant vitamins (vitamin E, 600 mg/day; vitamin C, 250 mg/day; and α-carotene, 20 mg/day) or placebo. Analyses are of the first occurrence of particular events, and compare all simvastatin allocated vs all placebo-allocated participants. These 'intention-to-treat' comparisons assess the effects of about two-thirds (85% minus 17%) taking a statin during the scheduled 5-year treatment period, which yielded an average difference in LDL cholesterol of 1.0 mmol/l (about two-thirds of the effect of actual use of 40 mg simvastatin daily).

The results showed that simvastatin led to a reduction in all-cause and vascular mortality, major coronary events, stroke, and revascularization (Table 16.16). Simvastatin and placebo did not differ for non-vascular mortality or cancer incidence. In contrast, antioxidants did not differ from placebo for any outcome measures.

For the first occurrence of any of these major cardiovascular events, there was a definite 24% (SE 3; 95% CI 19–28) reduction in the event rate (2033 [19.8%] vs 2585

Table 16.16 Simvastatin vs placebo in high-risk patients at mean 5-year follow-up

Outcomes	Simvastatin (n = 10 269)	Placebo (n = 10 267)	RR reduction (adjusted)	P value
All-cause mortality*	12.9%	14.6%	13%	0.0003
Vascular mortality*	7.6%	9.1%	17%	<0.002
Non-vascular mortality	5.3%	5.6%	5%	Not significant
Major coronary event†	8.7%	12%	27%	<0.0001
CHD death	5.7%	6.9%	17%	0.0005
Stroke	4.3%	5.7%	25%	<0.0001
Revascularization	9.1%	12%	24%	<0.0001

*Primary end-points; †Non-fatal MI or CHD death.
Source: Heart Protection Study Collaborative Group (2002c).

Table 16.17 Incidence of MI and stroke in diabetic patients without prior disease

Simvastatin (n = 2006)	Placebo (n = 1976)	Relative reduction (adjusted)	P value
279 (13.9%)	369 (18.7%)	28%	<0.0001

Source: Heart Protection Study Collaborative Group (2002c).

[25.2%] affected individuals; $P <0.0001$). During the first year the reduction in major vascular events was not significant, but subsequently it was highly significant during each separate year.

The effect on stroke was primarily driven by a reduction in ischaemic stroke, and there was no evidence of any increased risk of haemorrhagic stroke in the active treatment group. In diabetic patients without prior disease the results were as follows:

The proportional reduction in the event rate was similar (and significant) in each subcategory of participant studied, including: those without diagnosed coronary disease who had cerebrovascular disease, or had peripheral artery disease, or had diabetes; men and, separately, women; those aged either under or over 70 years at entry; and most notably, even those who presented with LDL cholesterol below 3.0 mmol/l (116 mg/dl), or total cholesterol below 5.0 mmol/l (193 mg/dl). The benefits of simvastatin were additional to those of other cardioprotective treatments. The annual excess risk of myopathy with this regimen was about 0.01%. There were no significant adverse effects on cancer incidence or on hospitalization for any other non-vascular cause.

The HPS (Heart Protection Study) is the most important lipid lowering trial since the first series of landmark statins studies such as the Simvastatin Scandinavian Survival Study (4S) and WOSCOPS (West of Scotland Coronary Prevention Study). HPS differs from these studies in that it was a mixed primary/secondary prevention study, aimed at the 'real-world' population, specifically targeting those at high risk,

Table 16.18 HPS: vascular event by prior LDL levels

Baseline LDL (mmol/l)	Statin ($n = 10\ 269$)	Placebo ($n = 10\ 267$)
<3.0 (116 mg/dl)	602	761
3.0–<3.5	483	655
≥3.5 (135 mg/dl)	957	1190
All patients	2042	2606

Source: Heart Protection Study Collaborative Group (2002c).

Table 16.19 HPS: vascular event by prior total cholesterol levels

Baseline total cholesterol (mmol/l)	Statin ($n = 10\ 269$)	Placebo ($n = 10\ 267$)
<5.0 (193 mg/dl)	361	476
5.0–<6.0	746	965
≥6.0 (232 mg/dl)	935	1165
All patients	2042	2606

Source: Heart Protection Study Collaborative Group (2002c).

Table 16.20 HPS: vascular event by LDL

Baseline LDL (mg/dl)	Statin (n = 10 269)	Placebo (n = 10 267)
<100	285	360
100–<130	670	881
≥130	1087	1365
All patients	2042	2607

Source: Heart Protection Study Collaborative Group (2002c).

regardless of their cholesterol levels. The study provided the strongest evidence to date that patients with normal or low cholesterol who are at high risk of CHD can benefit immensely from statin therapy. It also provided the first direct proof of the benefit of statins in people with diabetes and in the elderly. The question is whether statin achieved these impressive cardioprotective effects by lowering LDL cholesterol and raising HDL cholesterol, and/or by something else beyond, the answer is only of 'academic interest'. Practically, and simply, patients with established vascular disease or at high absolute risk of future cardiovascular events need a statin regardless of their initial cholesterol level.

An interesting statement made by Dr R. Colins (one of the principal investigators of HPS) says it all…. 'If people are at risk, we should lower their cholesterol and in the same way that we wouldn't measure platelets before giving someone aspirin maybe we don't need to take a cholesterol level before prescribing a statin.' Indeed, the editor of *The Lancet* has even advocated to 'tearing up the rule-book' on statin therapy. It may nevertheless be appropriate to monitor lipid levels during treatment to verify that cholesterol has been lowered to the degree expected, by about 30–35%.

Unlike previous trials such as the Cholesterol and Recurrent Events Trial (CARE) and the Long-Term Intervention with Pravastatin in Ischaemic Disease (LIPID), which has suggested a cholesterol 'threshold' of about 120 mg/dl (5.2 mmol/l), below which lowering cholesterol would not have any added benefit, HPS showed that there was no such cut-off level. However, trials that are designed to address specific-ally the 'threshold limit' question are still ongoing. These include: HPS-2 (also known as SEARCH, Study of the Effectiveness of Additional Reductions in Choles-terol and Homocysteine), which is comparing 80 mg of simvastatin with 20 mg of simvastatin in high-risk individuals; the Treat-to-New-Targets (TNT) study looking at atorvastatin 80 mg vs atorvastatin 10 mg; and the IDEAL (Incremental Decrease in Endpoints through Aggressive Lipid lowering trial), which pitches 80 mg of atorvastatin against 40 mg of simvastatin.

The negative findings that antioxidant intervention had no effect on CHD out-comes (or the incidence of cancer) was again disappointing, but not unexpected given the similar negative results of previous large randomized controlled trials, including the large HOPE study on vitamin E supplements in high and low doses in preventing CHD. |46| Therefore, antioxidants cannot be recommended for CHD prevention. Instead, greater efforts should be directed at implementing appropriate, proven preventive measures (use of aspirin, beta-blockers, ACEI and statins) in high-risk persons.

The findings from HPS support the need for change of treatment guideline to emphasize a strategy of treating high-risk, not high cholesterol.

References

1. Beevers DG. Beta-blockers for hypertension: time to call a halt? *J Hum Hypertens* 1998; **12**: 807–10.

2. ALLHAT Collaborative Research Group. Major cardiovascular events in hypertensive patients randomized to doxazosin vs chlorthalidone: the antihypertensive and lipid-lowering treatment to prevent heart attack trial (ALLHAT). *JAMA* 2000; **283**: 1967–75.

3. Psaty BM, Alderman MH, Applegate WB, Williamson JD, Cavazzini C, Furberg CD. Health outcomes associated with calcium antagonists compared with other first-line anti-hypertensive therapies: a meta-analysis of randomized controlled trials. *Lancet* 2000; **356**: 1949–54.

4. Hansson L, Lindholm LH, Niskanen L, Lanke J, Hedner T, Niklason A, Luomanmaki K, Dahlof B, de Faire U, Morlin C, Karlberg BE, Wester PO, Bjorck JE. Effect of angiotensin-converting-enzyme inhibition compared with conventional therapy on cardiovascular morbidity and mortality in hypertension: the Captopril Prevention Project (CAPPP) randomized trial. *Lancet* 1999; **353**: 611–16.

5. Hansson L, Hedner T, Lund-Johansen P, Kjeldsen SE, Lindholm LH, Syvertsen JO, Lanke J, de Faire U, Dahlof B, Karlberg BE. Randomised trial of effects of calcium antagonists compared with diuretics and beta-blockers on cardiovascular morbidity and mortality in hypertension: the Nordic Diltiazem (NORDIL) study. *Lancet* 2000; **356**: 359–65.

6. Lip GYH, Beevers DG. Calcium channel blockers in hypertension: the debate reawakens. *J Hum Hypertens* 2001; **15**: 85–7.

7. Beevers DG, Lip GYH. The protective effect of blocking angiotensin in both type I and type II diabetics with nephropathy. *J Hum Hypertens* 2001; **15**: 837–9.

8. Dahlöf B, Devereux RB, Kjeldsen SE, Julius S, Beevers G, de Faire U, Fyhrquist F, Ibsen H, Kristiansson K, Lederballe-Pedersen O, Lindholm LH, Nieminen MS, Omvik P, Oparil S, Wedel H. Cardiovascular morbidity and mortality in the Losartan Intervention For End-point reduction in hypertension study (LIFE): a randomized trial against atenolol. *Lancet* 2002; **359**: 995–1003.

9. Lindholm LH, Ibsen H, Dahlof B, Devereux RB, Beevers G, de Faire U, Fyhrquist F, Julius S, Kjeldsen SE, Kristiansson K, Lederballe-Pedersen O, Nieminen MS, Omvik P, Oparil S, Wedel H, Aurup P, Edelman J, Snapinn S. Cardiovascular morbidity and mortality in

patients with diabetes in the Losartan Intervention For Endpoint reduction in hypertension study (LIFE): a randomized trial against atenolol. *Lancet* 2002; **359**: 1004–10.

10. Yusuf S, Sleight P, Pogue J, Bosch J, Davies R, Dagenais G. Effects of an angiotensin-converting-enzyme inhibitor, Ramipril on cardiovascular events in high-risk patients. The Heart Outcomes Prevention Evaluation Study Investigators. *N Engl J Med* 2000; **342**: 145–53.

11. Sleight P, Yusuf S, Pogue J, Tsuyuki R, Diaz R, Probstfield J. Blood-pressure reduction and cardiovascular risk in HOPE study. *Lancet* 2001; **358**: 2130–31.

12. Svensson P, de Faire U, Sleight P, Yusuf S, Ostergren J. Comparative effects of ramipril on ambulatory and office blood pressures. A HOPE substudy. *Hypertension* 2001; **38**: e28–32.

13. PROGRESS Collaborative Group. Randomized trial of a perindopril-based blood-pressure-lowering regimen among 6,105 individuals with previous stroke or transient ischaemic attack. *Lancet* 2001; **358**: 1033–41.

14. Lip GYH, Beevers DG. ACE inhibitors in vascular disease: some PROGRESS, more HOPE. *J Hum Hypertens* 2001; **15**: 833–5.

15. Felmeden DC, Lip GYH. The renin–angiotensin–aldosterone system and fibrinolysis. *J Renin Angiotensin Aldosterone Syst* 2000; **1**: 240–4.

16. Li-Saw-Hee FL, Beevers DG, Lip GYH. Effect of antihypertensive therapy using enalapril or losartan on haemostatic markers in essential hypertension: a pilot prospective randomized double-blind parallel group trial. *Int J Cardiol* 2001; **78**: 241–6.

17. Le Noble FAC, Stassen FRM, Hacking WJG, Struijker Boudier HAJ. Angiogenesis and hypertension. *J Hypertens* 1998; **16**: 1563–72.

18. Belgore FM, Lip GY, Bareford D, Wadley M, Stonelake P, Blann AD. Plasma levels of vascular endothelial growth factor and its soluble receptor (SFlt-1) in essential hypertension. *Am J Cardiol* 2001; **87**: 805–7.

19. Ward HJ. Uric acid as an independent risk factor in the treatment of hypertension. *Lancet* 1998; **352**: 670–1.

20. Lip GYH, Edmunds E, Beevers DG. Should patients with hypertension receive anti-thrombotic therapy? *J Intern Med* 2001; **249**: 205–14.

21. Chin BS, Lip GYH. Blockade of the renin–angiotensin–aldosterone system with combination angiotensin receptor antagonist and ACE inhibitor therapy: observations from Val-HeFT and CALM. *J Hum Hypertens* 2001; **15**: 89–92.

22. Okin PM, Sverker J, Kjeldsen SE, *et al.* Regression of electrocardiographic left ventricular hypertrophy by losartan vs atenolol: The LIFE study. Program and abstracts from American Heart Association Scientific Sessions 2002, November 17–20, 2002; Chicago, Illinois. *Circulation* 2002; **106**(Suppl. II): II-477 (Abstract 2360).

23. Okin PM, Sverker J, Kjeldsen SE, *et al.* Regression of electrocardiographic left ventricular hypertrophy during antihypertensive treatment and the prediction of major cardiovascular events: The LIFE study. Program and abstracts from American Heart Association Scientific Sessions 2002, November 17–20, 2002; Chicago, Illinois. *Circulation* 2002; **106**(Suppl. II): II-573 (Abstract 2831).

24. The Joint National Committee on Prevention, Detection, Evaluation, And Treatment Of High Blood Pressure. The sixth report of the Joint National Committee on prevention, detection, evaluation, and treatment of high blood pressure. *Arch Intern Med* 1997; **157**: 2413–46.

25. Pitt S, Poole-Wilson PA, Segal R, Martinez FA, Dickstein K, Camm JA, Konstam MA, Riegger G, Klinger GH, Neaton J, Sharma D, Thiyagarajan B. Randomized trial of losartan versus captopril on mortality in patients with symptomatic heart failure: the losartan heart failure survival study – ELITE II. *Lancet* 2000; **355**: 1582–87.

26. Dickstein K, Kjekshus J and the OPTIMAAL Steering Committee. Effects of losartan and captopril on mortality and morbidity in high-risk patients after acute myocardial infarction: the OPTIMAAL randomized trial. Optimal Trial in Myocardial Infarction with Angiotensin II Antagonist Losartan. *Lancet* 2002 September 7: **360**(9335): 752–60.

27. Messerli FH, Grossman E, Goldbourt U. Are beta-blockers efficacious as first-line therapy for hypertension in the elderly? A systematic review. *JAMA* 1998; **279**: 1903–7.

28. Kjeldsen SE, Julius S, Brunner H, Hansson L, Henis M, Ekman S, Laragh J, McInnes G, Smith B, Weber M, Zanchetti A. Characteristics of 15,314 hypertensive patients at high coronary risk. The VALUE trial. The Valsartan Antihypertensive Long-term Use Evaluation. *Blood Press* 2001; **10**(2): 83–91.

29. Pfeffer M, McMurray J, Leizorovicz A, Maggioni A, Rouleau J, Van De Werf F, Henis M, Neuhart E, Gallo P, Edwards S, Sellers MA, Velazquez E, Califf R, and for the VALIANT investigators. Valsartan in acute myocardial infarction trial (VALIANT): rationale and design. *Am Heart J* 2000: **140**: 727–34.

30. Swedberg K, Pfeffer M, Granger C, Held P, McMurray J, Ohlin G, Olofsson B, Ostergren J, Yusuf S. Candesartan in heart failure-assessment of reduction in mortality (CHARM): rationale and design. *J Card Fail* 1999; **5**: 276–82.

31. Yusuf S. From the HOPE to the ONTARGET and the TRANSCEND studies: challenges in improving prognosis. *Am J Cardiol* 2002 Jan 24; **89**(2A): 18A–25A; discussion 25A–26A.

32. Brenner BM, Cooper ME, De Zeeuw D, *et al.* Effects of losartan on renal and cardiovascular outcomes in patients with type 2 diabetes and nephropathy. *N Engl J Med* 2001; **345**: 861–9.

33. Lewis EJ, Hunsicker LG, Clarke WR, *et al.*, for the Collaborative Study Group. Renoprotective effect of the angiotensin-receptor antagonist irbesartan in patients with nephropathy due to type 2 diabetes. *N Engl J Med* 2001; **345**: 851–60.

34. Parving HH, Lehnert H, Brochner-Mortensen J *et al.* The effect of irbesartan on the development of diabetic nephropathy in patients with type 2 diabetes. IRbesartan Micro-Albuminuria type 2 diabetes mellitus in hypertensive patients (IRMA II). *N Engl J Med* 2001; **345**(12): 870–8.

35. Adler AI, Stratton IM, Neil HA, *et al.* Association of systolic blood pressure with macrovascular and microvascular complications of type 2 diabetes (UKPDS 36): prospective observational study. *Br Med J* 2000; **321**: 412–19.

36. Devereux RB, Dahlof B, Kjeldsen SE, *et al.* Cardiovascular mortality in patients without pre-existing vascular disease in the Losartan Intervention For Endpoint reduction in hypertension study (LIFE). Abstracts from American Heart Association Scientific Sessions 2002, November 17–20, 2002; Chicago, Illinois. *Circulation* 2002; **106**(Suppl. II): II-475 (Abstract 2352).

37. Dalhof B, Hornestam B, Aurup P on behalf of the LIFE Study Group. Losartan decreases the risk of stroke in hypertensive patients with atrial fibrillation and left ventricular hypertrophy. 24th Annual congress of the European Society of Cardiology 2002, Berlin, Germany. *Eur Heart J* 2002; **23**(Suppl.): 412 (Abstract P2163).

38. Schiffrin EL, Park JB, Intengan HD, Touyz RM. Correction of arterial structure and endothelial dysfunction in human essential hypertension by the angiotensin receptor antagonist losartan. *Circulation* 2000; **101**: 1653–9.

39. Beevers DG, Ferner RE. Why are thiazide diuretics declining in popularity? *J Hum Hypertens* 2001; **15**: 287–9.

40. The ALLHAT Officers and Coordinators for the ALLHAT Collaborative Group. Major cardiovascular events in hypertensive patients randomized to doxazosin vs chlorthalidone: the antihypertensive and lipid-lowering treatment to prevent heart attack trial (ALLHAT). ALLHAT Collaborative Research Group. *JAMA* 2000; **283**: 1967–75.

41. Brown MJ, Palmer CR, Castaigne A, De Leeuw PW, Mancia G, Rosenthal T *et al.* Morbidity and mortality in patients randomized to double-blind treatment with a long-acting calcium-channel blocker or diuretic in the International Nifedipine GITS study: Intervention as a Goal in Hypertension Treatment (INSIGHT). *Lancet* 2000; **356**: 366–72.

42. Opie LH, Parving HH. Diabetic nephropathy: can renoprotection be extrapolated to cardiovascular protection? *Circulation* 2002 Aug 6; **106**(6): 643–5.

43. The Heart Outcomes Prevention Evaluation Study Investigators. Effects of ramipril on cardiovascular and microvascular outcomes in people with diabetes mellitus: results of the HOPE study and MICRO-HOPE substudy. *Lancet* 2000; **355**: 253–9.

44. Mogensen CE, Neldam S, Tikkanen I, *et al.* Randomized controlled trial of dual blockade of renin–angiotensin system in patients with hypertension, microalbuminuria, and non-insulin dependent diabetes: the candesartan and lisinopril microalbuminuria (CALM) study. *Br Med J* 2000; **321**: 1440–4.

45. Expert Panel on Detection, Evaluation, and Treatment of High Blood Cholesterol in Adults. Executive Summary of the Third Report of the National Cholesterol Education Program (NCEP). *JAMA* 2001; **285**: 2486–97.

46. Yusuf S, Dagenais G, Pogue J, Bosch J, Sleight P. Vitamin E supplementation and cardiovascular events in high-risk patients. The Heart Outcomes Prevention Evaluation Study Investigators. *N Engl J Med* 2000; **342**: 154–60.

List of abbreviations

11β-HSD	11β-hydroxysteroid dehydrogenase	CAPPP	Captopril Prevention Project study
4S	Simvastatin Scandinavian Survival Study	CARDIA	Coronary Artery Risk Development in Young Adults
AAMI	Association for the Advancement of Medical Instrumentation	CCA	common carotid arteries
		CCB	calcium channel blocker
AASK	African-American Study of Kidney Disease and Hypertension	CEE	conjugated equine oestrogen
		CFR	coronary flow reserve
		CFVR	Coronary flow velocity reserve
ABPM	ambulatory BP monitoring	CHARM	Candesartan in Heart Failure Assessment of Reduction in Mortality and Morbidity
ACE	angiotensin-converting enzyme		
ACEI	angiotensin-converting enzyme inhibitors		
ACh	acetylcholine	CHD	coronary heart disease
AGE	advanced glycation end-products	CHF	congestive heart failure
		CI	confidence interval
AGT	angiotensinogen gene	CVD	cardiovascular disease
AHA	American Heart Association	DBP	diastolic blood pressure
AIx	augmentation index	DM	diabetes mellitus
ALLHAT	Antihypertensive and Lipid Lowering to prevent Heart Attack Trial	DSMB	Data and Safety Monitoring Board
		EBT	electron beam tomography
Ang II	angiotensin II	ECG	electrocardiography
ANP	atrial natriuretic peptide	ECTIM	Etude Cas-Temoin de l'Infarctus Myocarde
APA	adrenal adenoma		
ARB	Ang II receptor blockers	EH	essential hypertension
ARR	aldosterone-to-renin ratio	ELSA	European Lacidipine Study on Atherosclerosis
ASCOT	Anglo-Scandinavian Cardiac Outcomes Trial		
		eNOS	endothelial nitric oxide synthase
AT1	angiotensin II receptor type 1	EPHESUS	EPlerenone's neuroHormonal Efficacy and SUrvival Study
ATP	Adult Treatment Panel		
BHS	British Hypertension Society	ERA	Estrogen Replacement and Atherosclerosis trial
BMI	body mass index		
BP	blood pressure	ERT	oestrogen replacement therapy
CA	cardiac arrythmias		
CAC	coronary artery calcification	ESC	European Society of Cardiology
CAD	coronary artery disease		

ESRIT	oEStrogen in the Prevention of ReInfarction Trial	INDANA	(Individual Data Analysis of Antihypertensive Intervention Trials)
ESRD	end-stage renal disease		
ESRF	end-stage renal failure	IR	insulin resistance
ET-1	endothelin-1	IRMA	IRbesartan MicroAlbuminuria trial
FBPP	Family Blood Pressure Program	ISH	isolated systolic hypertension
FH	family history of hypertension	IVUS	intravascular ultrasound
FIELD	Edinburgh Artery Study, and Fenofibrate Intervention and Event Lowering in Diabetes	JNC	Joint National Committee
		LDF	laser Doppler flowmetry
		LDL	low-density lipoprotein
FMD	flow-mediated dilatation	LIFE	Losartan Intervention For Endpoint study
FRS	Framingham risk score		
GENOA	Genetic Epidemiology Network of Atherosclerosis	L-NMMA	NG-monomethyl-L-arginine
		LV	left ventricular
GFR	glomerular filtration rate	LVEH	left ventricular ejection fraction
GTN	glyceryl trinitrate		
hANP	human atrial natiuretic peptide	LVH	left ventricular hypertrophy
		MAP	mean arterial pressure
HARVEST	Hypertension and Ambulatory Recording Venetia Study	MARVAL	MicroAlbuminuria Reduction With VALsartan study
HDL	high-density lipoprotein	MI	myocardial infarction
HERS	Heart and Estrogen/progestin Replacement Study	MICRO-HOPE	Microvascular Heart Outcomes Prevention Evaluation study
HF	heart failure	MLD	minimum lumen diameter
HHD	Hypertensive heart disease	MLR	mineralocorticoid receptor gene
HOPE	Heart Outcomes Prevention Evaluation study		
		MORE	Multiple Outcomes of Raloxifene Evaluation study
HPS	Heart Protection Study		
HR	heart rate	MPA	medroxyprogesterone acetate
HRT	hormone replacement therapy		
		MRFIT	Multiple Risk Factor Intervention Trial
HTR	heart transplant recipients		
HyperGEN	Hypertension Genetic Epidemiology Network	NCEP ATP III	National Cholesterol Education Program Expert Panel on Detection, Evaluation, and Treatment of High Blood Cholesterol in Adults
ICARUS	Insulin Carotids US Scandinavia		
IDEAL	Incremental Decrease in Endpoints through Aggressive Lipid lowering trial		
		NF	nuclear factor
		NHANES III	Third National Health and Nutrition Examination Survey
IDNT	Irbesartan Diabetic Nephropathy Trial		
IHD	ischaemic heart disease	NHLBI	National Heart, Lung, and Blood Institute
IMT	intima-media thickness		

NID	nitroglycerin-induced dilatation	RR	relative risk
NNT	numbers needed to treat	RUTH	Raloxifene Use for the Heart study
NO	nitric oxide	RWT	relative wall thickness
OHT	orthostatic hypertension	SAPPHIRe	Stanford Asian Pacific Program in Hypertension and Insulin Resistance study
OHYPO	orthostatic hypotension		
ONTARGET	Ongoing Telmisartan Alone and in Combination with Ramipril Global Endpoint Trial		
		SBP	systolic blood pressure
		SCI	silent cerebral infarct
OPTIMAAL	Optimal Trial In Myocardial Infarction with the Angiotensin II Antagonist Losartan	SDD	SD of differences
		SEARCH	Study of the Effectiveness of Additional Reductions in Cholesterol and Homocysteine
OR	odds ratio		
PA	primary aldosteronism	SEE	standard error of estimate
PAC	plasma aldosterone concentrations	SERM	selective oestrogen-receptor modulators
PE	pulmonary embolism	SHEP	Systolic Hypertension in the Elderly Program
PIUMA	Progetto Ipertensione Umbria Monitoraggio Ambulatoriale (study)	SHRSP	stroke-prone spontaneously hypertensive rats
PP	pulse pressure	SPSMQ	Short Portable Mental Status Questionnaire
PRA	plasma–renin activity		
PRESERVE	Prospective Randomized Enalapril Study Evaluating Regression of Ventricular Enlargement	SRH	skin reactive hyperaemia
		TEMI	transient episodes of myocardial ischaemia
		TIA	transient ischaemic attack
PROGRESS	Perindopril Protection Against Recurrent Stroke Study	TNT	Treat-to-New-Targets
		TOD	target organ damage
		TTDHE	transthoracic Doppler harmonic echocardiography
PWA	pulse-wave analysis		
PWV	pulse wave velocity	UACR	urine albumin/creatinine ratio
QCA	quantitative coronary angiography		
		UAER	urine albumin excretion
QoL	quality of life	UKPDS	UK Prospective Diabetes Study
RAAS	renin–angiotensin–aldosterone system		
		USPSTF III	Third US Preventive Services Task Force study
RAS	renin–angiotensin system		
RENAAL	Reduction of Endpoints in Non-insulin-dependent diabetes with the Angiotensin II Antagonist Losartan study	VALIANT	Valsartan in Acute Myocardial Infarction study
		VALUE	Valsartan Antihypertensive Long-term Use Evaluation trial
RH	refractory hypertension	VEGF	vascular endothelial growth factor
ROC	receiver operating characteristic		
		VHAS	Verapamil in Hypertension and Atherosclerosis Study
RPF	renal plasma flow		

WAVE	Women's Angiographic Vitamin and Estrogen trial	WISDOM	Women's International Study of Long Duration Estrogen after Menopause
WCH	white coat hypertension		
WEST	Women's Estrogen for Stroke Trial	WKY	Wistar-Kyoto rat
		WML	white matter lesion
WHI	Women's Health Initiative	WOSCOPS	West of Scotland Coronary Prevention Study
WHO	World Health Organization		

Index of papers reviewed

Aeschbacher BC, Hutter D, Fuhrer J, Weidmann P, Delacretaz E, Allemann Y. Diastolic dysfunction precedes myocardial hypertrophy in the development of hypertension. *Am J Hypertens* 2001; 14(2): 106–13. **242**

Ali S, Rouse A. Practice audits: reliability of sphygmomanometers and blood pressure recording bias. *J Hum Hypertens* 2002; 16(5): 359–61. **168**

Allayee H, de Bruin TW, Michelle Dominguez K, Cheng LS, Ipp E, Cantor RM, Krass KL, Keulen ET, Aouizerat BE, Lusis AJ, Rotter JI. Genome scan for BP in Dutch dyslipidaemic families reveals linkage to a locus on chromosome 4p. *Hypertension* 2001; 38(4): 773–8. **100**

Ansell BJ, Waters DD. Reassessment of National Cholesterol Education Program Adult Treatment Panel-III guidelines: one year later. *Amer J Cardiol.* 2002; 90(5): 524–5. **354**

Asai T, Ohkubo T, Katsuya T, Higaki J, Fu Y, Fukuda M, Hozawa A, Matsubara M, Kitaoka H, Tsuji I, Araki T, Satoh H, Hisamichi S, Imai Y, Ogihara T. Endothelin-1 gene variant associates with blood pressure in obese Japanese subjects: the Ohasama study. *Hypertension* 2001; 38(6): 1321–4. **113**

Aurigemma GP, Williams D, Gaasch WH, Reda DJ, Materson BJ, Gottdiener JS. Ventricular and myocardial function following treatment of hypertension. *Am J Cardiol* 2001; 87(6): 732–6. **262**

Barrett-Connor E, Grady D, Sashegyi A, Anderson PW, Cox DA, Hoszowski K, Rautaharju P, Harper KD; MORE Investigators (Multiple Outcomes of Raloxifene Evaluation). Raloxifene and cardiovascular events in osteoporotic post-menopausal women: four-year results from the MORE (Multiple Outcomes of Raloxifene Evaluation) randomized trial. *JAMA* 2002; 287(7): 847–57. **296**

Bartel T, Yang Y, Muller S, Wenzel RR, Baumgart D, Philipp T, Erbel R. Non-invasive assessment of microvascular function in arterial hypertension by transthoracic Doppler harmonic echocardiography. *J Am Coll Cardiol* 2002; 39(12): 2012–18. **34**

Bengtsson K, Melander O, Orho-Melander M, Lindblad U, Ranstam J, Rastam L, Groop L. Polymorphism in the beta(1)-adrenergic receptor gene and hypertension. *Circulation* 2001; 104(2): 187–90. **117**

Benetos A, Adamopoulos C, Bureau JM, Temmar M, Labat C, Bean K, Thomas F, Pannier B, Asmar R, Zureik M, Safar M, Guize L. Determinants of accelerated progression of arterial stiffness in normotensive subjects and in treated hypertensive subjects over a 6-year period. *Circulation* 2002; 105(10): 1202–7. **83**

Benetos A, Waeber B, Izzo J, Mitchell G, Resnick L, Asmar R, Safar M. Influence of age, risk factors, and cardiovascular and renal disease on arterial stiffness: clinical applications. *Am J Hypertens* 2002; 15(12): 1101–8. **76**

Black DM. A discussion of modalities for assessing regression and progression in vascular disease. *Am J Cardiol* 2002; 89(4A): 40–1B. **143**

Bohannon AD, Fillenbaum GG, Pieper CF, Hanlon JT, Blazer DG. Relationship of race/ethnicity and blood pressure to change in cognitive function. *J Am Geriatr Soc* 2002; 50(3): 424–9. **200**

Borghi C, Dormi A, Ambrosioni E, Gaddi A, On behalf of the Brisighella Heart Study Working Party. Relative role of systolic, diastolic and pulse pressure as risk factors for cardiovascular events in the Brisighella Heart Study. *J Hypertens* 2002; 20(9): 1737–42. **58**

Bosch J, Yusuf S, Pogue J, Sleight P, Lonn E, Rangoonwala B, Davies R, Ostergren J, Probstfield J; HOPE Investigators. Heart outcomes prevention evaluation. Use of ramipril in preventing stroke: double blind randomized trial. *Br Med J* 2002; 324: 699–702. **339**

Boutitie F, Gueyffier F, Pocock S, Fagard R, Boissel JP; INDANA Project Steering Committee. INdividual Data ANalysis of Antihypertensive intervention. J-shaped relationship between blood pressure and mortality in hypertensive patients: new insights from a meta-analysis of individual-patient data. *Ann Intern Med* 2002; 136(6): 438–48. **193**

Boutouyrie P, Tropeano AI, Asmar R, Gautier I, Benetos A, Lacolley P, Laurent S. Aortic stiffness is an independent predictor of primary coronary events in hypertensive patients: a longitudinal study. *Hypertension* 2002; 39: 10–15. **80**

Brem AS. Insights into glucocorticoid-associated hypertension: review. *Am J Kidney Dis* 2001; 37: 1–10. **8**

Budoff MJ, Yang TP, Shavelle RM, Lamont DH, Brundage BH. Ethnic differences in coronary atherosclerosis. *J Am Coll Cardiol* 2002; 39(3): 408–12. **215**

Campia U, Choucair WK, Bryant MB, Waclawiw MA, Cardillo C, Panza JA. Reduced endothelium-dependent and -independent dilation of conductance arteries in African-Americans. *J Am Coll Cardiol* 2002; 40(4): 754–60. **219**

Celentano A, Palmieri V, Di Palma Esposito N, Pietropaolo I, Arezzi E, Mureddu GF, de Simone G. Relations of pulse pressure and other components of blood pressure to preclinical echocardiographic abnormalities. *J Hypertens* 2002; 20(3): 531–7. **84**

Chelliah R, Sagnella GA, Markandu ND, MacGregor GA. Urinary protein and essential hypertension in black and in white people. *Hypertension* 2002; 39: 1064–70. **229**

Cherry N, Gilmour K, Hannaford P, Heagerty A, Khan MA, Kitchener H, McNamee R, Elstein M, Kay C, Seif M, Buckley H; ESPRIT team. Oestrogen therapy for prevention of reinfarction in post-menopausal women: a randomized placebo controlled trial. *Lancet* 2002; 360(9350): 1996–7. **292**

Corretti MC, Anderson TJ, Benjamin Celermajer D, Charbonneau F, Creager MA, Deanfield J, Drexler H, Gerhard-Herman M, Herrington D, Vallance P, Vita J, Vogel R; International Brachial Artery Reactivity Task Force. International Guidelines for the ultrasound assessment of endothelial-dependent flow-mediated vasodilation of the brachial artery: a report of the International Brachial Artery Reactivity Task Force. *J Am Coll Cardiol* 2002; 39(2): 257–65. **32**

Cosentino F, Bonetti S, Rehorik R, Eto M, Werner-Felmayer G, Volpe M, Luscher TF. Nitric-oxide-mediated relaxations in salt-induced hypertension: effect of chronic 1-selective receptor blockade. *J Hypertens*; 20(3): 421–8. **40**

Cruz ML, Huang TT, Johnson MS, Gower BA, Goran MI. Insulin sensitivity and blood pressure in black and white children. *Hypertension* 2002; 40: 18–22. **216**

Cushman WC, Brady WE, Gazdick LP, Zeldin RK. The effect of a losartan-based

Study. *Blood Press* 2001; 10(2): 74–82. **258**

Devereux RB, Bella JN, Palmieri V, Oberman A, Kitzman DW, Hopkins PN, Rao DC, Morgan D, Paranicas M, Fishman D, Arnett DK; Hypertension Genetic Epidemiology Network Study Group. Left ventricular systolic dysfunction in a biracial sample of hypertensive adults. The Hypertension Genetic Epidemiology Network (HyperGEN) Study. *Hypertension* 2001; 38: 417–23. **220**

Devereux RB, Palmieri V, Sharpe N, De Quattro V, Bella JN, de Simone G, Walker JF, Hahn RT, Dahlof B. Effects of once-daily angiotensin-converting enzyme inhibition and calcium channel blockade-based antihypertensive treatment regimens on left ventricular hypertrophy and diastolic filling in hypertension. The Prospective Randomized Enalapril Study Evaluating Regression of Ventricular Enlargement (PRESERVE) Trial. *Circulation* 2001; 104: 1248–54. **266**

Dickstein K, Kjekshus J and the OPTIMAAL Steering Committee. Effect of losartan and captopril on mortality and morbidity in high-risk patients after acute myocardial infarction: the OPTIMAAL randomized trial. *Lancet* 2002; 360(9335): 752–60. **341**

Diez J, Querejeta R, Lopez B, Gonzalez A, Larman M, Martinez Ubago JL. Losartan-dependent regression of myocardial fibrosis is associated with reduction of left ventricular chamber stiffness in hypertensive patients. *Circulation* 2002; 105: 2512–17. **274**

El-Gharbawy AH, Kotchen JM, Grim CE, Kaldunski M, Hoffmann RG, Pausova Z, Gaudet D, Gossard F, Hamet P, Kotchen TA. Predictors of target organ damage in hypertensive blacks and whites. *Hypertension* 2001a; 38: 761–6. **221**

El-Gharbawy AH, Nadig VS, Kotchen JM, Grim CE, Sagar KB, Kaldunski M,

Hamet P, Pausova Z, Gaudet D, Gossard F, Kotchen TA. Arterial pressure, left ventricular mass, and aldosterone in essential hypertension. *Hypertension* 2001b; 37(3): 845–50. **222**

Farsang C, Garcia-Puig J, Niegowska J, Baiz AQ, Vrijens F, Bortman G. The efficacy and tolerability of losartan vs atenolol in patients with isolated systolic hypertension. Losartan ISH Investigators Group. *J Hypertens* 2000; 18(6): 795–801. **323**

Feinstein SB, Voci P, Pizzuto F. Non-invasive surrogate markers of atherosclerosis. *Am J Cardiol* 2002; 89(5A): 31–43C. **142**

Ferrara A, Quesenberry CP, Karter AJ, Njoroge CW, Jacobson AS, Selby JV; Northern California Kaiser Permanente Diabetes Registry. Current use of unopposed estrogen and estrogen plus progestin and the risk of acute myocardial infarction among women with diabetes: The Northern California Kaiser Permanente Diabetes Registry, 1995–1998. *Circulation* 2003 Jan; 107(1): 43–8. **284**

Ford ES, Giles WH, Dietz WH. Prevalence of the metabolic syndrome among US adults. Findings from the Third National Health and Nutrition Examination Survey. *JAMA* 2002; 287: 356–9. **205**

Frantz S, Clemitson J-R, Bihoreau M-T, Gauguier D, Samani NJ. Genetic dissection of region around the *Sa* gene on rat chromosome 1: evidence for multiple loci affecting BP. *Hypertension* 2001; 38(2): 216–21. **116**

Frohlich ED. Local haemodynamic changes in hypertension: insights for therapeutic preservation of target organs. *Hypertension* 2001; 38(6): 1388–94. **126**

Galderisi M, Cicala S, Caso P, De Simone L, D'Errico A, Petrocelli A, de Divitiis O. Coronary flow reserve and myocardial diastolic dysfunction in arterial hypertension. *Am J Cardiol* 2002; 90(8): 860–4. **246**

Gallay BJ, Ahmad S, Xu L, Toivola B, Davidson RC. Screening for primary aldosteronism without discontinuing hypertensive medications: plasma aldosterone–renin ratio. *Am J Kidney Dis* 2001; 37(4): 699–705. **6**

Gandhi SK, Powers JC, Nomeir AM, Fowle K, Kitzman DW, Rankin KM, Little WC. The pathogenesis of acute pulmonary oedema associated with hypertension. *N Engl J Med* 2001; 344: 17–22. **248**

Gasowski J, Fagard RH, Staessen JA, Grodzicki T, Pocock S, Boutitie F, Gueyffier F, Boissel JP; INDANA Project Collaborators. Pulsatile BP component as predictor of mortality in hypertension: a meta-analysis of clinical trial control groups. *J Hypertens* 2002; 20: 145–51. **57**

Gerdts E, Papademetriou V, Palmieri V, Boman K, Bjornstad H, Wachtell K, Giles TD, Dahlof B, Devereux RB; Losartan Intervention For End (LIFE) point reduction in hypertension study. Correlates of pulse pressure reduction during antihypertensive treatment (losartan or atenolol) in hypertensive patients with electrocardiographic left ventricular hypertrophy (the LIFE study). *Am J Cardiol* 2002; 89(4): 399–402. **86, 300**

Glorioso N, Filigheddu F, Troffa C, Soro A, Parpaglia PP, Tsikoudakis A, Myers RH, Herrera VL, Ruiz-Opazo N. Interaction of α1-Na,K-ATPase and Na,K,2Cl-cotransporter genes in human essential hypertension. *Hypertension* 2001; 38(2): 204–9. **118**

Gokce N, Holbrook M, Hunter LM, Palmisano J, Vigalok E, Keaney JF Jr, Vita JA. Acute effects of vasoactive drug treatment on brachial artery reactivity. *J Am Coll Cardiol* 2002; 40(4): 761–5. **27**

Gomez-Cerezo J, Rios Blanco JJ, Suarez Garcia I, Moreno Anaya P, Garcia Raya P, Vazquez-Munoz E,

Barbado Hernandez FJ. Non-invasive study of endothelial function in white coat hypertension. *Hypertension* 2002; 40(3): 304–9. **35**

Gottdiener JS, Arnold AM, Aurigemma GP, Polak JF, Tracy RP, Kitzman DW, Gardin JM, Rutledge JE, Boineau RC. Predictors of congestive heart failure in the elderly: the Cardiovascular Health Study. *J Am Coll Cardiol* 2000; 35: 1628–37. **247**

Grady D, Herrington D, Bittner V, Blumenthal R, Davidson M, Hlatky M, Hsia J, Hulley S, Herd A, Khan S, Newby LK, Waters D, Vittinghoff E, Wenger N; HERS Research Group. Cardiovascular disease outcomes during 6.8 years of hormone therapy: Heart and Estrogen/Progestin Replacement Study Follow-up (HERS II). *JAMA* 2002; 288: 49–57. **282**

Guerin AP, Blacher J, Pannier B, Marchais SJ, Safar ME, London GM. Impact of aortic stiffness attenuation on survival of patients in end-stage renal failure. *Circulation* 2001; 103: 987–92. **74**

Hanson RL, Imperatore G, Bennett PH, Knowler WC. Components of the 'metabolic syndrome' and incidence of type 2 diabetes. *Diabetes* 2002; 51(10): 3120–7. **210**

Hasebe N, Kido S, Ido A, Kenjiro K, Angiographical Study in Angina with Hypertension Induced Insults (ASAHI) Investigators. Reverse J-curve relation between diastolic blood pressure and severity of coronary artery lesion in hypertensive patients with angina pectoris. *Hypertens Res* 2002; 25(3): 381–7. **201**

Hayward CS, Kraidly M, Webb CM, Collins P. Assessment of endothelial function using peripheral waveform analysis. A clinical application. *J Am Coll Cardiol* 2002; 40(3): 521–8. **132**

Heart Protection Study Collaborative Group. MRC/BHF Heart Protection Study of antioxidant vitamin supplementation in

20 536 high-risk individuals: a randomized placebo-controlled trial. *Lancet* 2002b; 360: 23–33. **355**

Heart Protection Study Collaborative Group. MRC/BHF Heart Protection Study of cholesterol lowering with simvastatin in 20 536 high-risk individuals: a randomized placebo-controlled trial. *Lancet* 2002c; 360: 7–22. **355**

Hengstenberg C, Schunkert H, Mayer B, Doring A, Lowel H, Hense HW, Fischer M, Riegger GA, Holmer SR. Association between a polymorphism in the G protein beta3 subunit gene (GNB3) with arterial hypertension but not with myocardial infarction. *Cardiovasc Res* 2001; 49(4): 820–7. **117**

Hermida RC, Calvo C, Ayala DE, Fernandez JR, Ruilope LM, Lopez JE. Evaluation of the extent and duration of the 'ABPM effect' in hypertensive patients. *J Am Coll Cardiol* 2002; 40(4): 710–17. **174**

Herrington DM, Howard TD, Hawkins GA, Reboussin DM, Xu J, Zheng SL, Brosnihan KB, Meyers DA, Bleecker ER. Estrogen-receptor polymorphisms and effects of estrogen replacement on high-density lipoprotein cholesterol in women with coronary disease. *N Engl J Med* 2002; 346: 967–74. **290**

Hilgers KF, Delles C, Veelken R, Schmieder RE. Angiotensinogen gene core promoter variants and non-modulating hypertension. *Hypertension* 2001; 38(6): 1250–4. **102**

Hlatky MA, Boothroyd D, Vittinghoff E, Sharp P, Whooley MA; Heart and Estrogen/Progestin Replacement Study (HERS) Research Group. Quality-of-life and depressive symptoms in post-menopausal women after receiving hormone therapy: results from the Heart and Estrogen/Progestin Replacement Study (HERS) trial. *JAMA* 2002; 287(5): 591–7. **288**

Horita Y, Inenaga T, Nakahama H, Ishibashi-Ueda H, Kawano Y, Nakamura S, Horio T, Okuda N, Ando M, Takishita S. Cause of residual hypertension after adrenalectomy in patients with primary aldosteronism. *Am J Kidney Dis* 2001; 37(5): 884–9. **14**

Hsu CY. Does treatment of non-malignant hypertension reduce the incidence of renal dysfunction? A meta-analysis of ten randomized, controlled trials. *J Hum Hypertens* 2001; 15(2): 99–106. **238**

Hulley S, Furberg C, Barrett-Connor E, Cauley J, Grady D, Haskell W, Knopp R, Lowery M, Satterfield S, Schrott H, Vittinghoff E, Hunninghake D; HERS Research Group. Non-cardiovascular disease outcomes during 6.8 years of hormone therapy: Heart and Estrogen/Progestin Replacement Study Follow-up (HERS II). *JAMA* 2002; 288: 58–66. **282**

Humphrey LL, Chan BKS, Sox HC. Post-menopausal hormone replacement therapy and the primary prevention of cardiovascular disease. *Ann Intern Med* 2002; 137: 273–84. **298**

Hunziker PR, Imsand C, Keller D, Hess N, Barbosa V, Nietlispach F, Liel-Cohen N, Weyman AE, Pfisterer M, Buser P. Bedside quantification of atherosclerosis severity for cardiovascular risk stratification: a prospective cohort study. *J Am Coll Cardiol* 2002; 39(4): 702–9. **82**

Ishikawa K, Baba S, Katsuya T, Iwai N, Asai T, Fukuda M, Takiuchi S, Fu Y, Mannami T, Ogata J, Higaki J, Ogihara T. T+31C Polymorphism of angiotensinogen gene and essential hypertension. *Hypertension* 2001; 37(2): 281–5. **104**

Jones DW, Frohlich ED, Grim CM, Grim CE, Taubert KA for the Professional Education Committee, Council for High Blood Pressure Research. Mercury sphygmomanometers should not be abandoned: an advisory statement from the Council for High Blood Pressure Research,

American Heart Association. *Hypertension* 2001; 37(2): 185–6. **167**

Jong P, Demers C, McKelvie RS, Liu PP. Angiotensin receptor blockers in heart failure: meta-analysis of randomized controlled trials. *J Am Coll Cardiol* 2002; 39(3): 463–70. **344**

Kahn DF, Duffy SJ, Tomasian D, Holbrook M, Rescorl L, Russell J, Gokce N, Loscalzo J, Vita JA. Effects of black race on forearm resistance vessel function. *Hypertension* 2002; 40(2): 195–201. **30**

Kaplan NM. Cautions over the current epidemic of primary aldosteronism. *Lancet* 2001; 357: 953–4. **4**

Kario K, Eguchi K, Hoshide S, Umeda Y, Mitsuhashi T, Shimada K. U-curve relationship between orthostatic blood pressure change and silent cerebrovascular disease in elderly hypertensives. Orthostatic hypertension as a new cardiovascular risk factor. *J Am Coll Cardiol* 2002; 40: 133–41. **196**

Khurana R, Martin JF, Zachary I. Gene therapy for cardiovascular disease. A case for cautious optimism. *Hypertension* 2001; 38(5): 1210–16. Review. **110**

Kikuya M, Chonan K, Imai Y, Goto E, Ishii M on behalf of the Research Group. Accuracy and reliability of wrist-cuff devices for self-measurement of blood pressure. *J Hypertens* 2002; 20(4): 629–38. **164**

Kingsbury M, Mahnke A, Turner M, Sheridan D. Recovery of coronary function and morphology during regression of left ventricular hypertrophy. *Cardiovasc Res* 2002; 55: 83–96. **269**

Kingwell BA, Waddell TK, Medley TL, Cameron JD, Dart AM. Large artery stiffness predicts ischemic threshold in patients with coronary artery disease. *J Am Coll Cardiol* 2002; 40(4): 773–9. **79**

Kinlay S, Creager MA, Fukumoto M, Hikita H, Fang JC, Selwyn AP, Ganz P. Endothelium-derived nitric oxide regulates arterial elasticity in human arteries *in vivo*. *Hypertension* 2001; 38: 1049–53. **136**

Kjeldsen SE, Dahlof B, Devereux RB, Julius S, Aurup P, Edelman J, Beevers G, de Faire U, Fyhrquist F, Ibsen H, Kristianson K, Lederballe-Pedersen O, Lindholm LH, Nieminen MS, Omvik P, Oparil S, Snapinn S, Wedel H; LIFE (Losartan Intervention for Endpoint Reduction) Study Group. Effects of losartan on cardiovascular morbidity and mortality in patients with isolated systolic hypertension and left ventricular hypertrophy. *JAMA* 2002; **288:** 1491–8. **320**

Knox SS, Hausdorff J, Markovitz JH; Coronary Artery Risk Development in Young Adults Study. Reactivity as a predictor of subsequent blood pressure: racial differences in the Coronary Artery Risk Development in Young Adults (CARDIA) study. *Hypertension* 2002; 40: 914–19. **217**

Kostis JB, Lawrence-Nelson J, Ranjan R, Wilson AC, Kostis WJ, Lacy CR. Association of increased pulse pressure with the development of heart failure in SHEP. Systolic Hypertension in the Elderly (SHEP) Cooperative Research Group. *Am J Hypertens*; 14(8 Pt 1): 798–803. **55**

Krum H, Nolly H, Workman D, He W, Roniker B, Krause S, Fakouhi K. Efficacy of eplerenone added to renin-angiotensin blockade in hypertensive patients. *Hypertension* 2002; 40(2): 117–23. **22**

Kumaran K, Fall CHD, Martyn CN, Vijayakumar M, Stein CE, Shier R. Left ventricular mass and arterial compliance: relation to coronary heart disease and its risk factors in South Indian adults. *Int J Cardiol* 2002; 83: 1–9. **225**

Laaksonen DE, Lakka HM, Niskanen LK, Kaplan GA, Salonen JT, Lakka TA. Metabolic syndrome and development of diabetes mellitus: application and validation of recently suggested definitions of the metabolic syndrome in a prospective cohort study. *Am J Epidemiol* 2002; **156**(11): 1070–7. **207**

Lakka HM, Laaksonen DE, Lakka TA, Niskanen LK, Kumpusalo E, Tuomilehto J, Salonen JT. The metabolic syndrome and total and cardiovascular disease mortality in middle-aged men. *JAMA* 2002; **288**(21): 2709–16. **208**

Lane D, Beevers M, Barnes N, Bourne J, John A, Malins S, Beevers DG. Inter-arm differences in blood pressure: when are they clinically significant? *J Hypertens* 2002; **20**(6): 1089–95. **176**

Lane D, Beevers DG, Lip GYH. Ethnic differences in blood pressure and the prevalence of hypertension in England. *J Hum Hypertens* 2002; **16**(4): 267–73. **213**

Lantelme P, Mestre C, Lievre M, Gressard A, Milon H. Heart rate: an important confounder of pulse wave velocity assessment. *Hypertension* 2002; **39**: 1083–7. **69**

Laurent S, Kingwell B, Bank A, Weber M, Struijker-Boudier H. Clinical applications of arterial stiffness: therapeutics and pharmacology. *Am J Hypertens* 2002; **15**(5): 453–8. **72**

Lebrun CE, Van Der Schouw YT, Bak AA, De Jong FH, Pols HA, Grobbee DE, Lamberts SW, Bots ML. Arterial stiffness in post-menopausal women: determinants of PWV. *J Hypertens* 2002; **20**(11): 2165–72. **73**

Lim PO, Donnan PT, MacDonald TM. Aldosterone to renin ratio as a determinant of exercise blood pressure response in hypertensive patients. *J Hum Hypertens* 2001; **15**(2): 119–23. **16**

Lim PO, Struthers AD, MacDonald TM. The neurohormonal natural history of essential hypertension: towards primary or tertiary aldosteronism? *J Hypertens* 2002; **20**: 11–15. **10**

Lim PO, Young WF, MacDonald TM. A review of the medical treatment of primary aldosteronism. *J Hypertens* 2001; **19**(3): 353–61. **7**

Lindholm LH, Ibsen H, Borch-Johnsen K, Olsen MH, Wachtell K, Dahlof B, Devereux RB, Beevers G, de Faire U, Fyhrquist F, Julius S, Kjeldsen SE, Kristianson K, Lederballe-Pedersen O, Nieminen MS, Omvik P, Oparil S, Wedel H, Aurup P, Edelman JM, Snapinn S; For the LIFE study group. Risk of new-onset diabetes in the Losartan Intervention For Endpoint reduction in hypertension study. *J Hypertens* 2002; **20**(9): 1879–86. **319**

Lindholm LH, Ibsen H, Dahlof B, Devereux RB, Beevers G, de Faire U, Fyhrquist F, Julius S, Kjeldsen SE, Kristiansson K, Lederballe-Pedersen O, Nieminen MS, Omvik P, Oparil S, Wedel H, Aurup P, Edelman J, Snapinn S; LIFE Study Group. Cardiovascular morbidity and mortality in patients with diabetes in the Losartan Intervention For Endpoint reduction in hypertension study (LIFE): a randomized trial against atenolol. *Lancet* 2002; **359**(9311): 1004–10. **316**

Little P, Barnett J, Barnsley L, Marjoram J, Fitzgerald-Barron A, Mant D. Comparison of acceptability of and preferences for different methods of measuring blood pressure in primary care. *Br Med J* 2002a; **325**(7358): 258–9. **170**

Little P, Barnett J, Barnsley L, Marjoram J, Fitzgerald-Barron A, Mant D. Comparison of agreement between different measures of blood pressure in primary care and daytime ambulatory blood pressure. *Br Med J* 2002b; **325**(7358): 254–7. **170**

London GM, Cohn JN. Prognostic application of arterial stiffness: task forces. *Am J Hypertens* 2002; **15**(8): 754–8. **62**

Lopez-Farre A, Rodriguez-Feo JA, Garcia-Colis E, Gomez J, Lopez-Blaya A, Fortes J, de Andres R, Rico L, Casado S.

natriuretic peptide) gene, albuminuria, and hypertension. *Hypertension* 2001; 37(6): 1416–22. **114**

Netea RT, Elving LD, Lutterman JA, Thien Th. Body position and blood pressure measurement in patients with diabetes mellitus. *J Intern Med* 2002; 251: 393–9. **169**

Novo S, Abrignani MG, Novo G, Nardi E, Dominguez LJ, Strano A, Barbagallo M. Effects of drug therapy on cardiac arrhythmias and ischaemia in hypertensives with LVH. *Am J Hypertens* 2001; 14(7 Pt 1): 637–43. **258**

O'Brien E, Waeber B, Parati G, Staessen J, Myers MG, on behalf of the European Society of Hypertension Working Group on Blood Pressure Monitoring. Blood pressure measuring devices: recommendations of the European Society of Hypertension. *Br Med J* 2001; 322(7285): 531–6. **159**

O'Leary DH, Polak JF. Intima-media thickness. A tool for atherosclerosis imaging and event prediction. *Am J Cardiol* 2002; 90(10C): 18–21L. **144**

O'Rourke MF. From theory into practice: arterial haemodynamics in clinical hypertension. *J Hypertens* 2002; 20(10): 1901–15. **62**

O'Rourke MF, Staessen JA, Vlachopoulos C, Duprez D, Plante GE. Clinical applications of arterial stiffness; definitions and reference values. *Am J Hypertens* 2002; 15(5): 426–44. **70**

Okin PM, Devereux RB, Jern S, Julius S, Kjeldsen SE, Dahlof B. Relation of echocardiographic left ventricular mass and hypertrophy to persistent electrocardiographic left ventricular hypertropy in hypertensive patients: the LIFE study. *Am J Hypertens* 2001; 14(8 Pt 1): 775–82. **256**

Okin PM, Wright JT, Nieminen MS, Jern S, Taylor AL, Phillips R, Papademetriou V,

Clark LT, Ofili EO, Randall OS, Oikarinen L, Viitasalo M, Toivonen L, Julius S, Dahlof B, Devereux RB. Ethnic differences in electrocardiographic criteria for left ventricular hypertrophy: the LIFE study. Losartan Intervention For Endpoint. *Am J Hypertens* 2002; 15(8): 663–71. **328**

Okumiya K, Matsubayashi K, Wada T, Fujisawa M, Osaki Y, Doi Y, Yasuda N, Ozawa T. A U-shaped association between home systolic blood pressure and four-year mortality in community-dwelling older men. *J Am Geriatr Soc* 1999; 47(12): 1415–21. **198**

Olsen MH, Wachtell K, Aalkjaer C, Dige-Petersen H, Rokkedal J, Ibsen H. Vasodilatory capacity and vascular structure in long-standing hypertension: a LIFE substudy. *Am J Hypertens* 2002; 15(5): 398–404. **137**

Olsen MH, Wachtell K, Borch-Johnsen K, Okin PM, Kjeldsen SE, Dahlof B, Devereux RB, Ibsen H. A blood pressure independent association between glomerular albumin leakage and electrocardiographic left ventricular hypertrophy. The LIFE Study. Losartan Intervention For Endpoint reduction. *J Hum Hypertens* 2002; 16(8): 591–5. **238**

Olsen MH, Wachtell K, Hermann KL, Frandsen E, Dige-Petersen H, Rokkedal J, Devereux RB, Ibsen H. Is cardiovascular remodeling in patients with essential hypertension related to more than high blood pressure? A LIFE substudy. *Am Heart J* 2002; 144(3): 530–7. **325**

Pachori AS, Huentelman MJ, Francis SC, Gelband CH, Katovich MJ, Raizada MK. The future of hypertension therapy: sense, antisense, or non-sense? *Hypertension* 2001; 37(2 part 2): 357–64. **111**

Palatini P, Frigo G, Vriz O, Bertolo O, Dal Follo M, Daniele L, Visentin P, Pessina AC; HARVEST Study Group. Early signs of cardiac involvement in

Rajagopalan S, Pitt B. Aldosterone antagonists in the treatment of hypertension and target organ damage. *Curr Hypertens Rep* 2001; 3(3): 240–8. **12**

Rehman A, Rahman AR, Rasool AH. Effect of angiotensin II on pulse wave velocity in humans is mediated through angiotensin II type 1 (AT1) receptors. *J Hum Hypertens* 2002; 16(4): 261–6. **87**

Rothermund L, Luckert S, Koßmehl P, Paul M, Kreutz R. Renal endothelin ETA/ETB receptor imbalance differentiates salt-sensitive from salt-resistant spontaneous hypertension. *Hypertension* 2001; 37: 275–80. **113**

Safar ME, Blacher J, Pannier B, Guerin AP, Marchais SJ, Guyonvarc'h PM, London GM. Central pulse pressure and mortality in end-stage renal disease. *Hypertension* 2002; 39(3): 735–8. **74**

Sawka AM, Young WF, Thompson GB, Grant CS, Farley DR, Leibson C, van Heerden JA. Primary aldosteronism: factors associated with normalization of blood pressure after surgery. *Ann Intern Med* 2001; 135(4): 258–61. **13**

Schannwell CM, Schneppenheim M, Plehn G, Marx R, Strauer BE. Left ventricular diastolic function in physiologic and pathologic hypertrophy. *Am J Hypertens* 2002; 15(6): 513–17. **244**

Schillaci G, Pasqualini L, Vaudo G, Lupattelli G, Pirro M, Marchesi S, Porcellati C, Mannarino E. Prognostic value of treatment-induced changes in twenty-four-hour mean and pulse pressures in adult hypertensive patients. *Am J Cardiol* 2002; 90(8): 896–9. **50**

Schillaci G, Pasqualini L, Verdecchia P, Vaudo G, Marchesi S, Porcellati C, de Simone G, Mannarino E. Prognostic significance of left ventricular diastolic dysfunction in essential hypertension. *J Am Coll Cardiol* 2002; 39(12): 2005–11. **243**

Schillaci G, Vaudo G, Pasqualini L, Reboldi G, Porcellati C, Verdecchia P. Left ventricular mass and systolic dysfunction in essential hypertension. *J Hum Hypertens* 2002; 16: 117–22. **262**

Schofield RS, Schuler BT, Edwards DG, Aranda JM Jr, Hill JA, Nichols WW. Amplitude and timing of central aortic pressure wave reflections in heart transplant recipients. *Am J Hypertens* 2002; 15(9): 809–15. **77**

Schram MT, Kostense PJ, Van Dijk RA, Dekker JM, Nijpels G, Bouter LM, Heine RJ, Stehouwer CD. Diabetes, pulse pressure and cardiovascular mortality: the Hoorn Study. *J Hypertens*; 20(9): 1743–51. **47**

Shargorodsky M, Leibovitz E, Lubimov L, Gavish D, Zimlichman R. Prolonged treatment with the AT(1) receptor blocker, valsartan, increases small and large artery compliance in uncomplicated essential hypertension. *Am J Hypertens* 2002; 15(12): 1087–91. **90**

Sidhu JS, Newey VR, Nassiri DK, Kaski J-C. A rapid and reproducible on line automated technique to determine endothelial function. *Heart* 2002; 88: 289–92. **26**

Sierra C, de la Sierra A, Pare JC, Gomez-Angelats E, Coca A. Correlation between silent cerebral white matter lesions and left ventricular mass and geometry in essential hypertension. *Am J Hypertens* 2002; 15(6): 507–12. **233**

Sigurjonsdottir HA, Franzson L, Manhem K Ragnarsson J, Sigurdsson G, Wallerstedt S. Liquorice-induced rise in blood pressure: a linear dose–response relationship. *J Hum Hypertens* 2001; 15(8): 549–52. **19**

Simon A, Gariepy J, Chironi G, Megnien JL, Levenson J. Intima-media thickness: a new tool for diagnosis and treatment of cardiovascular risk. *J Hypertens* 2002; 20(2): 159–69. **145**

General index

'4 E' study 23

A

ACE gene polymorphisms 100–1, 103–4
ACE inhibitors *see* angiotensin-converting
      enzyme inhibitors
acute pulmonary oedema, pathogenesis 248–9
α-adducin gene variant, effect on diuretic therapy
      345–6
adhesion molecule levels, effect of losartan 30
adrenal hyperplasia 7
      see also primary aldosteronism
adrenalectomy, persistence of hypertension in
      primary aldosteronism 13–15
β1-adrenergic receptor gene polymorphism 117
β2-adrenergic receptor stimulation, use in
      assessment of endothelial function 132–4
advanced glycation end-products (AGEs) 92–3
African American Study of Kidney Disease and
      Hypertension (AASK) 228–9, 349–51
Afro-Caribbeans
      prevalence of hypertension 216–17
      see also black population
age, influence on arterial stiffness 76–7
albuterol, use in assessment of endothelial
      function 132
aldosterone
      effects on heart and vasculature 12, 17
      interaction with excess salt 3
      relationship to BP and left ventricular
          geometry 222–3
      see also hyperaldosteronism; primary
          aldosteronism; tertiary aldosteronism
aldosterone-producing adrenal adenoma (ADA)
      3, 7, 23
      see also primary aldosteronism
aldosterone receptor antagonists 13
      effect in β-HSD hypertension 17–18
      see also eplerenone; spironolactone
aldosterone-to-renin ratio (ARR) 3, 23
      relationship to exercise systolic blood pressure
          16–17
      use in screening for primary aldosteronism 5–7
aldosterone synthase C-344 T polymorphism
      103, 104

aldosterone synthase gene 8
aldosterone synthesis escape 21, 23
ALLHAT *see* Antihypertensive and Lipid
      Lowering to prevent Heart Attack Trial
alpha-receptor, regulatory role on NO/cGMP
      relaxing system 139–40
ALT-711 45, 48, 92–3
ambulatory blood pressure monitoring 158,
      170–4
      pressor effect 174–6
      validation of devices 162–4
ambulatory pulse pressure 46–7
      prognostic value in older patients 50-2
American Heart Association, recommendations
      for HRT and CVD 286–8
American Society of Obstetricians and
      Gynaecologists, recommendations on
      HRT 301
amlodipine
      comparison with other antihypertensives
          (ALLHAT) 334–8
      effect on carotid atherosclerosis 150
      effect on renal disease (AASK) 349–51
amplification of pulse pressure 43–4, 68
angina *see* coronary artery disease
angiogenesis, relationship to hypertension 308
angiogenesis therapy 110–11
angiotensin II
      actions 125
      effect on pulse wave velocity 87–8
      interaction with nitric oxide 122–3
      role in end-organ damage 121–2, 127
angiotensin II receptor antagonists 307, 308
      combination therapy
          with ACE inhibitors 88, 89, 346–9
          with eplerenone 22, 23
      effect on arterial stiffness 45, 48, 88–92
      efficacy in heart failure 344
      in primary aldosteronism 8, 16
      renoprotection 318, 353
      see also candesartan; irbesartan; losartan;
          telmisartan; valsartan
angiotensin-converting enzyme gene
      polymorphism 103–5
      link to insulin resistance 101–2

KEEPING UP TO DATE IN ONE VOLUME

Subject matters dealt with in previous volume

The Year in Hypertension 2002

Basic science
Epidemiology
Risk factors

Hypertension and co-existing conditions
Stroke
Pregnancy and hypertension
Diabetes

Therapy
Current drugs
New developments in pharmacological therapy
Non-pharmacological therapy

Current practical issues
Clinical features
Clinical evaluation
Other issues

Clinical Publishing Services Ltd
Oxford Centre for Innovation
Mill Street
Oxford OX2 0JX, UK

T: +44 1865 811116
F: +44 1865 251550
E: info@clinicalpublishing.co.uk

KEEPING UP TO DATE IN ONE SERIES

"The Year in ..."

EXISTING AND FUTURE VOLUMES

The Year in Hypertension 2000	ISBN 0 9537339 0 4
The Year in Rheumatic Disorders 2001	ISBN 0 9537339 1 2
The Year in Neurology 2001	ISBN 0 9537339 5 5
The Year in Gynaecology 2001	ISBN 0 9537339 2 0
The Year in Hypertension 2001	ISBN 0 9537339 4 7
The Year in Diabetes 2001	ISBN 0 9527339 6 3
The Year in Dyslipidaemia 2002	ISBN 0 9537339 3 9
The Year in Interventional Cardiology 2002	ISBN 0 9537339 7 1
The Year in Rheumatic Disorders 2002	ISBN 0 9537339 9 8
The Year in Hypertension 2002	ISBN 1 904392 00 8
The Year in Gynaecology 2002	ISBN 1 904392 01 6
The Year in Allergy 2003	ISBN 1 904392 05 9
The Year in Neurology 2003	ISBN 1 904392 03 2
The Year in Diabetes 2003	ISBN 1 904392 02 4
The Year in Dyslipidaemia 2003	ISBN 1 904392 07 5

To receive more information about these books and future volumes,
or to order copies, please contact the address below:

Clinical Publishing Services Ltd
Oxford Centre for Innovation
Mill Street
Oxford OX2 0JX, UK

T: +44 1865 811116
F: +44 1865 251550
E: info@clinicalpublishing.co.uk
W: www.clinicalpublishing.co.uk